# Teaching Nursing: The Art and Science

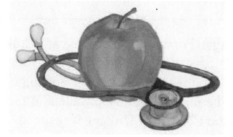

**Linda Caputi, MSN, EdD, RN**
Professor of Nursing
College of DuPage
Glen Ellyn, Illinois

**Lynn Engelmann, MSN, EdD, RN**
Professor of Nursing
College of DuPage
Glen Ellyn, Illinois

**Volume 2**
(Chapters 28 - 53)

**College of DuPage Press**

**College of DuPage Press**
425 Fawell Blvd.
Glen Ellyn, Illinois 60137

**Project Manager:** Joe Barillari
**Designer:** Janice Walker
**Typesetter:** Janice Walker
**CD Design:** Kevin Dudey
**Production Coordinator:** Dave Reifsnyder

**About College of DuPage**: For more than 15 years College of DuPage has been a leader in publishing educational materials for nursing education including multimedia computer programs, videos, books, and other print materials. We are committed to providing the highest quality products in the most appropriate format for our colleagues. Visit the College of DuPage website at www.cod.edu/software for information on all our products.

# Table of Contents

## Unit 3: Focus on Students

## Unit 4: Focus on Curriculum

# Unit 5: Focus on Critical Thinking

# Unit 6: Accreditation, Approval, and Certification

# Unit 7: Legal issues in Nursing Education

# Focus on Critical Thinking

Unit 5

# Chapter 28: AN INTRODUCTION TO DEVELOPING CRITICAL THINKING IN NURSING STUDENTS

Donna Ignatavicius, BS, MS, RN, Cm

*In this chapter, Donna Ignatavicius establishes a foundation for teaching critical thinking to nursing students. Subsequent chapters in the unit build on the foundation she establishes. A well-known educator, Ms. Ignativicius provides sound, practical advice from her many years of experience working with both nursing students and faculty. Also included in the chapter is information based on the ongoing research of Rosalinda Alfaro-LeFevre. We think readers will enjoy this fresh look at a very important concept – critical thinking. – Linda Caputi and Lynn Engelmann*

## Introduction

Critical thinking (CT) is not a new concept. Although mentioned in the educational literature over 30 years ago, critical thinking has only recently received increased attention in higher education. The National League for Nursing, and subsequently the National League for Nursing Accrediting Commission (NLNAC), has required nursing programs to develop critical thinking in their students for more than a decade. Furthermore, nursing programs have been expected to measure critical thinking development as a program outcome, using measurement tools that are reliable and valid. However, this standard was rescinded for all levels of undergraduate education programs in nursing in 2002. For programs accredited by the Commission on Collegiate Nursing Education (CCNE), critical thinking development is not a specified standard. Critical thinking has been and continues to be a difficult concept to measure.

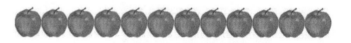

## Educational Philosophy

I have found that the most successful way to teach nursing students is to promote their learning through critical thinking and cooperative learning activities. Students are accountable for their own learning; faculty are accountable for facilitating student learning. – Donna Ignatavicius

In view of these accreditation criteria, three major issues have emerged:
- How to define critical thinking in nursing.
- How to measure critical thinking in nursing programs.
- How to develop critical thinking in nursing students.

## Defining Critical Thinking in Nursing and Exploring Critical Thinking Concepts

Numerous definitions of critical thinking are found in the educational and nursing literature, without a consensus on its definition. Some experts believe critical thinking is discipline-specific; others believe it is a universal phenomenon. In their extensive literature review of critical thinking definitions, Scheffer and Rubenfeld (2000) found that there are multiple interpretations of the term by nursing faculty, which poses a problem when communicating the construct to students and peers.

## Nursing Process and Critical Thinking

Some faculty believe critical thinking is synonymous with the nursing process, problem solving, or scientific method. However, most experts disagree because critical thinking is much more complex. Although the nursing process is a problem-solving approach to client problems and a precursor to CT, it is most likely not exactly the same as critical thinking, as shown below in Table 28.1.

Table 28.1 - Differentiating the Nursing Process and the Critical Thinking Process

| Nursing Process | Critical Thinking Process |
|---|---|
| Tends to be linear | Is more complex and helical |
| Requires sequential steps | Requires application of skills |
| Focuses on one problem at a time | Allows for visualization of the big picture |
| Steps can be standardized (e.g., NANDA diagnoses, Nursing Intervention Classification System) | Skills require creativity and thinking out of the box |
| Requires cognitive/intellectual ability | Has cognitive/intellectual and affective components |

# Definition/Description of Critical Thinking

Critical thinking has been defined by a number of experts, both in nursing and in higher education. Richard Paul (1992), the founder of the Foundation for Critical Thinking in California, posited several definitions, such as, "Critical thinking is the art of thinking about your thinking while you are thinking in order to make your thinking better" (p. 643). Although this definition may seem circular or vague, it points out that critical thinkers know how they think and think about how they think.

Rubenfeld and Scheffer (1999) used this habit of critical thinkers in their T.H.I.N.K. model of critical thinking. The K is for "knowing how you think." The acronym T.H.I.N.K. stands for:

- T – Total recall.
- H – Habit.
- I – Inquiry.
- N – New ideas and creativity.
- K – Knowing how you think.

The most comprehensive definition of critical thinking was offered by the American Philosophical Association under the direction of Facione (1990), in a large study seeking a universal definition and cognitive skills related to critical thinking. They concluded that critical thinking is a "purposeful, self-regulatory judgment which results in interpretation, analysis, evaluation, and inference as well as explanation of the evidential, conceptual, methodological, criteriological, or contextual considerations upon which judgment is based" (p. 2).

Alfaro-LeFevre (1999) viewed critical thinking as purposeful outcome-directed thinking that makes judgments based on knowledge that is derived from scientific principles or evidence. In her description of the construct, the critical thinker first considers what outcome or goal needs to be met and then develops options for arriving at the best solution for the situation, problem, or dilemma. Whatever option is selected is what the reflective thinker believes is the best fit for the situation. In other words, there is an affective or emotional part of critical thinking, not just a cognitive aspect.

In fact, most definitions adopted or developed by school-of-nursing faculty do include a cognitive, as well as an affective, component. Videbeck's (1997) survey of NLN-accredited BSN programs reported that 43 programs selected definitions that include both components; only 12 programs focused mainly on the cognitive or intellectual aspects. About half of these programs selected definitions from nursing literature.

In an attempt to derive a consensus definition and description of critical thinking, Scheffer and Rubenfeld (2000) conducted a study using the Delphi technique and an international panel of nurse experts. The experts agreed that critical thinkers use a cognitive skill set and an affective (habits of the mind) skill set. Each skill was defined in the last round of the study. The descriptors developed by consensus of 55 nurses are listed in Table 28.2.

Table 28.2 - Components of Critical Thinking

| Habits of the Mind (Affective Skills) | Cognitive Skills |
|---|---|
| Confidence | Analyzing |
| Contextual perspective | Applying standards |
| Creativity | Discriminating |
| Flexibility | Information seeking |
| Inquisitiveness | Logical reasoning |
| Intellectual integrity | Predicting and transforming knowledge |
| Intuition | |
| Open-mindedness | |
| Perseverance | |
| Reflection | |

## Critical Thinking Indicators

The consensus skills are similar to Alfaro-LeFevre's (2002) Critical Thinking Indicators (CTIs) – behaviors that demonstrate the knowledge, skills, and characteristics that help promote and develop critical thinking. The CTIs include many behaviors described by nurse experts in critical thinking as well as behaviors from the literature. Each CTI is described in terms of what the thinker does to illustrate the behavior. Examples of CTIs are illustrated in Table 28.3. A complete description and discussion of CTIs can be found in Alfaro-LeFevre's (2003) newest book, *Critical Thinking and Clinical Judgment: A Practical Approach.*

Table 28.3 is located on the CD-ROM accompanying this text for ease of use. Alfaro-LeFevre's website is also on the CD-ROM. Simply launch your internet browser, put the CD-ROM in the drive, go to Chapter 28 on the CD, and then click on the website address.

Table 28.3 - Examples of Critical Thinking Indicators (CTIs™)

# Examples of Critical Thinking Indicators™ (CTIs™)[1]

**Definition:** Critical Thinking Indicators™ (CTIs™) are evidence-based descriptions of behaviors that demonstrate the knowledge, characteristics, and skills that promote CT in clinical practice. CTIs™ give concrete descriptions and examples, and are listed in context of what's likely to be observed when a nurse is thinking critically in the clinical setting.[2] The complete list of CTIsTM and support material is available at www.AlfaroTeachSmart.com.

## CTIsTM Demonstrating Required Knowledge

**Clarifies:** nursing vs. medical responsibilities; manifestations of commonly encountered problems and complications; related anatomy, physiology, and pathophysiology; reasons behind interventions, medications, and diagnostic studies; policies and procedures and reasons behind them; nursing process and research principles; ethical and legal principles; spiritual and cultural concepts

## CTIsTM Demonstrating Characteristics/Attitudes of Critical Thinkers

- **Self-Confident:** expresses ability to think through problems and find solutions
- **Inquisitive:** seeks reasons, explanations, and new information
- **Honest and upright:** speaks and seeks the truth, even if the truth sheds unwanted light
- **Alert to context:** looks for changes in circumstances that may warrant a need to modify thinking or approaches
- **Open and Fair-Minded:** shows tolerance for different viewpoints; questions how own viewpoints are influencing thinking
- **Analytical and insightful:** identifies relationships; shows deep understanding
- **Logical and intuitive:** Draws reasonable conclusions (if this is so, then it follows that....because...); uses intuition as a guide to search for evidence.
- **Reflective and Self-Corrective:** carefully considers meaning of data and interpersonal interactions; corrects own thinking; observant for mistakes; identifies ways to prevent mistakes.
- **Sensitive to diversity:** Expresses appreciation of human differences related to values, culture, personality, or learning style preferences; adapts to preferences when feasible.

## CTIsTM Demonstrating Intellectual Skills/Competencies

**Nursing Process and Decision-making Skills:** assesses systematically and comprehensively; recognizes assumptions and inconsistencies; checks accuracy and reliability; identifies missing information; distinguishes relevant from irrelevant; supports conclusions with facts (evidence); sets priorities/makes decisions in a timely way; determines outcomes specific to each client; reassesses to monitor responses and outcomes

[1] Adapted with permission from: Critical Thinking IndicatorsTM . © 2003 R. Alfaro-LeFevre. Comprehensive list of CTIsTM . Available at: www.AlfaroTeachSmart.com. Critical Thinking IndicatorsTMand CTIsTM are registered trademarks of Rodalinda Alfaro-LeFevre.

[2] Alfaro -LeFevre, R. (2004). Critical thinking and clinical judgment: A practical approach, 3rd Ed. Philadelphia: WB Saunders.

# Measuring and Developing Critical Thinking

Any concept or construct requires multiple measures; one test does not reflect a student's ability to think critically. Most schools of nursing struggle with how to measure critical thinking in their students. Following are several ideas for measuring critical thinking.

## Constructing Tests that Measure Critical Thinking

Measurement is the process of gathering quantitative data that reflect student performance and abilities. Multiple measurements are then used to make judgments about student progress in the nursing program. Testing is a common method for measuring knowledge and the ability to apply that knowledge. See the chapter in this text titled *Test Construction and Analysis: Can I Do It?* by Susan Morrison for more information on testing.

One of the most difficult tasks for nursing faculty is constructing valid and reliable tests. For undergraduate education, multiple-choice tests are used primarily for clinical nursing courses that have a theoretical component, thereby preparing students for taking the NCLEX®-RN or PN examination.

In addition to measuring knowledge, these tests can also measure and foster critical thinking ability. Critical thinking is the construct, then, that is most important in testing. To establish evidence of construct-related evidence of measurement validity, faculty must develop questions that address critical thinking skills, such as those outlined by Facione (1990). Table 28.4 lists these evidence-based skills and examples of nursing content that can be tested.

Table 28.4 - Critical Thinking Skills That Can Be Measured

| Critical Thinking Skill | Example |
|---|---|
| Interpretation | Assessing data, such as lab results, client behavior, and physical findings |
| Analysis | Deriving "best fit" nursing diagnosis based on assessment data |
| Inference | Drawing conclusions about best practices |
| Explanation | Determining scientific rationale based on evidence |
| Evaluation | Determining if client outcomes have been met |

# Clinical Evaluation

Evaluation is the process of collecting and analyzing data through multiple measurements to make a judgment about the student being evaluated. The purpose of clinical evaluation is to identify student learning needs, assess student progress, and make decisions concerning student achievement. One of the major components of the clinical evaluation process is to determine a student's critical thinking ability. Alfaro-LeFevre's (2003) CTIs might be used as a basis for evaluation.

Using the skills delineated in Table 28.4 may be another way of determining whether or not a student can critically think during the clinical experience. See the chapter in this book titled *Operationalizing Critical Thinking* by Linda Caputi for additional tools for evaluating critical thinking in the clinical setting. In addition, a student who does self-evaluation demonstrates critical thinking through reflection and self-regulation. Despite these many attempts to objectively measure critical thinking, the evaluation process remains a subjective one.

## Progression of Critical Thinking Development

Critical thinking can be developed in anyone, but every person does not develop at the same rate.

### *First Stage in Developing Critical Thinking:*
### *Basic – Know Right from Wrong*

In the first stage of developing critical thinking, a person learns and practices right from wrong. These are the standards or rules that are applied for a situation, issue, or problem. For example, when nursing students are learning a new psychomotor skill, such as taking a blood pressure, they first learn one way.

### *Second Stage in Developing Critical Thinking:*
### *Complex – Realize that Alternative, Perhaps Conflicting,*
### *Solutions Exist*

Next, students realize the standard cuff does not fit every person. So some clients might require a large-sized cuff, and some might need a pediatric cuff. In this second stage of critical thinking development, the thinker realizes that the size of the cuff used depends on the size of the client's arm. So what size cuff should be used to take a blood pressure? It depends!

### *Third Stage in Developing Critical Thinking:*
### *Committed – Choose an Action or Belief Based on*
### *Alternatives Identified at the Complex Level*

The expert critical thinker knows there are many options for problems, issues, and dilemmas, and then selects one or more. For example, the student selects the cuff size believed to be the best for a particular client. At times, this third stage of critical thinking development requires more creativity. For instance, when managing a client with acute confusion, reality orientation may not reverse the problem. The higher-level thinker considers other options that might work for that individual client, such as music therapy.

Options in decision making are learned either in a formal education setting or from life or professional experiences. The role of the educator is to foster thinking about various options or thinking out of the box. The educator is the facilitator of the learning in the formal education environment.

## Enhancing Learning through Critical Thinking

Learning can occur only if the student's thinking is stimulated. The role of the nursing educator is to facilitate learning by arranging various learning activities; the role of the student is to learn. In other words, the student is accountable for the learning – not the faculty! Many learning activities are suggested throughout this book; only a few samples are described in this chapter.

Anderson (1996) described the "feeding" that nursing educators typically provide for their students when they teach. For example, they provide detailed syllabi with specific pages for readings rather than have the students use an index to locate the material in their books. She summarized her comments with the conclusion that "teaching is not feeding."

Adults are independent learners who are motivated by their experience to continue the learning process. When a person learns new content, each main concept is learned first. Then the subconcepts are learned in relation to the main concepts. Finally, the subconcepts are arranged in subordinate order and related to each other.

Although many educators focus on teaching, the goal should be learning instead. When learning is the focus, a paradigm shift occurs, and educators behave quite differently. O'Banion (1997) was one of the pioneers in helping colleges transition from teaching institutions to learning institutions. The tradition of teaching originated many centuries ago in England when higher education faculty lectured to students and students took notes on the lecture. Then the students studied their notes, hopefully to pass their tests. Long-term learning seldom occurs in this way because students are not stimulated to think, much less critically think, about what they are learning.

In a learning college, the focus is on student learning and how to make it happen. Barr and Tagg (1995) described several differences between teaching and learning, which are summarized in Table 28.5.

Table 28.5 - Differences in Teaching versus Learning

| Teaching | Learning |
|---|---|
| Lecture is the focus | Creating a learning environment is the focus |
| Efforts are to improve the quality of teaching | Efforts are to improve the quality of learning |
| Teachers have control | Students have control |
| Competition is fostered | Cooperation and collaboration are fostered |

## Cooperative Learning

As seen in Table 28.5, learning occurs using cooperative, collaborative strategies. Therefore, one of the best ways to develop critical thinking in students is to plan cooperative learning activities in the classroom, skills laboratory, and clinical setting that **replace** traditional lecture. As discussed throughout this book, students learn best when they are engaged as active learners. When working with each other, they often learn more than from the educator alone.

A number of books in general education have been written about the value of, and ideas for, cooperative learning strategies (Fuszard, 1995; Ignatavicius, 2001; O'Connor, 2001). Many of these activities can be used with any size group and take minimal time to implement. For example, the think-pair-share activity takes three to five minutes. The learning facilitator gives a topic or poses a question to the group and asks students to record their answers. Then each student pairs with another to share and compare the individual responses. The faculty can then ask what students learned from the experience.

Another approach for cooperative learning is cooperative testing. Although this strategy can be used a number of ways, one method is to have students take a test individually and then retake the same test in groups. The group discussion enhances learning and critical thinking because student discussion fosters critical thinking skills such as analysis, explanation, inference, and interpretation.

Sometimes educators need to be creative in planning ways to help students learn. For instance, to better understand fluids and electrolytes, students can be designated as either sodium, potassium, intracellular fluid, or extracellular fluid. Then these students come to the classroom and sit as they would find these substances in the body. During the class, volunteers demonstrate how substances move across a cell membrane. Although this exercise may seem simple, it can be chaotic at first. However, once the students get settled, they always remember, for example, which electrolyte is found primarily within the cells. Most students enjoy this type of interactive learning because it is fun and reinforces what they have learned.

## Written Assignments

Students should be required to complete written assignments for both the classroom and clinical experience. For theory, case studies, reaction papers, and research papers are examples of ways in which to develop critical thinking. In each of these activities, students must consider multiple concepts and put them together to meet the desired outcomes of the assignment. These assignments can be completed individually or in groups.

In the clinical setting, most faculty require traditional care plans. Although these are initially helpful to students in learning the nursing process, concept maps – also known as clinical correlation maps – should be used once the nursing process has been mastered. A concept map is a visual representation of subconcepts and their relationships. These maps may be used in the classroom, skills laboratory, or in the clinical setting as individual or group assignments. The chapter in this book titled *Using Concept Maps to Develop Critical Thinking* by Deanne Couey describes these learning tools for developing critical thinking in nursing students.

Journaling is another written assignment that can help students develop critical thinking. A journal should not be a diary of the student's experiences; rather, it should be a critical analysis of client care. Questions students might address include:
- What did I analyze during this clinical experience?
- What does this experience mean?
- How do I evaluate my performance today?
- Can I explain scientific evidence that supports my thinking?

Students may need guidelines on using this learning tool to reflect on practice.

## Skills Laboratory

Cooperative learning is not limited to the classroom. The skills laboratory and clinical setting are also ideally suited for this approach. Students can collaborate on how to perform skills and assessment techniques. They can evaluate each other's performance, as well.

Critical thinking is not enhanced, however, if students simply repeat and demonstrate the steps of a procedure. Rather, educators need to be creative in designing clinical-simulated situations within which skills can be performed. The clinical case below illustrates the use of simulation in the skills laboratory.

### *Critical Thinking Activity*

The nurse practitioner has ordered continuous tube feeding (Jevity©) at 50 mL/hr for a client who was transferred from acute care to your subacute care unit. At the present time, the client has a Keofeed® tube in place. An enteral feeding pump and open feeding bag system will be used for this client.

1. What physical assessment is needed before you start the client's enteral feeding?
2. How does a Keofeed® tube differ from a Levin® tube?  What is the most reliable way to initially ensure proper placement of either tube? Demonstrate the method you would use to check tube placement at frequent intervals.
3. Twelve hours after the feeding was started, the client becomes restless and experiences dyspnea. What should you do first and why?
4. Document your assessment and interventions that relate to this new situation above. Have another student or your faculty check your note for feedback. (Taken with permission from Ignatavicius, 2001.)

By participating in the above clinical simulation, the student develops critical thinking when asked to analyze and interpret the situation. Performing the skill is only part of the experience.

### Summary

This chapter introduced the concept of critical thinking and the importance of teaching that concept to nursing students. It presented some basic ideas and hopefully stimulated interest in how to teach critical thinking. The remaining chapters in this unit provide much more in-depth coverage on teaching critical thinking with many examples and suggested student assignments.

### Learning Activities

1. Review the components of critical thinking in Table 28.2.  Reflect on your own cognitive and affective skill ability, and place an S next to those abilities you believe are your strengths and an I next to those you would like to improve. Now think of ways that you could improve on each of the I designated skills.

2. Develop a clinical simulation scenario for students to help them learn how to perform an adult urinary catheterization. Be sure to include questions that will make them think!

3. What classroom learning activities could you use to promote critical thinking when planning a class on oxygenation concepts?

## References

Alfaro-LeFevre, R. (1999). *Critical thinking and clinical judgment: A practical approach* (2nd ed.). Philadelphia, PA: W. B. Saunders.

Alfaro-LeFevre, R. (2002). Sample of critical thinking indicators. Personal communication.

Alfaro-LeFevre, R. (2003). *Critical thinking and clinical judgment: A practical approach* (3rd ed.). St. Louis: W.B. Saunders-Elsevier Health Sciences.

Anderson, C. A. (1996). Teaching is not feeding. *Nursing Outlook, 14,* 257-258.

Barr, R., & Tagg, J. (1995, November/December). From teaching to learning: A new paradigm for undergraduate education. *Change,* 13-25.

Facione, P. A. (1990). *Critical thinking: A statement of expert consensus for purposes of educational assessment and instruction.* Millbrae, CA: California Academic Press.

Fuszard, B. (1995). *Innovative teaching strategies in nursing* (2nd ed.). Gaithersburg, MD: Aspen.

Ignatavicius, D.D. (2001). *A critical thinking approach to skill development and competency evaluation* (student guide and instructor's manual). Gatesville, TX: Medical Plastics Laboratory.

O'Banion, T. (1997). *A learning college for the 21st century.* Phoenix, AZ: Oryx Press.

O'Connor, A. B. (2001). *Clinical instruction and evaluation: A teaching resource.* Sudbury, MA: Jones & Bartlett.

Paul, R. (1992). *Critical thinking: What every person needs to survive in a rapidly changing world* (2nd ed., rev.). Santa Rosa, CA: The Foundation for Critical Thinking.

Rubenfeld, M. G., & Scheffer, B. K. (1999). *Critical thinking in nursing: An interactive approach* (2nd ed.). Philadelphia, PA: Lippincott.

Scheffer, B. K., & Rubenfeld, M. G. (2000). A consensus statement on critical thinking in nursing. *Journal of Nursing Education, 39,* 352-359.

Videbeck, S. L. (1997). Critical thinking: Prevailing practice in baccalaureate schools of nursing. *Journal of Nursing Education, 36,* 5-10.

## Bibliography

Facione, N. C., & Facione, P. A. (1996). Externalizing the critical thinking in knowledge development and clinical judgment. *Nursing Outlook, 14,* 129-136.

Paul, R., & Elder, L. (2001). *Critical thinking: Tools for taking charge of your learning and your life.* Upper Saddle River, NJ: Prentice Hall.

# Chapter 29: USING CONCEPT MAPS TO FOSTER CRITICAL THINKING

Deanne Couey, BSN, MS, RN

*Recently I was stopped by a group of students who were frantically studying for a test on pharmacology. One student said to me, "These just look like words on a page and I don't know anything anymore!" I shared with them how I might approach learning classifications and asked if they had recently cared for any clients who were prescribed any of the medications they were reviewing. I told them to think about the client situation that necessitated those medications, and to do some general drug cards with meaningful information to learn those particular classifications. They liked that idea and appreciated their new plan for how to learn the material. As I walked away, I couldn't help but think how use of concept maps involves the same type of approach, an approach that guides the learning process and fosters critical thinking.*

*Leading students to make associations between theory and practice is a critical factor in their development. Concept mapping allows students to actively examine their thoughts and actions as they relate to client care and the nursing process. Color and design lend to visual enhancement of concepts and encourages explanation of the facts presented. Concept mapping is a creative process that challenges students to go beyond the traditional column approach to writing a care plan. Not only do care maps facilitate student learning, they allow the teacher an opportunity to learn how the student is putting ideas and facts together. With a visual representation there is less chance for miscommunication between student and teacher and a better chance to intervene. A review of a care map allows the teacher to know what the student is thinking, highlighting what the student knows and doesn't know. This is essential if we are to foster an environment of learning. – Lynn Engelmann*

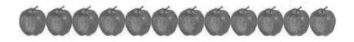

## Educational Philosophy

I respect each student nurse as a person and seek to facilitate the lifelong learning process by providing support and guidance throughout a multitude of opportunities that provide a foundation for practice as they begin the journey – Deanne Couey

# Introduction

The hallmark assignment in nursing school is the traditional student care plan. Briefly, this assignment consists of background information culminating with the standard five-column linear format. Many students complain about the amount of time they spend writing these care plans and fail to see the purpose of them or connections between components of the nursing process. They state writing care plans is frustrating, especially in proportion to the time invested. Once they master the steps of the nursing process, students often copy care plan content word for word from books, computerized care plans, or each other. The student care plan assignment then begins to lose effectiveness as a learning tool.

Concept maps have grown as a viable alternative to the traditional student care plan. Concept maps enhance learning through visual presentation and organization of data. They encourage critical thinking. Using concept maps, students link the steps of the nursing process and relate concepts. They concisely organize client information as they create a visual learning tool that is uniquely their own.

# Introduction to Concept Map Theory

The theory and development of Novak and Gowen's (1984) concept maps is based in part on the educational psychology of David Ausubel's (1968) assimilation theory developed in the 1960s and 1970s.

Ausubel proposed that new learning occurs by incorporating, relating, and subsuming new concepts and propositions into an existing knowledge base – incorporating concepts into one's existing cognitive makeup. This is different than simple memorization of new content. Rote memorization is not meaningful learning and does not promote critical thinking. Learning from the perspective of assimilation theory is meaningful as learners assimilate or make sense of new information based on their own unique, pre-existing cognitive schemes.

Novak and Gowen (1984) tested Ausubel's (1968) theory when studying how young children's knowledge of science is altered with learning. They coined the phrase **concept map**, referring to a detailed visual metacognitive tool used to organize knowledge in a hierarchical manner. Concepts or ideas are represented with geometric shapes, such as circles or squares, then labeled with symbols or words. A relationship between concepts is indicated with a line. Words on the lines state the specific relationship between the two concepts. Propositions – proposed relationships – are formed when the concepts are linked together. Crosslinks are creative connections used to demonstrate interrelationships among different parts of the concept map. See Figure 29.1 and 29.2 for an example of these concept map designs.

Figure 29.1 - A Concept map: Showing the Structure and Characteristics of Good Concept Maps.

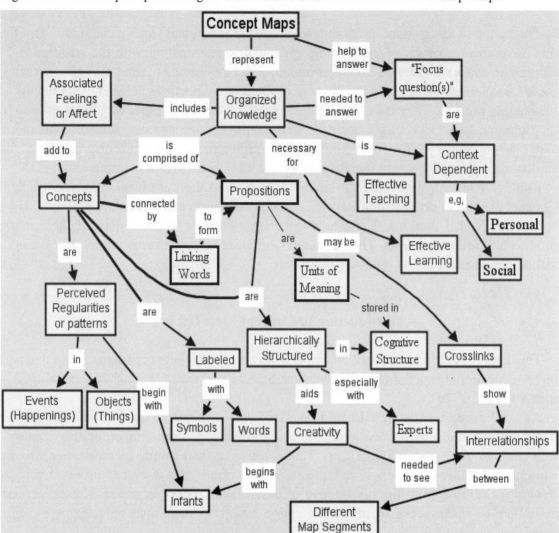

Reprinted with permission of Joseph Novak, copyright, 1990.

Figure 29.2 - Hybrid Map

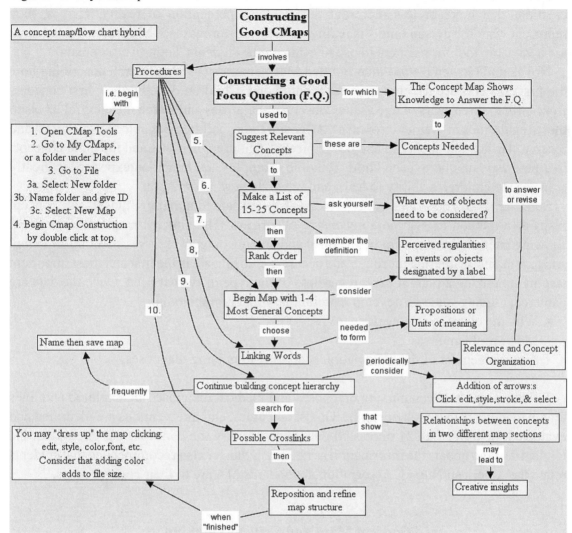

(Reprinted with permission, Joseph Novak, copyright 1990.)

Because concept maps represent a picture of what is in a person's mind, they are unique creations that more or less represent that person's perception of reality. That is, they represent what the person thinks is reality, so they may or may not be correct and, as such, are a valuable tool for teachers to use to evaluate the students' cognitive schemata.

Novak and Gowen (1984) incorporated MacNamara's (1982) research describing how the first concepts are developed in early childhood. Children develop their first concepts from birth to three years of age as they observe regularities and attach meaningful labels to these regularities in their environment. After age three, children begin to ask questions and receive clarification about old and new concepts. Children then link and integrate concepts in a new way, unique to each child. Tangible examples and hands-on experiences greatly enhance the children's ability to learn and integrate new information.

Schuster (2002) described concept maps as they relate to nursing. Students use concept maps as a method to plan comprehensive client care. The concept map becomes a tool showing interrelationships among medical and nursing diagnoses, assessment information, and treatments. Gathering thorough and accurate clinical data is the first and most important step in organizing a plan of care, regardless of the type of format used. Once the data are gathered, nursing students develop a preliminary diagram including:

- Why the client sought health care.
- Major problem areas.
- An arrangement of the information according to nursing diagnoses.

Relationships between nursing diagnoses and medical diagnoses are explored and lines drawn to indicate these relationships. Goals, outcomes, and interventions are identified and evaluated. Schuster (2002) suggested that students carry the concept map throughout the clinical day and update the information as needed. Schuster also recommended that students relate the American Nurses' Association's Standards of Care to their concept maps.

## Concept Maps and Critical Thinking

Beitz (1998) stated that concept mapping is a useful tool for developing critical thinking skills because students are able to visualize what they are thinking. Preliminary studies by Daley, Shaw, Balistrieri, Glasenapp, and Piacentine (1999) concluded that concept maps can significantly improve critical thinking abilities in nursing students when used in the clinical setting. Faculty can identify students' abilities to correctly or incorrectly document intricate relationships among client care concepts.

Daley et al. (1999) and Novak and Gowen's (1984) findings further support the idea that a concept map is not only a powerful learning tool but also is an important tool for evaluating critical thinking. Students' concept maps become more intricate and complex as they continue to construct subsequent maps. Daley et al. (1999) showed that students' scores on concept mapping significantly improved as students progressed through the nursing courses. This growth can be used as an outcome measure that demonstrates improved critical thinking abilities throughout the nursing curriculum.

Ignatavicius (2004) characterizes care plans as linear forms of documenting components of the nursing process. The ease of copying information directly from a care plan book does not encourage the nursing student in problem solving or to critically think. Nor does the multicolumnar care plan encourage the student to visualize or create different cross-links between components of the nursing process. Thus the relationships between different parts of the nursing process are not always apparent in a care plan as they are in a concept map.

In part, this may be because concept map development is a dynamic process which requires organizing client information in clusters. These clusters may be linked together with propositional phrases. Students see connections between information when they can move the concepts around the map and organize it in a way that makes sense to them. The students draw lines between propositions and connect each concept with descriptive words to show the connection. Students have the freedom to arrange and link the concept map together in many different ways and make connections that are not considered on a multicolumnar care plan. Cooperative learning strategies can occur when groups of students complete concept maps together as a team.

Daley et al (1999) found concept maps not only enhance critical thinking abilities in nursing students but also can be used as a tool to measure those abilities within the scope of nursing practice. Schuster (2000) suggests that concept maps are more helpful in increasing learning than traditional nursing care plans because when students develop concept maps they more clearly organize client data and plan nursing care.

Ignatavicius (2004) believes critical thinking occurs when students organize information and make connections between concepts in a unique way. The most difficult part of learning occurs when the student actually makes these connections between and among different, but related, concepts. The lecture driven, teacher-centered learning environment does not require or stimulate critical thinking. Developing concept maps is a form of active learning that develops critical thinking.

Students can also use concept maps to conduct a self-appraisal of their ability to understand relationships and document accurate, specific, client care. Student portfolios are an excellent mechanism for organizing this work and documenting progression in developing critical thinking skills from course to course.

## Constructing a Concept Map

Prior to implementation in the clinical setting, construction of concept maps may be discussed in the classroom setting. The first step in constructing a concept map is to select a particular client or another concept of interest. Topics currently under study in the course can serve as a guide in the selection process. The client care situation or concept is placed in the center of the paper, becoming the central point around which all concepts are related. Mueller, Johnston, and Bligh (2001) note that by placing the client in the center of the map, a nursing model of care rather than a medical model is projected, which imparts a holistic view. Students are encouraged to use pictures for the central concept to enhance the visualization aspect of concept mapping. See sample concept maps that may be accessed on the CD-ROM that accompanies this book.

The students then discuss how to begin mapping and making connections on the plan of care. Students identify key concepts and decide how to order or categorize each concept. This process begins with general concepts and advances to specific concepts.

Novak and Gowen (1984) stress the importance of students recognizing that all the concepts are related. Students should be selective in choosing cross-links and succinct in the wording used to connect the concepts. Novak and Gowen also state that providing students with a list of concepts is useful as the students begin the process of identifying some sort of hierarchy.

Key words related to the topic are placed on lines projecting from the central topic, resembling the spokes on a wheel. The structure may also take on the form of a flowchart. As the students gain experience in creating concept maps, the design tends to change.

Relationships among concepts are identified. Students draw lines with arrows connecting concepts and identifying their relationship. Students must include nursing diagnoses, goals and outcomes, nursing interventions, and evaluation of the client's response to nursing care. Often students forget or neglect to include the evaluation component of the nursing process.

Mueller et al. (2001) suggest using a color-coded system for better visual identification of the concepts represented on the map. All concepts with a common characteristic are given the same color or shape. What the colors and shapes signify is defined by the student. These colors and shapes help to sort and categorize the information and identify interrelationships. A key is included on the map to identify the coding system.

One possible coding system uses the colors red, yellow, and green. These colors take on the conventional meanings of danger, caution, and go forward. Red – a sign of danger – is used to denote anticipated signs and symptoms, absolute contraindications, or deadly aspects. Yellow is used as a cautionary color to represent nursing diagnoses or collaborative problems. Green, signifying "go ahead" or "making progress," is used to document nursing interventions.

General concepts are listed first and include both subjective and objective data located in the health history and the physical assessment. Other data can include allergies, medications, IV therapy, diagnostic tests, stages of growth and development, pain management, support services, nutritional information, activity level, and elimination patterns. Students can prioritize the collection of this data. Schuster (2002) suggests collecting information on medications and IV therapy as a priority because of the inherent danger if errors are made with these therapies. The students then fill in the map with specific client information, such as vital sign trends, side effects of medications, and specific laboratory values.

When initially teaching students how to develop a concept map, both non-nursing and nursing examples can be used. Schuster (2002) provides an example of a skeleton map with a client problem in the center and other related concepts projecting in a spoke-like wheel fashion. When students first begin to learn to construct concept maps, this type of skeleton can be provided with boxes already drawn. The students insert the concept names inside the boxes. Lines and boxes can be developed using a word processing program.

Computer software is available that can be used to develop concept maps. These programs ease the organization and movement of concepts around the map. Concepts with linking statements can be rearranged easily and the map restructured to add clearness. The size and type of font and the shapes containing the concepts can all be changed to improve the overall appearance of the concept map. Because it takes several revisions to complete a map, computer software is preferred over poster board, sticky notes, and markers. Student versions of these software programs are available with a free trial and reasonable pricing. Information about specific companies is listed at the end of this chapter. The school may also consider purchasing the software for campus use. A computer printout of a concept map provides a professional look for faculty to use in classroom presentations when role modeling how to organize concepts.

If software is not available or maps are developed in class, large items such as posterboard or butcher paper are used. Sticky notes represent a concept and are moved around until the design looks right to the student.

## Assisting Students in Developing Concept Maps

The primary role of the teacher is that of facilitator. The teacher gives support and encouragement fostering individual thinking and providing feedback to guide the student through the process. Teachers and students work together in a joint effort to promote each student's uniqueness. It is important that teachers be open to various approaches to concept map development. "Tell me about your concept map" is an opening remark that encourages students to discuss:

- How they organized client information.
- What client data is related and what data is not related.
- What connections are missing and how they should proceed.
- Validation of their thought processes related to client care.

As students "think out loud," teachers can correct any misperceptions related to the information the students share. Mueller et al. (2001) stated that concept maps are "thinking tools" – a work in motion.

Using concept maps, students' knowledge bases expand. Teachers facilitate this expansion of the knowledge base as the maps become more detailed and complex. It is this progression in sequential concept mapping throughout the nursing program that demonstrates the students' abilities to improve critical thinking skills.

## Using Concept Maps with Beginning Nursing Students

Instruction on developing concept maps can be successfully introduced in a fundamental nursing course after students demonstrate a beginning understanding about how to:
- Collect subjective and objective information.
- Cluster data to develop nursing diagnoses.
- Identify goals and outcome criteria.
- Incorporate specific nursing interventions into a plan of care.
- Evaluate client outcomes.

Applying the steps of the nursing process to these early concept maps is important. Knowledge of the nursing process is a prerequisite for developing a concept map in the clinical setting. Introducing concept mapping in the beginning nursing courses allows students to become familiar with the theory supporting the use of concept maps and the process of developing them.

## Teaching Concept Maps Using Small Groups

Students can work in small groups, brainstorming with peers to visualize the information. Small-group work leads students to better understand the process in preparation for individual development of concept maps. Groups of students working together foster collaboration and communication, both important skills for nursing students to master. Having students develop concept maps in small groups is one way to develop these skills. Learning is facilitated because students learn from each other and are actively involved in the process. Collaboration generates accomplishments, more constructive interpersonal student relationships, and better long-term retention of information. This type of group brainstorming does not happen when students write traditional student care plans. Topics for concept mapping with beginning nursing students can include simple case studies, a psychomotor skill, health history, physical assessment, pathophysiology, or medications as they relate to a specific client condition.

At this point, it is helpful for students to receive hands-on practice with faculty support and guidance. Group work in developing a concept map typically proceeds in the following way. Students select a specific client or a certain concept to review. Together, the group organizes the information on a diagram. The following are suggestions for guiding beginning nursing students in small-group work as they develop their initial concept maps.

- Give each group a piece of butcher's paper or poster paper and a variety of colored markers.
- Instruct each group to develop a concept map using the colored markers to develop a coding system as discussed earlier in this chapter.

The students work together to compare and evaluate the information, then consult and collaborate to formulate nursing diagnoses. They relate their understanding of the relationship between pathophysiology and clinical manifestations and begin making connections among all components in the nursing process. The students learn by creating meaningful relationships and eventually discovering the similarities and differences among concepts and ideas. This collaboration gives students an opportunity to link classroom knowledge with clinical practice, which improves critical thinking skills.

The groups then present their maps to the class. One member of each group explains how the information is connected, presents the selected case scenario, and leads the discussion about the concept map.

## Using Concept Maps in the Clinical Setting

Mapping the plan of care for an assigned client in the clinical setting is an exciting and meaningful way for students to organize information and see the bigger picture. The students collect all information contained on a traditional care plan, then sketch that information on a visual nursing care plan concept map. Students are able to see situations differently and make connections that are not as evident when using a traditional care plan layout.

Post-conference provides an opportunity for individual students to receive feedback from the entire group. Concept maps represent the students thinking out loud and making connections, all of which stimulate critical thinking (Mueller et al., 2001). Students explain how they are thinking and speculate how others might think and solve problems differently. These discussions provide links between classroom theory and clinical practice.

A roundtable discussion works well when discussing conceptual relationships. Students share their visions of how concepts relate and brainstorm various points of view. When students learn there is more than one way to complete a concept map, they begin to realize there is more than one way to approach a client situation – and each way can be uniquely different. Factors such as the students' interpretations of the information, the nature of the student-client relationship, and the students' views of the overall client situation all influence the way concepts are linked. Each concept map is innovatively different, in sharp contrast to traditional student care plans.

## Working with Nonvisual Learners

Assisting students in developing concept maps is important because not all students are visual learners. Some students prefer the multicolumn, traditional style student care plan and struggle with concept maps. Teachers can assist these students in developing mapping skills by cutting out the columns of the care plan and asking the student to paste the pieces around the most general concept. Teachers can assist students as needed in placing the components on the map and asking students questions about the relationships among the various concepts. Sticky notes in various colors and shapes can be used to move the concepts.

Some students become confused and overwhelmed at all the cross-link possibilities and have difficulty making even a single connection. These students may require additional time to complete the concept map. Students may choose to bring pieces of their concept map and discuss possible arrangement of concepts with faculty. This support demonstrates that faculty are open to various learning styles and function as facilitators of learning, partnering with the students to promote individuality in concept map development.

## Grading the Concept Map

Whether or not to grade concept maps is controversial among nursing educators. Some faculty want specific step by step guidelines, while others believe progression from week to week is evidence of improved critical thinking abilities by nursing students. Novak and Gowen (1984) selected grading criteria based on propositions, hierarchy, cross links, and examples. They propose the following grading criteria.
- When propositions between 2 concepts are meaningful, 1 point is given.
- If the map shows hierarchy, the student receives 5 points for each valid level.
- If the map shows meaningful cross links, the student receives 10 points if the cross links have both validity and significance, but only 2 points if one of these elements is missing.

- Creative cross links should be recognized and can receive extra points.
- Examples, not actual concepts, included on the map receive 1 point.

Daley et al (1999) used this scoring system to obtain mean group scores of nursing students as they introduced concept maps as a strategy to teach and evaluate critical-thinking. Comparison between the students' initial maps to the final maps showed a statistically significant difference, indicating the students' ability to increase conceptual thinking and critical thinking from using concept maps over the course of a semester.

Beginning maps should have all the components of the nursing process. Often students do not include evaluation of outcomes as part of the concept map. Early maps tend to show a more linear format; some students create maps resembling a spoke on a wheel. As the students continue to practice concept maps, it becomes obvious that new and creative relationships are seen as they draw lines from one concept to another. Each map, if properly completed, shows progression as the students come to a new understanding of the process.

Whatever method of evaluation used, the student will need to receive feedback about completed care maps. For many nursing faculty, providing such feedback may be a new experience. Fortunately, grading these maps is not difficult. If concept maps are new to the curriculum, faculty may consider assigning a pass/fail grade until a more formal grading process is developed.

To develop a formal grading process, faculty can review the maps as a group, discussing various map components, identifying the presence and relationship of each component in the nursing process, and looking for overall strengths and weaknesses. This exercise establishes consistency in both the nature of feedback and the assignment of a grade. The grading criteria for concept maps can then be developed. General grading criteria should be consistent throughout the curriculum, with specific criteria established for each level of nursing course to show progression. Finally, the criteria can be shared with students when the assignment is given. It is always prudent to include these criteria in the course syllabus.

The most effective way to grade concept maps is to have students verbally explain the connections and cross links between concepts. Mueller et al. (2001) suggested that the culminating benefit in constructing concept maps is not realized unless students can explain their reasoning for the organizational structure and connections. During the process of explaining their maps, students have the opportunity to verify the correctness of their thinking. This provides a rich learning experience for students.

As students progress through the nursing courses, their concept maps should become more complex and complete. Therefore, demonstration of progression is an important grading criterion. Some questions to address when evaluating progression include the following:

- Does each map improve upon the previous one?
- Does the map become more thorough?
- Is creativity evident in the concept map?
- Is the student showing relationships among concepts?
- Are the relationships valid?
- Are there more cross links each time a concept map is completed?
- Is all information complete and correct?

Concept map grades can be included in the clinical grade or as a classroom homework assignment. Beitz (1998) observed that students are motivated to earn a good grade by completing a thorough concept map. A thorough concept map is an important asset for helping students understand the big picture. Questions to guide evaluation of maps for completeness include the following:

- Are all components of the nursing process present?
- Is the assessment data complete?
- Is the client data grouped correctly to validate the nursing diagnoses?
- Are the side effects of medications connected to signs and symptoms or laboratory values?
- Are the abnormal laboratory values connected to a disease process or medication?
- Are goals supported and linked to nursing interventions?
- Are the nursing interventions specific, accurate, and supported by rationales?
- Has the client progressed toward short-term and long-term goals?
- Was the student able to evaluate the effectiveness of care?
- Is there a teaching component included?

## Student Evaluation of Concept Maps as a Learning Tool

It is helpful for faculty to have students evaluate the use of concept maps as a learning tool. This section summarizes responses to various questions asked by the author when working with a clinical group of students completing concept maps every one to two weeks in a critical care clinical setting during the final semester of an associate degree nursing program. The first question was, "How did concept maps clarify client information?" Student comments included:

- "It put pieces of a puzzle together."
- "It considered aspects of the nursing process and client care that get overlooked on a busy day."
- "I saw connections I hadn't seen before."
- "It was a good visual picture."

- "I saw relationships with drugs, why they were taken, the adverse effects of them, and how they affect lab values."
- "It did clarify the information but took a lot of time."

One student preferred completing traditional care plans and commented, "It was confusing to me; I am used to a linear form of work."

The second question involved the time required to construct a concept map. Student responses included that time was a major issue, especially for those who had trouble joining things together. The time factor varied from 1 to 10 hours to complete a map. One student commented, "One map each week stressed me out."

It is obvious that some students spend many hours organizing and revising their concept map. However, other students may display minimal effort and produce very simple concept maps. In these cases, faculty can require the student to continue to revise the concept map until the connections among concepts are made. With each subsequent concept map, the time required to complete the assignment should decrease.

The third question asked what steps the students took in developing a concept map for the clinical setting. Their answers included:

- "I would pick my topic, then find the signs and symptoms, the medical management, nursing care, lab values, client education, rationales, and goals. Each part really first needed to be researched to find out what should be done."
- "Data came from the chart; textbooks to organize and finalize."
- "Data came from the nursing shift report and client information gathered throughout the clinical day; I tried to work it in the concept map."
- "I started with a general diagnosis and included all clinical data, adding the nursing diagnoses; then I fine-tuned it, reorganized, and looked for connections and relationships."
- "I gathered information on the disease, taped it on a board, and analyzed the connections."
- "I did a rough draft first; a care plan outline helped me get going."

The fourth question asked students if they found the process of developing concept maps beneficial. They gave a resounding yes! Some specific responses included:

- "I loved the concept maps."
- "A wonderful learning tool."
- "It helped me look at every aspect of my client!"
- "It was a great learning experience."
- "I could piece things together."
- "I could picture the map in my head when I thought about the subject during a test."
- "It requires us to use critical thinking skills to gather information and put it all to-

gether. My assessment skills and history-taking skills are greatly improved as a result. It brought the entire nursing process together for me."
- "It solidified the concepts."
- "I looked at the client as a whole."
- "It was a visual way to see how it all relates."

The fifth question asked students to compare and contrast a concept map with a traditional student care plan.
- "It was a different way to look at things."
- "Different formats, same information."
- "The concept map was a 3-D care plan."
- "Care plans can be done just opening a book; concept maps require you to **think** in order to form relationships between all aspects of care."
- "The concept map was a more visual learning tool."
- "You could see the care that was needed for the client [with the concept map]."
- "The concept map was more creative, in an expanded form."
- "The concept maps connect different medications, assessment data, and nursing care together in a way I did not see when doing care plans."

The group was very positive about developing a concept map and preferred the concept map over traditional care plans. Some additional responses included:
- "I wish we could have done them from day one. Thank you!"
- "I like the option of expanding on a concept map from one week to the next."
- "This really helped me."

## Educating Faculty about Concept Maps

Because the traditional student care plan has long been regarded as the norm for developing care plans, there may be resistance to changing to concept maps. It may take time to integrate this assignment into the curriculum framework. Faculty may need to be educated on how to use concept maps as an effective learning strategy. It is important that faculty understand the theoretical basis for concept mapping and how to construct a concept map so they can teach students the skill. This information is also important to ensure consistency in grading. Consistency in grading is essential if concept maps are used to measure critical thinking as an expected outcome.

## Conclusion

Concept maps, although not new to education in general, are relatively new to nursing education. When introducing or extending the use of concept maps in a curriculum, faculty may want to address the following questions:

- When is the best time to introduce concept maps into the nursing curriculum?
- What is the best way to grade the concept maps?
- When used in the clinical, what is the best time to have the students present this information, pre-planning or post-conference?
- How do we get all faculty to use concept maps?
- Can we use concept maps to measure critical thinking outcome criteria?
- Do students have improved test scores after implementing concept maps?

Faculty may not be able to answer all the above questions but can use them to stimulate creative curriculum planning. Many of these questions provide rudimentary research ideas for nursing faculty to explore in the future.

## Examples of Student Concept Maps

The CD-ROM accompanying this book contains examples of actual concept maps developed by students in the clinical setting at at North Arkansas College in Harrison, Arkansas during their last semester in an Associate Degree Nursing program. These maps can be found under chapter 29 on the CD-ROM.

## Discussion: Should Concept Maps Be Graded?

Under Chapter 29 on the CD-ROM accompanying this book are responses from nurse educators when the question, " I am looking for different grading criteria/tools for concept maps to foster critical thinking skills in nursing students. Does anyone have an example to share?" was posted on the Nurse Educator's listserv. Their comments were in response to an invitation to share their thoughts in this chapter.

## Contact Information for Purchasing Concept-Mapping Software

Inspiration software can be downloaded for a 30-day free trial and is available for about $70 for a single license. It is quite user friendly and provides a visually pleasing concept map. For more information about Inspiration software concept mapping, contact inspiration.com.

Joseph Novak (2002) has concept mapping software available at IHMC Concept Map Software for about $80. For more information on Novak's software, check the website http://cmap.coginst.edu/info.

KnowledgeManager is an international website for help with concept mapping and knowledge management, and it is located at http://www.knowledgemanager.us/KM-KnowledgeManager-eng.htm. The software purchase price is listed in Euros.

Numerous websites on concept mapping can be searched for various examples of concept maps, accessing software for easier development of a concept map, and theory behind concept mapping for a better understanding on why it works so well. Search with key words – concept map or mind map– to locate the many websites for additional information. For your convenience, these website addresses are included under Chapter 29 on the CD-ROM accompanying this book.

## Learning Activities

1. Make a concept map on a topic covered in class, i.e. hematology. As you discuss the lesson, refer to your concept map. The components of the blood, normal laboratory values, blood transfusions, and nursing actions are all interrelated concepts within hematology. Give each student a copy of your concept map as a reference. This helps the students see how the components of the map are linked and how to begin building their own concept maps. On an exam, include valid test items over the content in the concept map.

2. Design a skeleton concept map filling in some/none of the concepts and some/all of the linking words for students to complete as a quiz grade, as a way to prepare for class, or as a homework assignment. The skeletal concept map could also be used as a tool to measure assessment of classroom learning to see if students were grasping the information presented.

3. Display your students' concept maps for all to see. Have a prize for the most creative concept map each week. Make copies of exceptional concept maps and give to other students to use an example. Laminate the exceptional concept maps and use with subsequent classes as student examples.

# References

Ausubel, D. P. (1968). *Educational psychology: A cognitive view.* New York: Holt, Rinehart, and Winston.

Beitz, J. M. (1998). Concept mapping: Navigating the learning process. *Nurse Educator, 23*(5), 35-41.

Daley, B. J., Shaw, C. R., Balistrieri, T., Glasenapp, K., & Piacentine, L. (1999). Concept maps: A strategy to teach and evaluate critical thinking. *Journal of Nursing Education, 38*(1), 42-47.

Ignatavicius, D. (Jan. 2004 in press). From Traditional Care Plans to Innovative Concept Maps. In Oermann, M. & Heinrich, K. *Annual review of nursing education.* Springer Publishing Company, New York.

Macnamara, J. (1982). *Names for things: A study of human learning.* Cambridge, MA: MIT Press

Mueller, A., Johnston, M., & Bligh, D. (2001). Mind-mapped care plans: A remarkable alternative to traditional nursing care plans. *Nurse Educator, 26*(2), 75-80.

Novak, J. D. (2002). *The theory underlying concept maps and how to construct them* [online]. Retrieved April 4, 2002. Available: http://cmap.coginst.uwf.edu/info

Novak, J. D., & Gowen, D. B. (1984). *Learning how to learn.* New York: Cambridge University Press.

O'Banion, T. (1997). *A learning college for the 21st century.* American Association of Community Colleges. Oryx Press.

Schuster, P. (2000). Concept mapping: Reducing clinical care plan paperwork and increasing learning. *Nurse Educator, 25*(2), 76-81.

Schuster, P. (2002). Concept mapping: *A critical-thinking approach to care planning.* Philadelphia, PA: F. A. Davis Company.

# Bibliography

Anderson, C. A. (1996). Teaching is not feeding. *Nursing Outlook, 14*(6), 257-258.

Ausubel, D. P., Novak, J. D., & Hanesian, H. (1978). *Educational psychology: A cognitive view* (2nd ed.). New York: Holt, Rinehart, & Winston.

Barr, R., & Tagg, J. (1995, November/December). From teaching to learning: A new paradigm for undergraduate education. *Change,* 13-25.

Baugh, N. G., & Mellott, K. G. (1998). Clinical concept mapping as preparation for student nurses' clinical experiences. *Journal of Nursing Education, 37*(6), 254-256.

Cravener, P. A. (1997). Promoting active learning in large lecture classes. *Nurse Educator, 22*(3), 21-26.

Daley, B. (1996). Concept maps: Linking nursing theory to clinical nursing practice. *Journal of Continuing Education in Nursing, 27*(1), 17-27.

Johnson, D. W., Johnson, R. T., & Smith, K. A. (1991). *Cooperative learning: Increasing college faculty institutional productivity* (ASHE-ERIC Higher Education Report No.4). Washington, DC: George Washington University, School of Education and Human Development.

Novak, J. D. (1990). Concept maps and vee diagrams: Two metacognitive tools to facilitate meaningful learning. *Instructional Science, 19*, 29-52.

Yensen, J. (2002). *Strategies for learning: From concept maps to learning objects and books to works* [online]. Retrieved June 15, 2002. Available: http://www.langara. bc.ca/vnc/ojni.htm

# Chapter 30: CRITICAL THINKING IN PROGRESSIVE STUDENT LABORATORY EXPERIENCES

Arlene Morris, BSN, MSN, RN

*Faculty and staff educators need to ensure that students and practicing nurses can perform nursing skills at a competent level, and typically use the return demonstration method for this type of evaluation. The psychomotor skills laboratory is often seen as a place to apply rote memorization of a lock-step approach to skill return demonstrations. However, over the years many visionary educators have struggled to develop a plan for using the skills laboratory in a more creative and productive manner. Arlene Morris offers such a plan. – Linda Caputi and Lynn Engelmann*

## Introduction

Nursing simulation laboratories have traditionally been used for teaching psychomotor skills. Students practice the skill on a mannequin, and then are evaluated on the accurate and safe performance of that skill. Variations may occur, such as:

- Validation of certain skills at differing points in the nursing curriculum, such as medication administration during the first term, invasive procedures such as urinary catheterization or tracheostomy suctioning during more advanced semesters.
- Group practice followed by validation of one group member representing the skill performance of all members of the group (personal communication at Creative Teaching for Nurse Educators workshops, March 2001 and March 2002).

### Educational Philosophy

My teaching philosophy includes two core values that are also inherent in my nursing philosophy: the dignity of the individual and an emphasis on quality. I believe the individual student brings personal attributes and experiences to the learning environment. Nurse educators are challenged to build on these to assist the student in developing both a commitment to learning and a self-expectation of providing the highest quality nursing care. A potential for transformation in both student and faculty occurs through collaboration as students are actively engaged in seeking their highest level of knowledge and professional nursing performance. – Arlene H. Morris

Acceptable skill performance for a specific nursing skill is typically validated only once in the simulation laboratory setting during the student's nursing education. Further opportunity to perform that specific skill depends upon client needs during the student's clinical rotations.

Another, more recently developed system of skill validation is the use of videotaped return demonstrations (Aronson, et al, 1997). Johnson, et al (1999) included scenarios and telephone simulations with skills validation videotaping. A telephone interview of faculty from ten randomly selected baccalaureate level nursing schools in Alabama, Arkansas, Georgia, Kentucky, Mississippi, North Carolina, and Tennessee revealed mixed opinions regarding videotaped skill performances (personal communication, May, 1997). Some faculty stated their nursing program would continue the use of videotaped performances because it seemed to decrease student anxiety. Others, however, were planning to discontinue use of videotaped return demonstrations because it was difficult to observe all aspects of the skill being performed by the student and there was no opportunity to question the student's thinking during the videotaped performance.

This chapter discusses the problems and limitations of these traditional approaches to psychomotor skill validation. A different approach is offered using practice-based learning. Incorporating client scenarios, this approach provides a more realistic environment and focuses on critical thinking skills often required when performing the skill during client care.

## Problems with the Traditional Approach

The traditional approach suffers from recurring problems. The following accounts exemplify a few of these problems:

- Student nurses discuss the process of psychomotor skill evaluations. Comments such as "Try to get (name of instructor) to validate your performance. This person is not as concerned if you do it right as if you know why you are doing it." Another student comments, "But if you validate with (name of instructor), you will get so many tips for how to hold the equipment." A third student states, "It is on mannequins not real clients, so it doesn't really matter. Just get it over with so we can go study for tomorrow's test."

- A student nurse memorizes the steps to perform a psychomotor skill, such as urinary catheterization, and confidently performs the skill in the simulation laboratory. However, when this same student is called upon to insert a urinary catheter during client care, the student becomes anxious and overwhelmed. Extraneous factors in the environment specific to the individual client confound the performance of the skill. For example, the student must incorporate therapeutic communication and client teaching, while remembering the correct procedure for catheterization. This leads to statements by the student such as, "That was not **anything** like what we practiced in lab."

- A student nurse completing the final weeks of the senior year is called upon to perform a skill learned during the first term of the nursing program. The student states, "I know I learned that, but I'm just so unsure of myself because it has been such a long time and I've never really gotten to do it on a **real** client in my clinical experiences."

The preceding accounts may ring very familiar to many readers. The purpose of this chapter is to present an approach to teaching psychomotor skills that can address the problems presented in these examples. It offers ways the nursing simulation laboratory of a school of nursing or of a healthcare institution's nursing education department can provide the setting for assessing all domains of learning: psychomotor, cognitive, and affective (Bloom, 1956). This approach is beneficial to both students and practicing nurses.

The following overall goals can be achieved by using the approach offered in this chapter:

- The steps in psychomotor skill performance can be validated.
- Cognitive understanding of the steps in the procedure as well as application to a situation requiring critical thinking can be evaluated.
- The affective components of responding, valuing, and making judgments can be integrated.
- Scenarios are used that promote progression from simple to more complex learning.
- Faculty or nursing staff educators are afforded a heightened awareness of students' needs.

Communication of these needs can then be facilitated between faculty and student or among faculty to assist students in meeting their needs.

## Psychomotor Skill Performance

Before explaining the practice-based skill validation process, it may be helpful to review how students progress through the attainment of acceptable performance of a psychomotor skill. Expectations for the psychomotor skill performance progress from simple to complex. Oermann and Gaberson (1998) offer an understanding of this concept with their taxonomy of psychomotor skill performance:

1. **Imitation** — Skills are learned in the beginning after they have been demonstrated, whether directly by the teacher or by observation of the process on a film, videotape, or slide tape sequence. The performance lacks neuromuscular coordination or control and, hence, is generally in a crude and imperfect form (i.e., impulse, overt repetition).

2. **Manipulation** — In this level, the learner follows a prescription as outlined on a procedure sheet, learning to follow instructions, performing selected actions and fixing performance through necessary practice.

3. **Precision** — Performance has reached a level of refinement and can be carried out without a set of directions or a model, and performance is characterized by accuracy, i.e., exactness with reduction in errors.

4. **Articulation** — Performance is coordinated in a logical sequence of activities that reflects harmony and consistency among the activities. The time dimension is added here, for speed and time must be within a realistic expectation.

5. **Naturalization**—Skill represents a high degree of proficiency, which has become an automatic response to appropriate situational cues. Performance is efficient and meets criteria for professional competence (p. 17).

They then go on and apply performance criteria to each level of their psychomotor skill taxonomy:

1. **Imitation**
   - Observed actions are followed.
   - Movements are gross.
   - Coordination lacks smoothness.
   - Errors are present.
   - Time and speed are based on learner need.

2. **Manipulation**
   - Written instructions are followed.
   - Coordination of movements is variable.
   - Accuracy is in terms of the written prescription.
   - Time and speed are variable.

3. **Precision**
   - A logical sequence of actions is carried out.
   - Coordination is at a high level.
   - Errors are minimal and do not involve critical actions.
   - Time and speed are variable.

4. **Articulation**
   - A logical sequence of actions is carried out.
   - Coordination is at a high level.
   - Errors are generally limited.
   - Time and speed are within reasonable expectations.

5. **Naturalization**
   - Sequence of actions is automatic.
   - Coordination is consistently at a high level.

- Time and speed are within reality.
- Performance reflects professional competence (p. 17-18).

## Skill Performance Levels of Attainment

An adaptation of this psychomotor taxonomy for the junior and senior years of a baccalaureate level nursing program follows. Other adaptations may be indicated for different types of nursing education programs, depending on the sequencing of psychomotor skill performance.

1. **Imitation** (expectation for junior level – first term, practice sessions only)
   Initially skills are learned following demonstration, whether directly by the teacher or by observation of the process on a film, videotape, or slide sequence. The performance lacks neuromuscular coordination or control and, hence, is generally in a crude and imperfect form. Time and speed are based on learner need.

2. **Manipulation** (expectation for junior level – first term, evaluation)
   The learner follows a prescription as outlined on a procedure sheet, learning to follow instructions, performing selected actions and fixing performance through necessary practice. Coordination of movements is variable. A time frame of at least one week has elapsed from initial imitation to the evaluation of the student at a manipulation level.

3. **Precision** (expectation for junior level – second term, evaluation)
   Performance reaches a level of refinement and can be carried out without a set of directions, and performance is characterized by accuracy. Coordination is at a high level.

4. **Competency** (expectation throughout senior level)
   Skill represents a high degree of proficiency, which has become an automatic response to appropriate situational cues. Coordination is consistently at a high level. Performance is efficient and reflects professional competence.

## A Practice-Based Approach to Laboratory Skills Evaluation

A practice-based approach to laboratory skills evaluation builds on the previous discussion of psychomotor skill attainment. With this practice-based approach, scenarios are written based on client-care situations. These scenarios present situations similar to those encountered in various areas of nursing practice and provide support for student preparation prior to beginning specific clinical rotations. A progression of scenarios is developed that incorporates increasingly complex situations as the student progresses through the nursing courses. These provide a simulated practice-based environment, in which the student can apply critical thinking and clinical judgment in addition to validating psychomotor skill performance throughout the curriculum.

Use of a scenario which resembles anticipated client situations in the approaching clinical experience promotes much more than a routine skill validation. Students are presented with situations that prompt critical thinking and reasoning. They are asked to determine if planned nursing interventions are appropriate, and what adaptations or modifications should be made to the standard skills procedures. For example, urinary catheterization of an infant requires modification from the standard procedures used for an adult client. Incorporating an opportunity for the student to verbalize rationales for modifying a procedure for a client described in a scenario allows discussion and refinement of the student's thinking prior to actual experiences in the clinical setting. Using a practice-based approach, students have voiced comments such as, "It is good to go through this in the lab. I feel that I am more prepared for what we will do next week in clinical."

For a video example of a Junior level practice-based skills validation, refer to the CD-ROM accompanying this book. Under Chapter 30, view the video clips titled *Junior Example*. There are 3 clips to this example.

Additionally, use of a scenario allows for integration of subtle differences often observed in various clinical practice settings. For example, a scenario can be contrived in which a previously dry wound dressing now has drainage, chest tubes that are maintained inaccurately, and pupil responses which are unequal. These variations promote astute observation of the client and surroundings. Incorporating an error for the student to observe, such as oxygen set at a level different than ordered, expired medication bottles, orders for medications to which the client has an allergy for a similar medication are all examples that can be integrated into the practice-based scenarios.

An especially memorable scenario used with students included the presence of a family member in the client's room. Upon close examination, it was determined the family member was not breathing, necessitating the student to determine the priority action!

Scenarios are written to promote communication with clients, families, or other healthcare staff, and when making referrals to other agencies or services. The level of the student influences the communication expected in the scenario. At first it may be difficult for students to communicate with a plastic mannequin. However, the faculty evaluator may briefly enter into the communication process in the role of family member or member of the interdisciplinary healthcare team providing interaction or prompts requiring a student response.

An additional benefit of using a practice-based validation procedure each term is that students who are returning to school following an absence have the opportunity to refresh their skill performance including an evaluation of critical thinking skills applied to client care. These returning students have an opportunity to get back on the same level as their classmates who were enrolled in classes the prior term, and prepare for situations similar to those they will be encountering during the forthcoming term.

## Incorporating Critical Thinking

Consider the following:
- Staff nurses state, "Your graduates are well prepared, but it takes them quite a bit of time to learn how to prioritize and manage multiple clients. Couldn't you work on that while they are still in school?"
- After many years on one unit, a staff nurse transfers to a different area of practice. The subtle differences of clients in this area are unfamiliar to the nurse who is now challenged to use different cognitive and psychomotor skills. This nurse has several options:
    - Seek assistance from the nursing education department or other staff members.
    - Return to the school of nursing to discuss issues of concern with previous faculty members.
    - With time, develop the needed skills.

The above examples demonstrate the need for students and staff to apply critical thinking to nursing skills. Incorporating the evaluation of critical thinking during psychomotor skill performance allows a level of evaluation far beyond the traditional format for evaluating critical thinking – multiple-choice exams. In addition to the performance of the skill, the student's understanding of the rationale for the intervention can be evaluated and feedback provided. Evaluating the student's understanding of the rationale for interventions, prioritization of nursing interventions, and creative use of self enhances the student's formation of clinical judgment. Critical thinking, in its application to nursing, must be developed (Alfaro-LeFevre, 1999).

Practice-based skills validation provides a venue for praise of accurate and effective thinking, discussion of possible alternatives, and clarification of misunderstandings. Faculty feedback in the safe setting of the simulation laboratory can decrease performance anxiety that often accompanies initial performance of skills in the clinical setting. An attitude of "the lab is a place for learning, for practice, and for positive, constructive feedback" encourages collaboration between faculty and student while meeting the learning needs of the student, thereby promoting formation of student knowledge and critical thinking.

### *Expectations for Critical Thinking in Practice-Based Skills Validation*

Expectations for student performance in critical thinking moves from simple to complex.

Incorporating more than one psychomotor skill during a validation session provides the student an opportunity to prioritize interventions to best meet client needs. For example, in the first semester, a simple scenario may involve a client in need of assistance with a bed bath and bed change. For this scenario, the student determines that assistance with the bath should precede changing the linens to prevent moisture on the bed, which in turn can cause client discomfort and a risk for skin breakdown. An addition to this scenario could easily include wound care or colostomy irrigation. See Figures 30.1 and 30.2 for example scenarios. Because students who are validating the same skill may receive different scenarios, informing students which skills may be included allows time for practice of the skills. If time or personnel constraints exist, the student can verbally prioritize interventions then validate only one intervention chosen by the faculty. Prioritization of actions can be written or verbalized by the student immediately prior to skill validation.

Figure 30.1 – Sample Scenario

Scenario for Bath, ROM, Restraints, and Bed Making (option for wound care addition)

G. Gore was admitted to the nursing home 3 weeks ago for generalized weakness and confusion. Skills to be performed today include:

Change occupied bed
Provide complete bed bath (perform on one side of body and state for other side)
Perform ROM to right arm and leg
Apply vest restraint

**Faculty Guidelines for Evaluating Student Performance (to be included on faculty page, but not on student page)**
- The student should choose to complete the bed bath prior to changing the bed linens. Not touching contaminated linens should be emphasized. If the student mentions assessing for type of isolation versus standard precautions, compliment that thinking!
- ROM could be performed during the bath, or if you wish to state that the client is tired and weak, the student should allow a rest before the ROM. Throughout the bath and ROM, the student should be using acceptable communication techniques with the confused client, and assessing physical and cognitive functioning.
- The student should verify current orders and the need for the restraint, and assure that the restraint is the least restrictive method of providing client safety. The student should be able to recall alternative to restraint use from class discussion.

Figure 30.2 – Scenario for Wound Care

---

A. Adams is 2 days post-operative following a colon resection and has an abdominal incision. Physician orders are to clean the incision with NS and apply a dry sterile dressing. Observe universal precautions.

**Faculty Guidelines for Evaluating Student Performance (to be included on faculty page, but not on student page)**

The wound care scenario may be included following wound care instruction and added to the scenario presented in Figure 30.1 as an additional client assignment. In that case, the student should verbalize rationale for selected order of actions. Assure that the student incorporates therapeutic communication with the client during the procedure, and seeks opportunity for teaching.

---

The student should begin by identifying which aspects of the scenario require intervention, then gathering the necessary supplies for all needed interventions to be performed at one time. Performing multiple psychomotor skills during one validation session requires planning ahead for all needed supplies and the order in which these supplies will be needed. Presenting scenarios with a client who has multiple needs or two clients with varying needs encourages the student to prioritize care. Transferring this skill of prioritizing should be evident in the student's clinical experience. For example, when the student informs the clinical teacher a skill is to be performed, all the supplies should be gathered before entering the client's room.

More complex scenarios promote critical thinking at progressive levels. Figure 30.3 provides an example of a complex scenario. For a video example of a complex scenario, refer to the CD-ROM accompanying this book. Under Chapter 30, view the video clips titled *Senior Example*. There are 6 clips to this example.

Students are expected to plan and prioritize nursing interventions, solve problems, and use effective communication, which may include client or family teaching.

Communication and discussion with students during these more complex scenarios slightly prolongs the skill validation process. To save time, students can briefly write pertinent information prior to beginning the skill validation. This sheet is attached to the evaluation form as a record of the student's performance at this point in the curriculum. See Figure 30.4 for an example of a pertinent information sheet for a medication administration validation. Note the item labeled SCENARIO USED. This item is included because there may be many scenarios written for any individual skill. This prevents students from discussing with each other what questions will be asked during the skill validation process that might encourage students to memorize answers rather than apply their own critical thinking skills.

Figure 30.3 – Sample Complex Scenario

---

### NG, Urinary catheterization, IM, SC, ID Medication Administration

At 0800 you receive a new admission to the unit. Mrs. Sweet is 48 years old and admitted with a GI bleed due to chronic alcoholism. Mrs. Sweet also has a severe UTI and a history of well-controlled diabetes x 10 years. **Vital signs:** 103.6, 84, 22,134/82. **Physical findings:** Alert and oriented x 3. Skin warm and dry. Denies pain at this time. Reports nausea. States unable to void.

**Physician's orders**:
Admitting diagnosis: GI bleed, UTI, diabetes mellitus
Diet: NPO
Activity: bed rest
VS q 4h
Allergies: PCN (penicillin)
Foley catheter to BSD (bedside drainage)
Obtain urine for C&S
NG tube to low continuous suction
Schedule KUB in AM
FSBS q 4 hr
Medications:
10u Humulin R and 15u Humulin N SQ before breakfast & dinner
Bactrim 1 po bid
Phenergan 25 mg IM q 4-6h prn
PPD ID today

**Faculty Guidelines (to be included on faculty page, but not on student page)**

Student should consider client risk and comfort factors. As a faculty, you should verbalize for the client when the student assesses for severity of nausea versus abdominal discomfort or bladder distention to determine the priority need for either relief of nausea or for catheterization. The student should determine the risk for hypoglycemia if the insulin has been administered and the client is on NPO status without an IV. The priority action may be to assess blood sugar levels. The student may also state that the stress or infection may cause elevation of the blood sugar. The prioritization order of skill performance could realistically be: FSBS (state that the blood sugar is 125 at this time); then either the foley insertion, NG tube insertion (should have chosen Salem sump type for suction) or phenergan administration (depending on how you relate the client's current feelings). The student should state that the urine C & S can be obtained at time of foley insertion and should be collected prior to Bactrim administration. The student should recognize and discuss the conflict of PO Bactrim and the client is NPO, and problem solving should ensue, such as contacting physician for revision or order for route of medication. Following catheterization, state that 800 cc cloudy amber urine drained into the bag. The student should question administration of insulin in relation to NPO status without an order for an IV. You may role play the physician and provide an order for an IV of D5 ½ NS following catheterization, for the student to have opportunity to mix and administer the insulin. Note that the medications are P.O., S.C., IM, and ID routes. The TB test (PPD) should be the last priority. Additionally, the student may mention a concern regarding the chronic alcoholism and possible withdrawal symptoms. Compliment the student's thinking during this validation. If areas of concern were not noticed by the student, discuss them at completion of the skills validation.

Figure 30.4 – Pertinent Information Sheet

Attachment for student completion prior to medication administration

List the five (5) rights of medication administration: _____

_____

_____

List the three times you check the medication label: _____

_____

Describe some precautions to use when preparing a liquid medication for administration:

_____

Write the needle length and maximum amount of solution to administer via:

Intradermal_____

Subcutaneous_____

Intramuscular_____

Demonstrate the location of intradermal, subcutaneous, and intramuscular injection sites. Name the anatomical landmarks used for each.

Nurses' Notes: _____

_____

_____

_____

_____

_____

Student self-evaluation:

_____

_____

_____

Signature_____     Date_____

SCENARIO USED_____     Demonstration attempt #_____

Scoring:  Critical thinking_____, Assessment_____, Planning_____,

            Implementation_____, Evaluation_____

Overall EVALUATION (E, S, or  U) _____ for _____SKILL

E =  Excellent, S = Satisfactory, U = Unsatisfactory

Faculty evaluator comments:

_____

_____

_____

_____

Signature_____     Date_____

## Variations in Skill Validation Procedures

Variations in the skill validation procedure are possible. Some of these variations provide an opportunity for students to collaborate. Following are some suggestions:

- Students may form pairs to practice the psychomotor skill procedure steps.
- Students may role play the client.
- An effective collaboration between RN to BSN students in the Leadership/Management course and junior level baccalaureate students provides an opportunity for the RN to BSN student to practice evaluating the baccalaureate student. The RN to BSN student can incorporate management theory in providing constructive feedback.
- The faculty role-plays the client, while evaluating the management skills of the upper level student (Dearman, et al, 1999). Educator creativity expands the bounds and application of this approach, limited only by time.

At an advanced level, students are expected to include management skills such as delegation and referrals. Student rationale for priorities can be verbal or written. Figure 30.5 provides an example of a form for student completion during an advanced level course in which all scenarios depicted clients from vulnerable populations. That course involved care of clients with multiple needs such as homeless, victims of abuse, multiple chronic illnesses, etc. It was offered the same term as the leadership-management course. In an attempt to correlate application from the two courses, the student evaluation section of the form depicted in Figure 30.5 was created.

This form includes a section for Student Evaluator comments. This section can be used in one of two ways. The student can complete this section as a self-evaluation in which areas of needed improvement are self-identified along with areas in which the student feels strongly competent. Alternatively, the Student Evaluator section can be used for a RN-to-BSN student to practice evaluation of a beginning nursing student. The RN-to-BSN student should incorporate both positive comments and constructive criticism in identifying areas for improvement needed by the beginning student. This use enables application of leadership and management theory by the RN-to-BSN student in providing feedback to another healthcare team member. If the Student Evaluator section is used for the RN-to-BSN student completion, the Faculty Facilitator comment section should include if the faculty agrees with the RN-to-BSN student's evaluation comments.

Figure 30.5 – Sample form for Scenarios Depicting Clients from Vulnerable Populations

---

Student Name_____

### VULNERABLE POPULATION EVALUATION

Scenario_____

Evaluator:  Please comment on effectiveness in each area.  Give examples when possible.

I. Communication (Privacy provided, non-judgmental attitude, open-ended questions, nonverbal message, etc.)

_____
_____
_____
_____

II. Prioritization  (Appropriateness, rationale stated)

_____
_____
_____
_____

III. Referrals (Appropriate, realistic)

_____
_____
_____
_____

IV. Management (Delegation of tasks, time management, etc)

_____
_____
_____
_____

Student Evaluator comments:

_____
_____
_____
_____

Signature:_____  Date:_____

Faculty Facilitator comments:

_____
_____
_____

Signature:_____  Date: _____

---

## Psychomotor Skill Performance Simulating Clinical Practice

As previously mentioned, a review of traditional psychomotor skill guides reveals step-by-step instruction of a procedure, often with areas for checking accomplishment of each of the steps in the procedure. However, performance in the clinical environment requires more than carrying out predetermined steps of a procedure. Many variables impact the performance of a skill in the clinical environment, including:

- Critical thinking.
- An awareness of the rationale for implementing nursing actions in a particular manner at a particular time.
- Problem-solving.
- Communication.
- Creative use of self.
- Delegation.
- Making referrals.

Incorporating performance of these variables into the psychomotor skill evaluation in a simulated nursing skills laboratory creates a more realistic and more interesting psychomotor skill evaluation for both student and faculty evaluator. Figure 30.6 presents a critical thinking evaluation tool that can be used in conjunction with specific skill evaluation guides. This tool for evaluating critical thinking in progressive scenarios can be used by students in future learning. Areas that are identified as not completed are then viewed as areas needing improvement in performance. For example, the area not completed may be critical thinking (such as ability to verbalize rationales for care), or may be in the actual intervention (steps in performance of the psychomotor skill). The student receives a copy of this Skill Evaluation Tool. If the validation did not include completion of all critical (italicized) behaviors, the student will need to schedule a time for another evaluation attempt. The student's copy of the Skill Evaluation Tool can then be used by the student as a reminder of areas needing additional work. Each term, the Skill Evaluation Tool is filed in the student's color-coded clinical folder. If areas are identified in which the student has not been able to successfully complete during recurrent validation attempts, remediation with the student can be done in these areas. For example, a student who repeatedly has difficulty maintaining a sterile field during evaluations will need to schedule practice sessions in which sterile technique is practiced. Alternately, a student who repeatedly has difficulty accurately determining priority nursing actions will need to schedule remediation work (possibly with computer-assisted instruction) to assist in the critical thinking skill of prioritization.

Figure 30.6 – Critical Thinking Evaluation Tool

| Skill Evaluation Tool | | | | |
|---|---|---|---|---|
| Student Name_____ Date_____ Skill (s)_____ Scenario_____ Demonstration attempt #____ Time for Documentation_____ | | | | |
| **Critical Thinking  (Designate skill being performed in boxes to the right.)** | | | | |
| *1.  Incorporation/application of case situation.*<br>*Assess client to determine that the intervention is still appropriate.*<br>**Assess client's level of consciousness, ability to cooperate, and need for explanation and/or psychological support.** | | | | |
| *2.  Prioritization of client needs and care to be given.* | | | | |
| *3.  Verbalization of rationales for care.* | | | | |
| **4.  Problem-solving (Includes appropriate interdisciplinary involvement, referrals, using community resources.)** | | | | |
| **5.  Therapeutic use of self / creativity in skill (communication with client, innovative approaches to client care.)** | | | | |
| Assessment | | | | |
| *1.  Verify physician's order.* | | | | |
| *2.  Identify client by room number, armband, and having client state name.* | | | | |
| 3.  Perform focused assessment on system related to skill being performed. | | | | |
| Planning | | | | |
| 1.  Identify expected outcomes. | | | | |
| *2.  Obtain equipment (all needed supplies are to be brought to room prior to skill and organized for use.)* | | | | |
| Intervention | | | | |
| *1. Identify client by room number, armband, and having client state name.* | | | | |
| *2.  Introduce yourself to the client, including both name and title/role, and explain what you plan to do and why, in terms the client can understand.  Provide client teaching about intervention and allow for questions.* | | | | |
| *3.  Wash hands for at least 10 seconds.* | | | | |
| *4.  Perform needed assessment prior to skill implementation.* | | | | |
| *5.  Raise bed to appropriate working height and maintain client safety and comfort throughout procedure.* | | | | |
| *6.  Verify allergy to iodine or latex if applicable.*<br>*Verify verbal allergy to medications.* | | | | |
| *7.  Perform skill in logical manner, maintaining communication with client.* | | | | |
| *8.  Maintain sterile technique if applicable (sterile field at waist level, arms remain above waist level, does not cross over sterile field, touches only sterile areas with sterile gloves, does not contaminate sterile areas.)* | | | | |
| *9.  Reassess client's respiratory and cardiovascular status if needed.* | | | | |

Figure 30.6 – Critical Thinking Evaluation Tool cont.

| | | | | |
|---|---|---|---|---|
| **Following any procedure:** | | | | |
| *1. Position client for comfort.* | | | | |
| *2. Be certain client has a way to call for help and knows how to use it.* | | | | |
| *3. Lower the bed to the lowest position and raise the side rails if indicated.* | | | | |
| *4. Discard supplies in appropriate area.* | | | | |
| *5. Wash hands for at least 10 seconds after client contact and after removing gloves.* | | | | |
| **Evaluation** | | | | |
| *1. Documentation (neat, legible, and concise).*<br>  *a. Client status at assessment.*<br>  *b. Steps performed in the skill and supplies used.*<br>  *c. Client's response (with expected and unexpected outcomes) and status at the end of interaction.* | | | | |
| **2. Revise nursing care plans as necessary.** | | | | |
| **Excellent:** Completion of ALL behaviors     **Satisfactory:** *Completion of critical (italicized) behaviors* | | | | |

Many factors influence the students' ability to perform a psychomotor skill. Figure 30.7 shows a schema for practice-based learning. This figure depicts the concept that the student initially approaches learning psychomotor skills from integration of prior knowledge and experience and the influence of new learning gained in the beginning nursing courses. The point of application of the learning is the practice-based scenario, in which the student must apply both the knowledge of the psychomotor skill performance and the critical thinking components that vary with different scenarios. The schema continues to reflect the influence of the student's lifelong learning and continual application of the learning in future situations throughout the individual's nursing profession.

Students bring their prior knowledge and experience to the learning environment. Faculty, videotaped demonstrations, nursing textbooks, classroom discussion of nursing practice, and computer-assisted instruction all influence the student's understanding of the need for, and method of, performing psychomotor skills. These influences converge at the point of application, when the student performs the skill. For some students, understanding may not be achieved until the action is applied to a scenario. At this point, faculty can provide feedback about the student's performance of the skill and the student can verify understanding regarding the skill and its application in the scenario.

Ideally, students will encounter further opportunities in various settings to perform the skill after validation in the skills lab. Each opportunity provides unique features requiring slight modifications as the student performs the skill. The influence of each new application promotes greater understanding of the variations in skill performance and heightens awareness

Figure 30.7 – Schema for Practice-Based Learning

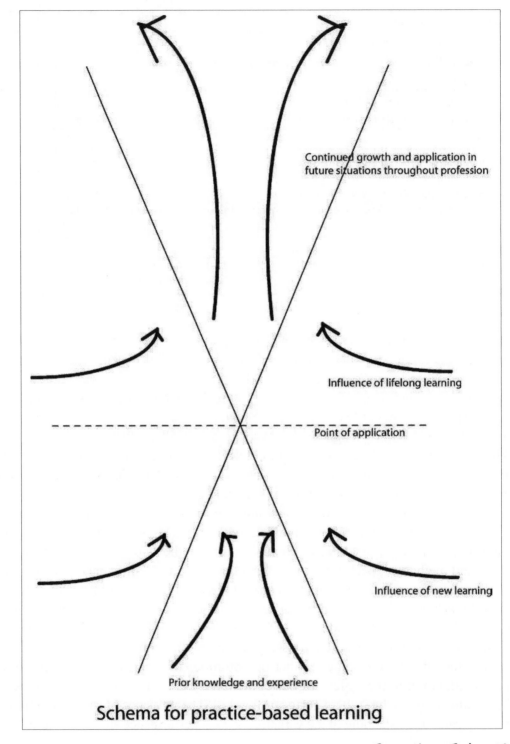

Continued growth and application in future situations throughout profession

Influence of lifelong learning

Point of application

Influence of new learning

Prior knowledge and experience

Schema for practice-based learning

of critical thinking skills needed in differing situations. This model for learning psychomotor skills can become a pattern for approaching learning of new psychomotor skills. Not all psychomotor skills that nurses perform in their practice can be taught in nursing school. Therefore, it is helpful that the student has learned to approach the learning of a psychomotor skill by initially considering the purpose of the skill and if it is still appropriate for the client's needs. This is followed by the critical thinking task of prioritizing this skill in light of other client needs. The student is able to consider the rationales for the intervention in the prioritization process, and plan for any adaptations that will be needed by a particular client. Therapeutic use of self and/or creativity may be involved. Following this critical thinking process, the student will verify the order, assure client identification, and assess the client to assure that the intervention is still needed. Expected outcomes will be determined, and all needed equipment obtained. At this point, the actual performance of the nursing intervention occurs. Standard procedures listed in the intervention section are applicable to nearly all psychomotor skills, and should be included in performance of skills the student has not performed in prior situations. Following nursing interventions, evaluation of the effectiveness is a necessary action, and documentation is needed to record the action and client response.

## Adapting the Practice-Based Model in Nursing Education

Faculty in schools of nursing at any level as well as nurse educators in practice settings can adapt this model of practice-based skills validation to their needs. Identification of specific student needs is a necessary first step in implementation. Suggested questions regarding this type of learning **activity** follow:

1. How can the simulation laboratory become most like the actual clinical environment, reflecting multiple needs of multiple clients occurring simultaneously?
2. How can student involvement/engagement in the learning activity be increased?
3. How can the simulation laboratory be used to better prepare students for situations they will encounter in clinical experiences in the upcoming term?
4. How can learning of selected psychomotor skills form the basis for approaching learning of new skills throughout basic nursing education and throughout lifelong learning in practice?

A brief overview of possible answers to these questions may prompt adaptation of practice-based skills validation to various educational settings.

## Consideration of the Learning Activity

### 1. How can the simulation laboratory become most like the actual clinical environment, reflecting multiple needs of multiple clients occurring simultaneously?

The use of simple to complex scenarios enables progression of experiences from beginning to senior level student. Scenarios that reflect anticipated client situations typical of the unit or institutional setting enables orientation and validation of skills needed by practicing nurses. Scenarios that include clients with multiple needs, or multiple clients, increases the realism of the skill validation.

### 2. How can student involvement/engagement in the learning activity be increased?

As adult learners, students want to know how the learning experience relates to their needs. Each student is aware of requirements for clinical experiences. When the validation of the skill relates to the need to prepare for clinical experiences, students are more likely to be active in their learning. For example, students arrive at the nursing simulation laboratory 30 minutes prior to the scheduled evaluation time, dressed in their uniforms as if they were preparing for the clinical setting. A laboratory assistant gives the student their assignment for the day which involves a written scenario of one or more clients (much like the client assignments they receive in the clinical environment). The student spends the 30 minutes reading the scenario(s), learning about any unfamiliar medications, and prioritizing actions. A beginning student receives a very simple scenario with at least two psychomotor skills to prioritize. At the end of the 30 minutes, the student takes the scenario to the faculty evaluator and states the prioritization of care, and the rationales (usually takes less than 5 minutes). In beginning semesters, if the prioritization is incorrect, the student is allowed to complete performance of the skill procedure. When the student has completed the skill, the faculty guides the student in understanding pertinent information regarding prioritizing. This decreases anxiety for the beginning student. However, by the end of the junior year, if the students' prioritization is incorrect – with no logical rationale for their thinking – students are asked to return for a second skill validation attempt with a different scenario. Recording the title of the scenario and demonstration attempt number on the Documentation/Evaluation Form is helpful in tracking these attempts. See Figure 30.8 for a sample Documentation/Evaluation Form.

### 3. How can the simulation laboratory better prepare students for situations they will encounter in clinical experiences in the upcoming term?

One method is for faculty to discuss usual occurrences in clinical practice with fellow educators. Personal experiences with challenging practice situations provide a rich source of scenarios. Identification of typical client needs and incorporation of unique client situations can be recorded to represent individual clients in contrived scenarios. In another approach

Figure 30.8 – Documentation/Evaluation Form

*Skill performance level of attainment:*

**Imitation***:* Junior fall practice; **Manipulation:** Junior fall evaluation;
**Precision:** Junior spring; **Competency:** Throughout Senior Year

**Documentation/Evaluation Form for Skills Validations**

Time skill began: _____          Time skill ended: _____
Documentation time: _____

Student's self-evaluation:_____
_____
_____
_____Signature_____

Scenario Used:_____ Demonstration attempt #_____

Circle student Attainment Level: *imitation / manipulation / precision / competency*

| *Skill* | | | | |
|---------|--|--|--|--|
| Critical thinking | | | | |
| Assessment | | | | |
| Planning | | | | |
| Implementation | | | | |
| Evaluation | | | | |
| *Cumulative score* | | | | |

Faculty Evaluator Comments: _____
_____
_____
_____

Faculty Signature: _____          Date: _____

Nurses' Notes for Student Documentation:_____
_____
_____
_____
_____
_____

**Excellent:  Completion of ALL Behaviors  Satisfactory: Completion of *critical (italicized) behaviors***

Auburn University Montgomery School of Nursing Skills Evaluation Guide students are asked to write a scenario representative of skills needed at their level. These can be used with future students as a critical thinking skill validation for similar clinical environments. Figure 30.9 presents a scenario written by students.

### 4. How can learning of selected psychomotor skills form the basis for approaching learning of new skills throughout basic nursing education and throughout lifelong learning in practice?

This can be accomplished by providing a pattern of learning in which critical thinking becomes the foundation for approaching all learning of psychomotor skills – determining the need for nursing intervention, rationale, and priority for performing the intervention. Effective communication skills for therapeutic communication, interdisciplinary communication, and client/family teaching are integrated throughout the skills laboratory experience. From this foundation, an approach to the actual skill performance follows the nursing process of assessment, problem identification, planning and intervention, and evaluation.

### Considerations Regarding Learning Outcomes

Suggested questions regarding the learning **outcomes** include:
1. What critical thinking components can be evaluated in conjunction with each psycho-motor skill performance?
2. How can levels of skill attainment progress from simple to complex?
3. How can consistency in faculty evaluation be promoted?
4. How can evaluation and tracking tools be used to record the students' progress for benchmarking data collection?

Answers to the above questions may include the following:

### 1. What critical thinking components can actually be evaluated in conjunction with psychomotor skill performance?

There are basic critical thinking skills that can be evaluated with each psychomotor skill. Figure 30.10 repeats the first five items from the Critical Thinking Evaluation Tool presented in Figure 30.6. These skills can be incorporated in each validation session.

### 2. How can levels of skill attainment progress from simple to complex?

Students and faculty should be made aware of the expected level of skill attainment for the specific practice session or term. A very simple imitation level of skill performance is expected for beginning nursing students during their initial practice sessions. However,

Figure 30.9 – Sample Scenario Written by Students

Scenario- Neonate Addicted to Cocaine

A 27-year-old woman, 34 weeks gestation, just gave birth to a premature baby girl weighing 3 lbs. The baby was intubated and sent to the NICU. She tested positive for cocaine. The baby is experiencing tachycardia, hyperirritability, vomiting and diarrhea, and showing signs of Respiratory Distress Syndrome. She has not quit crying since she was born. She has a poor sucking reflex and will not feed from the bottle. Breast-feeding is contraindicated in this situation.

Vital Signs: T 97.4, RR 60, HR 235, BP 40/32

Physician's Orders:
Thermoregulation (according to protocol)
IV .45 NaCl at cc/hr *KVO*
Administer erythromycin ointment OU
0.5 mL Vit. K IM
0.5 mL HBV IM
Monitor respiratory status q 15 minutes
NG tube
Place on ventilator with 1L supplemental Oxygen
Administer Survanta 100mg/kg (Intratracheal) q 6 hours for first two days of life.

**Faculty Guidelines (to be included on faculty page, but not on student page)**
Perform head-to-toe perfunctory assessment upon initiating care. Check patency of airway before giving intratracheal meds. 5 Rights and 3 checks before giving any meds. High priority is thermoregulation.

Auscultate bowel sounds and check patency of nares before inserting NG tube. Check placement upon insertion of NG tube. Since the infant is constantly crying and restless, give consideration to positions that comfort the baby while discouraging dislodgement of NG tube or IV line.

Communication: Since this infant is too young to understand the treatments, explain to the mother treatments and why meds are being used, taking into account the mother's developmental level, physical and emotional status at the time. Encourage her to ask questions about her baby's condition and do not be judgmental.

Prioritization: Order of skills would be: 1. IV 2. Administer medications 3. NG Insertion

Rationales: Respiratory status is monitored due to respiratory distress syndrome. Survanta is given because it is a pulmonary surfactant and helps the newborn's immature lungs. Vit. K is given because this is low in newborns and is essential in the coagulation cycle. Erythromycin is mandated as a prophylactic against Chlamydia trachomatis and to prevent opthalmia neonatorum. HBV is now recommended for newborns within 48 hours due to the rise in hepatitis in recent years. An IV is started to keep baby hydrated and for easy access for emergency drugs. NG placement is for feeding purposes. Ventilator and supplemental oxygen are needed in RDS.

Management: Care for this infant should be scheduled to minimize stimulation and reduce irritability. Coordination between social workers, respiratory therapists, pediatricians, and the mother is essential to improve the health status and future of this infant.

Referral Skills: Know how to refer pregnant clients to substance abuse treatment programs and

Figure 30.9 – Sample Scenario Written by Students cont.

> social agencies that can aid in obtaining proper prenatal care and in stopping the use of cocaine. Since this infant is addicted at birth referral to appropriate social work agencies, home health, and developmental specialists would be appropriate.

Figure 30.10 – Critical Thinking Components from the Critical Thinking Evaluation Tool

| |
|---|
| *1. Incorporation/application of case situation.* **Assess client to determine that the intervention is still appropriate. Assess client's level of consciousness, ability to cooperate, and need for explanation and/or psychological support.** |
| *2. Prioritization of client needs and care to be given.* |
| *3. Verbalization of rationales for care.* |
| **4. Problem-solving (Includes appropriate interdisciplinary involvement, referrals, using community resources.)** |
| **5. Therapeutic use of self / creativity in skill (communication with client, innovative approaches to client care.)** |

with successive terms, increased nursing knowledge from class and clinical experiences promotes the expectation of a more precise or competent level of skill performance. Increased complexity of scenarios in successive terms of the nursing curriculum promote an increased level of critical thinking. Similarly, increased exposure to psychomotor skill performance will enable more precise performance.

### 3. How can consistency in faculty evaluation be promoted?

Written scenarios that include notes for faculty are helpful in promoting consistency among faculty evaluators. Meetings of all faculty involved in validating student performance are scheduled prior to the beginning of the term to discuss issues and reach an agreement regarding issues such as:

- Guidelines for student practice.
- Guidelines for faculty evaluation of skills.

Providing written guidelines regarding expectations is helpful for both faculty and students. Written guidelines such as those presented in Figure 30.11 – Skills Evaluation Overview – can be given to faculty and students at the beginning of each term.

Figure 30.11 – Skills Evaluation Overview

## I. STUDENT INSTRUCTIONS
- The student will bring a copy of the evaluation guide for each evaluation attempt.
- The student will document appropriately and complete the self-evaluation portion, then submit the completed documentation for evaluation.
- Following each evaluation and prior to leaving the nursing lab, the student will photocopy the pages of documentation and evaluation for each skill and submit to the evaluator for filing in the lab office.

## II. EVALUATOR INSTRUCTIONS
- Circle the skill performance level of attainment (see descriptors below).
- When evaluating a student's skill demonstration using a case scenario, you are in the role of **evaluator**, not **teacher**.
- Refrain from any verbal or non-verbal prompting.
- Objectively record the student's demonstration on the provided form, checking boxes to the right of the behaviors.
- While the student is documenting and self-evaluating, enter the name of the case scenario, specify first or second demonstration attempt, and tally the scoring for each category. After receiving the student documentation, tally the evaluation portion of the procedure. A score of at least a Satisfactory is required for evaluation as a successful skill performance. Satisfactory is completion of all critical (italicized) behaviors.
- Complete the evaluator comment portion, specifying areas needing improvement. Date and mark through unused lines.
- Briefly provide verbal feedback following completion of the evaluation.

## III. SKILL PERFORMANCE LEVELS OF ATTAINMENT
I. Imitation (expectation for junior level, fall semester practice sessions only)
Initially skills are learned following demonstration, whether directly by the teacher or by observation of the process on a film, videotape, or slide sequence. The performance lacks neuromuscular coordination or control and, hence, is generally in a crude and imperfect form. Time and speed are based on learner need.

2. Manipulation (expectation for junior level, fall semester evaluation)
The learner follows a prescription as outlined on a procedure sheet, learning to follow instructions, performing selected actions and fixing performance through necessary practice. Coordination of movements is variable. A time frame of at least one week has elapsed from initial imitation to the evaluation of the student at a manipulation level.

3. Precision (expectation for junior level, winter quarter or spring semester)
Performance reaches a level of refinement and can be carried out without a set of directions, and performance is characterized by accuracy. Coordination is at a high level.

4. Competency (expectation for senior level, all semesters)
Skill represents a high degree of proficiency, which has become an automatic response to appropriate situational cues. Coordination is consistently at a high level. Performance is efficient and reflects professional competence.

## 4. How can evaluation and tracking tools be used to record the students' progress for benchmarking data collection?

A computer program such as Excel® or Access® provides a grid format for recording individual student performance (see Figure 30.12 – Specific Skills Experiences). This form can be placed in a color-coded folder for all students in the beginning term. As students progress through the curriculum, validation experiences are scheduled that relate to the skills needed in subsequent terms. If the student does not progress with the beginning cohort, the color-coded file can be placed with files of the next beginning class as a reminder to provide that student with additional opportunity to practice skills at the beginning of the next term.

At the completion of each term, or year, a tally of students performing the skills validation at an **excellent** level, **satisfactory** level, or **unsatisfactory** level provides benchmarking data. The number of validation attempts for students who have performed at the unsatisfactory level is also recorded. Specific information can be obtained by filing the Documentation/Evaluation Form in the student's individual folder throughout the curriculum to identify specific patterns of need.

Figure 30.12 – Specific Skills Experiences

| Specific Skills Experiences | | | | | | | | | | |
|---|---|---|---|---|---|---|---|---|---|---|
| Student Name: | Jr. Fall | | Jr. Spring | | Jr. Summer | | Sr. Fall | | Sr. Spring | |
| Skill | Lab | Clin. | Lab | Clin. | Lab | Clin. | Lab | Clin. | Lab | Clin. |
| AM care | | | | | | | | | | |
| Isolation | | | | | | | | | | |
| Restraint | | | | | | | | | | |
| Transfer | | | | | | | | | | |
| Sterile technique | | | | | | | | | | |
| Wound care | | | | | | | | | | |
| Central line dressing | | | | | | | | | | |
| IV: Start | | | | | | | | | | |
| Maintain | | | | | | | | | | |
| IVPB | | | | | | | | | | |
| Meds: PO | | | | | | | | | | |
| SC | | | | | | | | | | |
| ID | | | | | | | | | | |
| IM | | | | | | | | | | |
| Catheter: Insert | | | | | | | | | | |
| Removal | | | | | | | | | | |
| Colostomy care | | | | | | | | | | |
| Enema | | | | | | | | | | |
| Trach: Suction | | | | | | | | | | |
| Care | | | | | | | | | | |
| NG: Insertion | | | | | | | | | | |
| Lavage | | | | | | | | | | |
| Gavage | | | | | | | | | | |

# Conclusion

Ongoing refinement of practice-based skills validation continues. Some lessons learned that educators may find helpful include the following:

- Designate specific times for practice versus validation.
- Faculty must assume the role of evaluator and not coach during validation sessions.
- Student self-evaluation promotes student awareness of own learning needs.
- Faculty evaluation should include positive reinforcement and suggestions.
- Practice-based skills validation promotes students' thinking on their feet.

Teaching nursing is a multi-faceted endeavor. Accurate performance of psychomotor skills required by nurses in routine interventions for client care must be assessed as students progress through nursing education programs. Evaluation of specific psychomotor skills may be accomplished at varying points in the nursing curriculum to correlate with skills expected to be encountered in specific clinical experiences. Feedback must be presented to students in such a manner that the student is able to progress in competent performance; both verbal and written feedback promotes student understanding and retention of areas needing improvement. Suggested evaluation tools have been presented in this chapter to facilitate feedback to the student as well as to enable tracking for curricular benchmarking.

A major addition to the rote step-by-step skill performance is the use of scenarios based on realistic clinical situations. This approach enables the student to relate the performance of psychomotor skills to expected clinical experiences. Moreover, critical thinking skills such as prioritization, verbalization of rationales for the intervention or modifications of the intervention, problem-solving, therapeutic communication, and creativity can be evaluated. Individual student progress can be tracked to assist in identifying patterns of individual student need and providing experiences to meet student learning needs prior to actual client care in the clinical environment.

Faculty commitment to the practice-based approach is necessary. Creation of practice-based scenarios can be fun and promote faculty dialogue regarding which skills need evaluation in varying settings, and which components of skill performance are critical. One outcome can be increased communication between faculty and between faculty and students. Other very important outcomes can be the increased engagement of students in their own learning and the increased level of understanding of nursing concepts and skills. This then leads to a higher level of student performance and impacts provision of client care at a higher standard.

## Learning Activities

1. Identify a clinical setting in which student nurses will be working during the first term in the nursing curriculum. Create a beginning level scenario in which students will need to perform two or more psychomotor skills. Structure the scenario such that one of the skills has a higher priority than the other. Write a faculty notes page to accompany the scenario that specifies expected behavior and prioritization, with expected rationales. Present this scenario to nursing faculty for feedback. Then present the refined scenario to beginning nursing students as the format for a practice-based psychomotor skill validation.

2. Identify a clinical setting in which advanced nursing students will be working. Consider past experiences in this setting, and create a scenario in which the client in the scenario experiences difficulty similar to that experienced by actual clients in this setting. This difficulty may be in multiple needs arising simultaneously or in need for therapeutic communication or referral to other members of the health care team. Write a faculty notes page to accompany the scenario that specifies expected behavior and prioritization, with expected rationales. Present this scenario to nursing faculty for feedback. Then present the refined scenario to advanced nursing students as the format for a practice-based psychomotor skill validation.

3. Determine which clinical skills are imperative for psychomotor validation in the nursing setting in which you are involved. Refine the examples in Figure 30.8 and 30.12 to correspond to the skills you have identified. Identify a percentage of students that will successfully validate each skill as a benchmark level. Use these tools to track one cohort of students and record the benchmark attainment.

# References

Alfaro-LeFevre, R. (1999). *Critical thinking in nursing: A practical approach* (2nd ed.). Philadelphia: Saunders.

Aronson, B. S., Rosa, J. M., Anfinson, J., & Light, N. A simulated clinical problem-solving experience. *Nurse Educator,* 22 (6), 17-19.

Bloom, B. (1956). *Major categories in the taxonomy of educational objectives.* Retrieved May 10, 2002 from the World Wide Web: http://faculty.washington.edu/krumme/guides/bloom.html.

Carnevali, D. L. (1993). *Diagnostic reasoning and treatment decision making in nursing.* Philadelphia: Lippincott.

Conrick, M., Dunne, A., Skinner, J. (1997). Learning together: Using simulation to foster the integration of theory and practice. *The Australian Electronic Journal of Nursing Education,* 1, 1.

Dearman, C, Lazenby, R. B., Faulk, D., & Coker, R. (2001). Simulated clinical scenarios: Faculty-student collaboration. *Nurse Educator, 26 (4), 167-169.*

Gijselaers, W. H. (1996). *Bringing problem-based learning to higher education: Theory and practice.* San Francisco: Jossey-Bass.

Johnson, J. H., Zerwic, J. J., & Theis, S. L. (1999). Clinical simulation laboratory: An adjunct to clinical teaching. *Nurse Educator,* 24 (5), 37-41.

Kataoka-Yahiro, M., & Saylor, C. (1994). A critical thinking model for nursing judgment. *Journal of Nursing Education,* 33 (8), 351-356

Linn, R. L., & Gronlund, N. E. (2000). *Measurement and assessment in teaching* (8th ed.). Upper Saddle River, NJ: Prentice-Hall.

Lunney, M. (2001). *Critical thinking and nursing diagnosis: Case studies and analyses.* Philadelphia: North American Nursing Diagnosis Association.

Maynard, C. A. (1996). Relationship of critical thinking ability to professional nursing competence. *Journal of Nursing Education,* 35 (1), 12-18.

Miller, M. A., & Babcock, D. E. (1996). *Critical thinking applied to nursing.* St. Louis: Mosby.

Oermann, M. H., & Gaberson, K. (1998). *Evaluation and testing in nursing education.* New York: Springer.

Sloan, R. (1999). Evaluation in graduate nursing programs using practice based learning. *Assessing Program Outcomes: Fourth National conference for Nurse Educators.* Indiana University School of Nursing, Indianapolis, IN, November 10.

Wilson, M. (1999). Using benchmarking practices for the learning resource center. *Nurse Educator,* 24 (4), 16-20.

Youngblood, N., & Beitz, J. M. (2001). Developing critical thinking with active learning strategies. *Nurse Educator,* 26 (1), 39-42.

# Bibliography

Gaberson, K., & Oermann, M. H. (1999). *Clinical teaching strategies in nursing education.* New York: Springer.

# Chapter 31: TEACHING THE CRITICAL THINKING SKILLS OF DELEGATING AND PRIORITIZING

Lynn M. Derickson, BS, MS, RN, CNS and Linda Caputi, MSN, Ed D, RN

*I recently attended a nurse educator's conference where Lynn Derickson, along with two colleagues, was presenting on the topic of preparing nursing students to delegate client care. The room was packed – standing room only! The topic was of great interest to the conference attendees. The presentation was excellent. With this level of interest, I believed it important to include a chapter on this topic in this book. – Linda Caputi*

## Introduction

Models of nursing care delivery continue to change. In many client care environments, nursing care is provided by a mix of licensed and unlicensed assistive personnel (UAPs). This new skill mix requires the nurse to assume the role of delegator of various aspects of client care. Nursing faculty are challenged to educate students not only to be providers of nursing care but to be managers of client care in the midst of the revolutionary changes that have occurred in the healthcare industry over the past several decades (Nursing Crisis Commission, 2003).

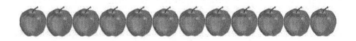

## Educational Philosophy

I believe that the desire to learn is burning in all of us. Each of us brings a special quality to the field of nursing. It is our responsibility, as nursing educators, to nurture that desire and those qualities so that the profession will grow. – Lynn M. Derickson

My educational philosophy is succinct: Give the best educational experience possible. I feel faculty should continuously challenge themselves to provide creative, interesting, and sound education - students soon learn that education doesn't have to be boring; they become self-motivated, enthusiastic, and interested.....learning then follows. – Linda Caputi

The National Council of State Boards of Nursing, Inc. (NCSBN) (2001) reported in its practice analysis of newly licensed registered nurses that these nurses are responsible for delegating, prioritizing, and managing client care. These responsibilities require use of high-level critical thinking skills and strategies. It is imperative that educators provide instruction whereby new graduates can safely and competently carry out these functions. The intent of this chapter is to provide educators with ideas and instructional strategies to use when teaching both nursing students and graduate nurses delegation skills.

## Delegation Theory

Delegation is defined as the accomplishment of desired tasks or objectives through the use of other personnel and through allocation of authority or responsibility (Grohar-Murray & DiCroce, 2003). Healthcare reform and changes in healthcare delivery have affected the way nurses deliver care. Nurses are required to delegate to a variety of healthcare personnel, both licensed and unlicensed. Some of these personnel possess minimal skills and knowledge, making the task of delegation even more challenging.

As managers of client care, nurses are required to delegate specific tasks to UAPs. It is imperative that delegation theory be taught throughout a nursing program if graduate nurses are to be comfortable with this aspect of client care management. Delegation must be addressed both as a process and as a legal entity. Nurses must be aware that delegating a task involves much more than just asking someone else to do something. It requires a thorough understanding of the process of delegation of a task and the legal aspects of empowering another person to carry out that task.

## Why Teach Delegation Theory

Turnover rates for nurses are highest in the first year of employment (Prior, Cottington, Kolski, & Shogan, 1990). During this time, nurses report higher levels of stress and job dissatisfaction than do experienced nurses (Shader, Broome, West, & Nash, 2001). Factors influencing retention include staffing levels, agency help, management support, work schedules, heavy workloads, and insufficient autonomy (Strachota, Normandin, O'Brien, Clary & Krukow, 2003). Nurses frequently become overwhelmed, resulting in burnout and stress. Many ultimately leave the profession.

It may be possible that if students are provided with opportunities to learn to delegate effectively, some of these factors may produce less stress for graduate nurses. Preparing new nurses to be confident in assuming a leadership role in managing client care may be a proactive way to retain nurses in the profession.

Anthony, Standing, and Hertz (2001) identified that most nurses believed that it was experience that prepared them best for their delegation role. Nurses believed that they had not been adequately prepared in the art of delegation by their nursing programs. This suggests that faculty must incorporate actual clinical experiences that provide students an opportunity to apply delegation theory.

However, throughout nursing school, there may be minimal opportunity for students to manage the care of a group of clients. Because students typically care for clients using a "case study" approach, they are responsible for total care of several clients rather than delegating some of that care to others. This approach to student clinical experiences provides little opportunity to learn or practice delegation skills. Without these opportunities as students, new graduates may be asked to manage clients without the necessary delegation skills. The ability to delegate enables nurses to maintain personal integrity and to survive in the ever-changing healthcare environment (O'Mara, 1999).

## Integrating Delegation Theory into the Curriculum

What may appear to be a simple task – asking someone to do something – is actually quite complex and requires time to master. As such, teaching delegation should be integrated throughout the curriculum. Then, as new skills are introduced, the following questions relative to delegation are addressed:
- What scope of practice includes this responsibility?
- To whom might this task be delegated?
- How does one know that the individual possesses the knowledge or the skills to complete this task?
- Where do accountability and responsibility lie for the proper completion of this task?
- What are the steps to effective delegation relative to this task?

## Delegation Content

Just as the five rights of medication administration have become a gold standard for nursing, so must the "rights" of delegation. Hansten and Washburn (1992) listed the following four rights:
1. The right task: the task that can be delegated.
2. The right person: the person qualified to do the job.
3. The right communication: a clear, concise description of the objectives and expectations when performing the task.
4. The right feedback: evaluation in a timely manner, during and after the performance

of the task.

The NCSBN (1995a) revised these four rights, adding a fifth:
1. Right task: one that is delegable for a specific client.
2. Right circumstances: appropriate client, setting, available resources, and other relevant factors.
3. Right person: the right person is delegating the right task to the right person to be performed on the right person.
4. Right direction/communication: clear, concise description of the task, including its objective, limits, and expectations.
5. Right supervision: appropriate monitoring, evaluation, intervention, and feedback.

These "rights" of delegation can serve as an organizing scheme for teaching delegation theory. Students can use them as a checklist when applying delegation theory to client care.

## Basic Management Skills Necessary for Effective Delegation

Delegation is a high-level cognitive activity that requires the use of other thinking skills. Both interpersonal and intrapersonal skills are required. These skills are not used alone, but work in synergy. For example, an essential interpersonal skill for effective delegation is conflict resolution. Conflict resolution theory is taught so the nurse is able to work with staff, clients, and families to resolve interpersonal conflicts that may influence the delegation process.

Intrapersonal skills important for effective delegation include stress management, effective time management, and prioritization of client care. These are necessary for managing the nurse's own professional life. Stress management is essential for dealing with change and preventing burnout as a leading cause of nurses leaving the profession or as a reason for diminished quality of client care (Arnold, 1999; Lachman, 1983). Time management skills contribute to a feeling of control and to reducing stress and anxiety often experienced in the workplace.

Prioritization of client care is essential for providing safe, effective nursing care. For the new graduate, one of the most frustrating and intimidating responsibilities is to ensure care for a large group of clients. It is important that the nurse be skilled in prioritizing care for this group of clients so all identified needs are met. When prioritizing, the nurse identifies which tasks might be delegated to others. Both prioritizing and delegating contribute to time management.

Many additional elements are needed for effective delegation. These include:
- Client teaching.
- Effective communication.
- Ethical decision making.
- Professional practice, applying guidelines from the American Nurses Association Code for Nurses and the Nurse Practice Act.
- Career management. (Wywialowski, 1997).

All concepts of delegation, ethics, professionalism, and time management must be incorporated throughout the curriculum as a base for the delegation experience during the final term of the nursing program. This enables the graduating nurse to assume the role of a professional with skills in leadership and management. These skills enable graduates to effectively manage a client load and to manage their personal careers.

Although each of these elements may be introduced at various times throughout the nursing curriculum, it is important to demonstrate how all these elements relate. One approach is to provide a synthesis course that puts them all together. This course integrates all the skills needed by the nurse as a direct care giver, manager of care, teacher, communicator, and member of the profession, and then provides a clinical experience that allows practical application (Wor-Wic, 2002). Figure 31.1 provides a content outline of a sample synthesis course.

Figure 31.1 - Sample Content Outline for a Synthesis Course

**ADVANCED NURSING II: MANAGEMENT**

| Unit I | Roles of the RN in Management |
|---|---|
| Unit II | Understanding the Environment |
| Unit III | Conflict Resolution |
| Unit IV | Giving and Receiving Shift Report and Transcribing Physician's Orders |
| Unit V | Theories of Human Motivation;  Management vs Leadership |
| Unit VI | Delegation, Supervision, and Evaluation |
| Unit VII | Ethics, Spirituality, and the Law; Managing Your Career |

(Wor-Wic Community College, 2003)

# Learning Experiences

How can these learning opportunities best be provided? Because the organizational environment, educational preparedness, and personal characteristics of nurses affect future job satisfaction, organizational commitment, and plans for continuing in nursing (Ingersoll, Olsan, Drew-Cates, Devinney, & Davies, 2002), it is suggested that these learning opportunities be provided through carefully planned experiences in the classroom, skills laboratory, and clinical practicum.

Course and program evaluation tools should solicit feedback relative to outcomes that measure graduates' ability to delegate. Course evaluations completed by students, program evaluations completed by institutions that hire program graduates, and NCLEX® results can all provide valuable information when planning curriculum interventions relative to delegation.

## *Classroom Lecture/Discussion*

As with most management concepts, examples of actual clinical experiences make difficult or complex concepts clearer. Using examples from practice is an excellent method to explain, clarify, and substantiate concepts during classroom lectures and discussions. This method supports visualization and understanding of the issues being explained (deTornyay & Thompson, 1987).

Lectures and discussions are designed to generate dialogue and questions regarding the process and responsibilities of delegation. Through lecture and discussion and a thorough exploration of the five rights of delegation (Wywialowski, 1997), it becomes clear that to assume responsibility for a group of clients, it is necessary to manage resources and to delegate responsibly. This is a concept that is best introduced in the initial nursing courses and reinforced throughout the program.

Concurrently, it is important to connect the processes and responsibilities of delegation with ethical and legal issues surrounding client care. Complex issues entailed with the Health Insurance Portability and Accountability Act (HIPAA) (Calloway & Venegas, 2002), advanced directives, beneficence, non-maleficence, veracity, justice, confidentiality, and accountability are explored and discussed in detail. Students are encouraged to provide examples from their own practices and personal observations how these issues might impact decisions to delegate.

In addition to in-depth exploration of the above topics, simple "drill and practice" activities can spark discussion. One such activity might involve presenting students with brief clinical scenarios and asking if one of the five rights of delegation has been violated. Figure 31.2 provides a few examples for use with this type of drill and practice activity.

Figure 31.2 - Drill and Practice Activity #1

---

- Scenario: A client has returned to the surgical unit following a nephrectomy. The nurse is working with a nursing assistant. The nursing assistant is a senior in the nursing program at a local university. The nurse quickly assesses the client, then says to the nursing assistant, "I assessed the client very quickly. Keep an eye on her and let me know if there are any problems. Hang a new IV bag at 4 P.M. Thanks!" Discussion is centered on the idea that an unlicensed nursing assistant cannot hang an IV.

- Scenario: A nurse working with a nursing assistant says, "Please ambulate the client this morning. Thank you." Discussion may focus on the lack of clear communication regarding how far to ambulate the client, what information to report about the client's tolerance of the activity, etc.

- Scenario: The nurse caring for a client with congestive heart failure administered an antidiuretic medication through the intravenous line. The nurse asks the nursing assistant to check the urinary output and lung sounds in 15 minutes. Discussion may focus on the specific tasks the nurse delegated.

---

Another "drill and practice" activity involves brief situations with the students to decide if a skill can be delegated to another person. Figure 31.3 gives examples that can be used in this activity.

These types of activities provide client-centered examples of delegation and open discussion regarding all aspects of the delegation process.

Figure 31.3 – Drill and Practice Activity #2

---

- The client is to receive a Neomycin enema as a bowel prep. Can the registered nurse delegate this task to a nursing assistant? To a licensed practical/vocational nurse?

- The client is one day postoperative following an open cholecystectomy and is receiving patient-controlled analgesia. The client needs help with the bath. Can a nursing assistant provide this help with the bath?

- A client returned to the medical unit following a colonoscopy with conscious sedation. Can a nursing assistant perform the general assessment when the client arrives on the unit?

---

## *Skills Laboratory Experiences*

Clinical case scenarios are provided during sessions in the skills laboratory. As each new psychomotor skill is introduced, case scenarios are used to integrate delegation theory related to the performance of the skill. Case scenarios may be developed by individual faculty or purchased from commercial resources (College of DuPage, 2003; MEDS Publishing, 2002a). Additional resources include videos, journal articles, and instructor manuals from various nursing texts (Tomey, 2000; Wywialowski, 1997; Yoder-Wise, 2003).

In fundamentals courses, as the skills are practiced, teachers may clarify and reinforce by asking if skills can be delegated and to whom, as well as reviewing client stability and assessment. As higher level skills are introduced, variations in client conditions may be used as examples of delegation decisions. For example, students may have one answer when asked if a nursing assistant can independently turn a client who is one-day postoperative following an abdominal hysterectomy, yet a quite different answer if the client is one-day postoperative following a total hip replacement.

## *Test Questions*

Throughout the nursing education program, tests and quizzes with questions requiring critical thinking should include items relative to delegation. Working through these types of questions in class helps students learn the process of reading, analyzing, and answering a critical thinking question. Figure 31.4 is a sample question that can be used for this purpose.

Figure 31.4 – Sample delegation question

---

**Question:** A nurse on an obstetrics unit is in charge of a group of clients. Which of the following interventions can the nurse assign to the nursing assistant?

    A.  Provide a warm blanket and perform postpartum checks to a stable client who is 30 minutes post delivery and experiencing intense shaking. Then report back to the nurse.
    B.  A primigravida client states she is beginning to feel a slight urge to push. Ask the nursing assistant to assist this client to push.
    C.  Monitor a client who has just arrived on the unit and is very anxious. She is not experiencing contractions, but the bag of water has ruptured.
    D.  Assess a laboring client to determine if she is fully dilated.

Rationales:
    A.  Correct. Shakiness after giving birth is a typical occurrence and the nursing assistant may provide this care.
    B.  No. The nursing assistant should not be asked to assist the client to push.
    C.  No. The nurse must first assess this client prior to delegating any care to the nursing assistant.
    D.  No. It is not appropriate to delegate the task of performing a vaginal examination to a nursing assistant.

---

Additionally, to reinforce a firm base of knowledge and practice, questions on delegation, ethics, and professional practice must become a part of every exam throughout the nursing program.

### *Clinical Experience with Managing Client Care*

The clinical practicum is a vital part of the management experience. Clinical experience has always been an important part of nursing education because it facilitates student ability to do – as well as know. Applying classroom theory in the clinical setting stimulates the use of critical thinking skills to problem solve using actual client situations (Dunn & Burnett, 1995).

During the final clinical nursing course, the objective of the management component is to apply the nursing process to problem solve with a group of clients and staff. Students learn that the management process and the nursing process are similar and to use both as they manage care for a group of clients (Marquis & Huston, 2003). Students must communicate effectively and then evaluate their ability to do so. Using appropriate resources, such as the Nurse Practice Act, policies and procedures, standards of licensing and certification, position descriptions, mission statements, and philosophy statements, students learn to practice within the ethical and legal framework of nursing.

In addition to the content on delegation, theoretical content for a final term management course can incorporate content on the roles of the nurse (Wywialowski, 1997), the difference between management and leadership, types of organizations and organizational structures, and a historical account of nursing service delivery patterns. Important to understanding how organizations work are components such as mission and philosophy statements, goals, values of organizations, position descriptions, and performance appraisals. The students also become familiar with the components of a performance appraisal. They practice their role in preparing for both giving and receiving the performance appraisal.

## *An Example Clinical Experience*

As is often the case in nursing education, a simple to complex approach can be taken when providing students with delegation experiences. Therefore, first efforts to facilitate delegation experiences might take place in a long-term care environment. This environment provides a stable even-paced setting in which students can practice newly acquired management skills. Following is a discussion of how this has been accomplished in one nursing program (Wor-Wic, 2003).

Groups of six to eight students are assigned to a clinical area. Each student is designated a specific day to experience the role of a charge nurse. On this day, students assign groups of clients to their fellow students, who perform assessments and provide care. The student charge "shadows" the agency charge nurse, assuming responsibility for following up on assignments, client assessments, change of condition reports, 24-hour shift reports, narcotic counts, tube feedings, tube medications, communications, and assessments of all clients – activities that have been delegated to other personnel.

The charge experience is new to most nursing students. For many, it is the first experience they have with giving colleagues assignments and taking charge of a group of both staff and clients. They are required to plan the day, using time management skills to organize and plan activities. They conduct brief, initial assessments of clients at the beginning of the shift and prioritize client needs. They must assign clients and nursing tasks using the principles of delegation when deciding which clients and which functions to assign to whom. Adjustments to time organization must be made as emergencies arise or priorities change (Sullivan & Decker, 2001; Wywialowski, 1997; Yoder-Wise, 2003).

Each student attends a preconference where assignments, expectations, and guidance are given and questions are answered. The clinical day focuses on application of the delegation process. Students must have knowledge of and be able to apply the Nurse Practice Act and the various job descriptions of the agency. Figure 31.5 is a sample delegation worksheet that students may use.

Figure 31.5 – Delegation Worksheet

| **Delegation Worksheet** | | |
|---|---|---|
| Client_____  Room #_____ | | |
| | Check if task delegated | Delegated to whom |
| Vital signs q _____ | | |
| Assist with meals | | |
| Measure and record I&O | | |
| IV infusing | | |
| Activity | | |
| Hygiene | | |
| Dressing Change | | |
| Assessments:<br>    Weight<br>    Abdominal Girth<br>    Pulse Oximetry<br>    Finger Stick Glucose<br>    Telemetry | | |
| Specimens:<br>    Collect Urine Specimen<br>    Blood Draw for CBC | | |

The NCSBN (1997a, 1997b) offers additional tools helpful in clinical practice. The *Delegation Decision-Making Grid* and the *Delegation Decision-Making Tree* are two tools that can be found at their website (www.ncsbn.org).

During postconference, observations and problems are discussed in a group setting. The teacher facilitates as the students solve problems, discuss positive outcomes of the day, and make suggestions for changing interventions that did not have positive outcomes. If a student makes a recommendation for a change in a routine or procedure at the facility, that student must present a clear picture of the suggested change, documentation from the literature to support the change, and an explanation of why the change would be beneficial.

Additionally, students are required to identify a staff need in the clinical setting and provide teaching to staff. This process results in the application of critical thinking for the students and the development of collaborative, positive changes in client care routines and teaching tools for the staff at the clinical agency. The goal of proposing possible solutions when a problem is addressed teaches students how to have a positive influence on change. Figure 31.6 provides a sample teaching project assignment.

Figure 31.6 – Sample Teaching Project Assignment

WOR-WIC COMMUNITY COLLEGE
NURSING DEPARTMENT
NURSING 252
MANAGEMENT

MANAGEMENT TEACHING PROJECT

This is a group project. As a clinical group, you will assess a problem on the unit to which you are assigned. You will research that problem, and be able to provide evidence that will support your teaching points. (Example: Skin care – you will provide a reference list that will support your approach to skin care, and develop a teaching tool that will promote change to affect skin care.) You will then present, as a group, your project as a staff in-service education.

This is a graded project. It will count as 12.5% of your clinical grade. It will be graded by the 2 clinical faculty. Areas that will be graded include: self evaluation, group work, evidence to support teaching information (at least 5 references), content, and presentation.

## *Evaluating Performance*

Student charge nurses objectively evaluate their fellow students' performance when in the charge nurse role. The student charge nurse is also evaluated as a manager of client care. Figure 31.7 is a sample of the tool used by faculty to evaluate students in the charge nurse role.

Figure 31.7 – Faculty Evaluation of Charge Experience

---

### FACULTY EVALUATION OF CHARGE EXPERIENCE

SCORE EACH AREA UP TO 10 POINTS:

1. Assignments were made according to staff licensure, experience and qualifications. _____

2. Student charge was able to assess clients and prioritize needs. _____

3. All required unit functions were completed accurately. _____

4. Student charge was able to focus on the needs of the client group, rather than on individual clients, and allowed staff to focus on the individual clients. _____

5. Student charge was effective as a manager of client care. _____

6. Student charge was able to direct staff. _____

7. Student charge was able to resolve conflict as it occurred. _____

8. Student charge was approachable by staff. _____

9. Student charge accepted input from peers, and was able to identify areas for improvement/change.

_____

10. All pertinent information was included in change of shift report. _____

Total _____

Final grade:
(25% self evaluation, 25% peer evaluation average, 50% faculty evaluation) _____

---

## *Delegation in the Acute Care Setting*

Ideally, following the long-term care experience, students return to the acute-care facility and further apply client management theory. Students take on the role of staff nurse and specifically focus on the delegation of client care to UAPs. Job descriptions for UAPs in the acute-care environment are compared and contrasted with those in the long-term care facility.

The Delegation and Prioritization Tool located in the chapter of this book titled *Operationalizing Critical Thinking* by Linda Caputi can be used in the acute-care setting. This tool can be used both as a learning experience for students refining their delegation skills and to evaluate students' strengths and weaknesses.

## *Evaluating the Organization*

An additional clinical assignment involves the student evaluating the organizational environment. This evaluation includes identifying components of the organization that drive the entity, such as values statements, a vision statement, mission, philosophy, and goals of the organization. Postconference discussions focus on how these components fit together to make a statement about the organization. This helps prepare students to look at these components of an organization when considering employment. Students are also encouraged to look at the culture of the organization and the subcultures that exist within it, then evaluate how the organization is affected by those subcultures (Sullivan & Decker, 2001). Students can then compare and contrast long-term care facilities with acute-care institutions.

## Conclusion

The purpose of incorporating the management of client care in a final nursing course is to solidify all the pieces of management and delegation that have been taught and experienced in the earlier nursing courses. In this final course, the students are able to practice the skills of delegation, conflict resolution, problem identification, problem solving, and time management. Students begin to master some of these skills so they can indeed move from novice to advanced beginner (Benner, 1984) upon graduation and entry into practice. Because these are complex skills, they must be taught and applied throughout the nursing curriculum. The final nursing course is a synthesis course to reinforce and practice all these skills in a variety of situations.

# Learning Activities

1. Analyze the curriculum of a nursing program. Identify where delegation is taught and how delegation theory is applied to clinical practice.
2. Add to the drill-and-practice scenarios presented in this chapter. Use these with students and note the discussions that ensue.

# References

Anthony, M. K., Standing, T. S., & Hertz, J. E. (2001). Nurses' beliefs about their abilities to delegate within changing models of care. *Journal of Continuing Education in Nursing. 32*(5), 210-215.

Arnold, E. (1999). Communicating with clients in stressful situations. In E. Arnold & K. Underman Boggs (Eds.), *Interpersonal relationships: Professional communication skills for nurses* (3rd ed.) (pp. 445-475). Philadelphia: Saunders.

Benner, P. E. (1984). *From novice to expert: Excellence and power in clinical nursing practice.* Upper Saddle River, NJ: Prentice-Hall.

Calloway, S. D., & Venegas, L. M. (2002). The new HIPAA law on privacy and confidentiality. *Nursing Administration Quarterly, 26*(4), 40-54.

College of DuPage. (2003). *Critical thinking case studies and more.* Glen Ellyn, IL: Author.

de Tornyay, R., & Thompson, M. A. (1987). *Strategies for teaching nursing* (3rd ed.). Albany, NY: Delmar Publishers.

Dunn, S. V., & Burnett, P. (1995). The development of a clinical learning environment scale. *Journal of Advanced Nursing, 22*, 1166-1173.

Grohar-Murray, M. E., & DiCroce, H. R. (2003). *Leadership and management in nursing* (3rd ed.). Upper Saddle River, NJ: Prentice Hall.

Hansten, R., & Washburn, M. (1992, April). How to plan what to delegate. *American Journal of Nursing,* 71-72.

Ingersoll, G., Olsan, T., Drew-Cates, J., Devinney, B., & Davies, J. (2002). Nurses' job satisfaction, organizational commitment, and career intent. *Journal of Nursing Administration. 32*(50), 250-263.

Lachman, V. D. (1983). *Stress management: A manual for nurses.* New York: Grune & Stratton, Inc.

Marquis, B. L., & Huston, C. J. (2003). *Leadership roles and management functions in nursing: Theory and application* (4th ed.). Philadelphia: Lippincott Williams & Wilkins.

MEDS Publishing. (2002a). *Learning system RN* (Version 3.0). Burtonsville, MD: Author.

MEDS Publishing. (2002b). *Test-taking RN* (Version 3.0). Burtonsville, MD: Author.

National Council of State Boards of Nursing [NCSBN]. (1995a). Delegation: Understanding the concepts and decision-making process. Retrieved April 30, 2003 from http://www.ncsbn.org/public/regulation/delegation_documents_delegati.htm

National Council of State Boards of Nursing [NCSBN]. (1995b). A model nurse practice act. Retrieved August 2002 from http://www.ncsbn.org/public/regulation/nursing_ practice_model_practice_act.htm

National Council of State Boards of Nursing [NCSBN]. (1997a). Delegation decision-making grid. Retrieved April 30, 2003 from www.ncsbn.org

National Council of State Boards of Nursing [NCSBN]. (1997b). Delegation decision-making tree. Retrieved April 30, 2003 from www.ncsbn.org

National Council of State Boards of Nursing [NCSBN]. (2001). National council detailed test plan for the NCLEX-RN® examination. Chicago: NCSBN.

Nursing Crisis Commission. (2002). Maryland Board of Nursing. Retrieved February 28, 2003 from http://www.mbon.org/nursingcrisiscommission/june52002presentation

O'Mara, A. (1999). Communicating with other health professionals. In E. Arnold & K. Underman Boggs (Eds.), *Interpersonal relationships: Professional communication skills for nurses* (3rd ed.) (pp. 496-523). Philadelphia: Saunders.

Prior, M. M., Cottington, E. M., Kolski, B. J. & Shogan, J. O. (1990). Nurse turnover as a function of employment, experience and unit. *Journal of Nursing Management, 21*(7), 27-28.

Shader, K., Broome, M. E., West, M. E., & Nash, M. (2001). Factors influencing satisfaction and anticipated turnover for nurses in an academic medical center. *Journal of Nursing Administration. 31*(4), 210-216.

Strachota, E., Normandin, P., O'Brien, N., Clary, M., & Krukow, B. (2003). Retention is directly related to job satisfaction. *Journal of Nursing Administration. 33*(2), 111.

Sullivan, E. J., & Decker, P. J. (2001). *Effective leadership and management in nursing* (5th ed.). Upper Saddle River, NJ: Prentice Hall.

Tomey, A. M. (2000). *Guide to nursing management and leadership* (6th ed.). St. Louis: Mosby.

Wor-Wic Community College. (2002). *Catalog.* Salisbury, MD: Author.

Wor-Wic Community College. (2003). Nursing program: NUR 101, NUR 151, NUR 202, NUR 252, course syllabi. Salisbury, MD: Author.

Wywialowski, E. F. (1997). *Managing client care* (2nd ed.). St. Louis: Mosby.

Yoder-Wise, P. S. (2003). *Leading and managing in nursing* (3rd ed.). St. Louis: Mosby.

# Bibliography

American Nurses Association. (1985). *Code for nurses with interpretive statements.* Washington, DC: American Nurses Publishing, American Nurses Foundation/American Nurses Association.

Anonymous. (2002). HHS predicts growing nurse shortage. *Healthcare Financial Management, 56*(10), 24.

Barney, S. M. (2002). The nursing shortage: Why is it happening? *Journal of Healthcare Management. 47*(3), 153-155.

DeYoung, S., Bliss, J., & Tracy, J. P. (2002). The nursing faculty shortage: Is there hope? *Journal of Professional Nursing, 18*(6), 313-319.

Dreyfus, S. E., & Dreyfus, H. L. (1980). *A five-stage model of the mental activities involved in directed skill acquisition.* Unpublished report supported by USAF (Contract F49620-79-C-0063). Berkeley, CA: University of California.

Maryland Board of Nursing. (2003). *Nurse Practice Act* (Annotated code of Maryland: Health occupations article, Title 8: Code of Maryland regulations: Title 10 subtitle 27).

Nelson, R. (2002). U.S. nursing shortage a "national concern." *The Lancet. 360*(9336), 855.

# Chapter 32: OPERATIONALIZING CRITICAL THINKING

Linda Caputi, MSN, EdD, RN

*Critical thinking is an extremely complex process. So often we say to students, "You must use critical thinking in your approach to this situation." Does the student really know what we mean? Many students have never had critical thinking explicitly modeled, so how can we, as educators, expect students to engage in critical thinking if they are not even sure what critical thinking is? – Linda Caputi*

## Introduction

"Critical thinking" is a term frequently used in nursing education. It describes the thinking skills nurses are expected to develop and use in their professional endeavors. Because the ability to think critically increases with experience, faculty need to provide students with as many critical thinking activities as possible.

Teaching critical thinking is different from teaching other skills of nursing. For example, psychomotor skills are easily taught, observed, and evaluated. Critical thinking, however, is abstract; it is a process in which the actual events are not discernible until the outcomes of decisions are evident. As such, critical thinking is difficult to teach and difficult to learn. Nursing faculty are continuously searching for ways to ensure that critical thinking is taught in their courses.

This chapter offers a definition of critical thinking, descriptions of critical thinking skills and strategies, and examples of activities for nursing students to foster the development of critical thinking. After reading this chapter, nursing faculty are encouraged to develop critical thinking activities specifically for their students.

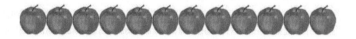

## Educational Philosophy

My educational philosophy is succinct: Give the best educational experience possible. I feel faculty should continuously challenge themselves to provide creative, interesting, and sound education - students soon learn that education doesn't have to be boring; they become self-motivated, enthusiastic, and interested.....learning then follows. – Linda Caputi

# Definition of Critical Thinking

Paul and Elder (2001) asserted that critical thinking is developed as part of larger contextual issues, not as a set of technical skills. Critical thinking needs to be learned in a dialectical way, as arguments in relation to counter-arguments that are examined and reformulated until a conclusion is reached.

**Key concept: Critical thinking involves thinking about your thinking while you are thinking in order to make your thinking:**
- **Better.**
- **More clear.**
- **More accurate.**
- **More defensible.**

McPeck (1990) defined critical thinking as thinking with skepticism about a subject or field. The thinker possesses the skills associated with practitioners in that field. Critical thinking includes certain aspects of problem-solving and other thinking skills. McPeck argued that critical thinking can be taught using drill and practice but not with just any drills. The drills need to encourage the use of critical thinking. These drill and practice activities must use critical thinking skills within the context of the discipline.

**Key concept: Thinking skills are best developed when applied to actual or simulated practice.**

Ennis (1992) noted that critical thinking is disciplined, self-directed thinking. It is thinking that displays a mastery of intellectual skills and abilities. Ennis believed that reasonable, reflective thinking is focused on deciding what to believe or do.

**Key concept: Critical thinking requires disciplined, self-directed thinking and is based on mastery of intellectual skills and abilities.**

Hatcher (1995) contended that critical thinking requires thinkers to evaluate an argument, which involves asking the basic questions of logic:
- Are the claims made in the premises and conclusion clearly understood?
- Do the premises support the conclusion?
- Are the premises themselves true or acceptable?
- What evidence does the learner have for believing them?
- Are there examples that counter the claims made in the premises?
- Are any common fallacies committed?
- Are there alternative accounts that need to be considered?

**Key concept: Critical thinkers apply logic to evaluate their thinking and decisions.**

Following is a working definition of critical thinking drawn from the key concepts of each of these theories (Caputi, 2003a):

Critical thinking is a complex thinking process that:

- Is disciplined and self-directed.
- Is based on mastery of many thinking skills and abilities.
- Is best developed when applied to actual or simulated real-world situations.
- Involves thinking about the thinking process as it is occurring.
- Evaluates a decision or problem solution against a standardized set of criteria.

## Critical Thinking Skills and Strategies

Many thinking skills are used in the process of critical thinking (Alfaro-LeFevre, 1999; Kozier, Erb, Berman, & Burke, 2000; McDonald, 2002). This section contains many of the critical thinking skills and strategies explained in the *Critical-Thinking Tutorial* (Caputi, 2003a), a computer-assisted education program that teaches nursing students critical thinking skills and strategies with many examples and practice situations.

This list can be used to operationalize the abstract concept of critical thinking. When reading through this list, think of assignments that can help students sharpen their ability to use these thinking skills. Please note that this is not a complete, exhaustive list of all the thinking skills and strategies used in critical thinking but rather a representative list of 23 commonly used thinking skills and strategies.

The critical thinking skills listed below are grouped into four categories:

- Basic-level thinking skills.
- Gathering data.
- Providing nursing care.
- Evaluating responses.

These categories are used for teaching purposes and to provide concrete examples. However, all the skills listed may be applied in many different contexts, and many of these skills are used concurrently.

When reading through this section, it may become apparent that most of these thinking skills are used in everyday life; the challenge is to apply them to nursing situations. Students become more proficient in using these thinking skills in nursing as their knowledge base of nursing increases and as they encounter additional clinical experiences.

While reading about these individual thinking skills and strategies, also consider ways to encourage students to use these skills in client-care situations. For example, develop a one-minute assignment®. A one-minute assignment® is a small exercise focused on helping students apply a specific critical thinking skill or strategy. These are small assignments that are carried out in the clinical setting.

The following is an example of a quick, one-minute assignment® addressing the thinking skill of **determining relevant from irrelevant data**. Many times students do not relate preoperative conditions with the immediate postoperative care of a client. The student may report a high blood pressure reading, and not relate that reading to the fact that the antihypertensive medication was not restarted after surgery. Therefore, a one-minute assignment may be to ask the student to read the client's history and physical, including previous surgeries, medical history, and medications taken prior to admission. The student should then discuss which information will have an impact on the client's recovery from surgery.

This type of assignment may actually take more than one minute to complete, but should not exceed more than 5 minutes. The purpose of these assignments is to provide opportunities for students to apply an isolated thinking skill to client care. A series of these assignments builds on one another until finally the student moves intuitively from one thinking skill to the next – engaging in a total critical thinking modus operand.

As educators it is apparent that critical thinking involves all the thinking skills and strategies discussed in this chapter. And, as experts, faculty know how to gingerly move from one to another. This is where students become overwhelmed! However, if students are afforded the practice of using individual thinking skills prior to being required to engage in critical thinking about the total care of a client, the task of thinking critically becomes achievable. This method of teaching critical thinking applies the theoretical approach of teaching from simple to complex.

### *Basic-Level Thinking Skills*

Students need a solid knowledge base from which to draw information for answering questions requiring higher-level thinking. Knowledge refers to information committed to memory as well as knowing how to find needed information. Students also must be aware of all the resources available that can be used to find the information needed to solve problems and make decisions related to client care. The skills in this category provide this foundation.

Basic-level thinking skills include:
- Identifying signs and symptoms.
- Recalling knowledge about diagnostic tests.
- Understanding the physiology of body systems.

### *Identifying Signs and Symptoms*

An ability to identify signs and symptoms of disease, side effects of drugs, and a host of other causes is based on knowledge of normal functioning. Higher-order thinking skills, such as comparing and contrasting, are used to differentiate normal signs and symptoms from abnormal ones.

### Recalling Knowledge About Diagnostic Tests

Laboratory and diagnostic tests provide a window into the client's internal environment. These studies provide critical information necessary for an accurate assessment, the basis for the subsequent steps of the nursing process. Nurses must be aware of all aspects of diagnostic testing. This knowledge is necessary for properly scheduling tests, ensuring the most accurate results, and carrying out post-procedure care so no harm comes to the client as a result of the testing.

### Understanding the Physiology of Body Systems

Understanding the physiology of body systems serves as a foundation for performing an accurate and complete physical assessment. Knowing what is normal is key to detecting abnormalities. This knowledge is necessary for recognizing signs and symptoms of disease, diagnosing actual and potential problems, and evaluating the effect of nursing interventions.

### Gathering Data

Each of the thinking skills listed in this category is commonly used when a nurse gathers data. These skills include:
- Assessing systematically and comprehensively.
- Checking accuracy and reliability.
- Clustering related information.
- Collaborating with co-workers.
- Determining the importance of information.
- Distinguishing relevant from irrelevant information.
- Gathering complete and accurate data and then acting on that data.
- Judging how much ambiguity is acceptable.
- Recognizing inconsistencies.
- Using diagnostic reasoning.

### Assessing Systematically and Comprehensively

Assessing systematically and comprehensively is a critical thinking strategy applied to all areas of nursing practice. Nurses use a systematic method such as a body-systems or a head-to-toe approach so no areas are forgotten.

A systematic and comprehensive approach is also used when collecting data during a shift report. Most nurses use a specific format for gathering client data to ensure that all important areas of information are noted.

### *Checking Accuracy and Reliability*

Nurses must make judgments about the accuracy and reliability of information. Decisions about what nursing actions to take are based on this information. Problems can develop or even harm can come to a client if care is based on information that is not accurate and reliable.

### *Clustering Related Information*

Clustering related information refers to grouping together information with a common theme. This is the process used when formulating nursing diagnoses. Related signs and symptoms are clustered together to form the basis for a nursing diagnosis.

### *Collaborating with Co-workers*

The critical thinking needed to solve problems seldom happens when working alone; many people can be involved. In soliciting information and suggestions from others, new perspectives on a problem are realized. Various approaches and solutions may be suggested.

Present-day health care is a complex environment requiring the input and cooperation of many members working as a team. Team members engage in a critical thinking process when they examine delivery of care, noting compliance with standards of care and adherence to accepted protocols. This team approach, with all members collaborating and working together, strengthens client care and fosters positive outcomes.

### *Determining the Importance of Information*

Nurses have a myriad of information to sort through for every client. This information may change often throughout the course of a day. Therefore, nurses must be able to determine the importance of information, act on that which is important, and disregard that which is not.

## Distinguishing Relevant from Irrelevant Information

The thinking skill of distinguishing relevant from irrelevant information refers to the nurse deciding which information is pertinent or connects with the matter at hand. All information about a client may be important for the client's overall care, but the nurse must sort out which information is relevant to a particular problem or situation currently under consideration.

## Gathering Complete and Accurate Data then Acting on That Data

Gathering complete and accurate data is fundamental to critical thinking. Data is collected from all sources available to the nurse. The data is then used as the basis for solving problems and making decisions, so it is important that data collection is complete and accurate.

## Judging How Much Ambiguity is Acceptable

"Ambiguous" refers to a situation that is unclear, uncertain, or vague. Ambiguity occurs when factors relating to a situation make it somewhat unclear or gray rather than "black and white." Many situations appear similar on the surface but actually differ when all factors are carefully considered.

## Recognizing Inconsistencies

The beginning point of the nursing process is assessment. Throughout the assessment, both subjective and objective data are collected. In reviewing all this data, nurses are cognizant of any inconsistencies that may indicate additional problems that may not be readily apparent.

## Using Diagnostic Reasoning

The word "reasoning" refers to using critical thinking to solve problems and make decisions. Generally speaking, reasoning can be used as a synonym for critical thinking. Diagnostic reasoning applies this type of thinking to clinical practice. Specifically, it refers to the formulation of nursing diagnoses about a client's health status.

Diagnostic reasoning is a complex process that takes into account many factors about the client, such as current health status, family history, prior illnesses, and a host of other factors. When using diagnostic reasoning, it is always important to consider how the client is coping with the situation or problem. Although helpful with the diagnostic process, assessing the client's coping is often an overlooked aspect of data collection.

## Providing Nursing Care

Each one of the thinking skills in this category is commonly used when nurses provide care to clients. These skills include:
- Applying the nursing process to develop a treatment plan.
- Communicating effectively.
- Predicting and managing potential complications.
- Resolving conflicts.
- Resolving ethical dilemmas.
- Setting priorities.
- Teaching others.

### Applying the Nursing Process to Develop a Treatment Plan

The nursing process is the framework for providing safe, effective, and humanistic nursing care. This process is applied systematically by all nurses and serves as the basis for all nursing actions.

Students may think of the nursing process as labor intensive, based on their experience writing student care plans. It is helpful for them to learn that the nursing process is used continuously throughout the day as a way of thinking. Consider the nurse's response to a client's report of pain. The nurse immediately:
- Assesses all characteristics of the pain.
- Formulates a goal and outcome criteria.
- Develops a plan for controlling the pain.
- Implements the plan.
- Follows up with the client to evaluate the effectiveness of the interventions.

All this happens within a matter of minutes. It is automatic and second nature to expert nurses.

### Communicating Effectively

Communicating effectively is a highly complex process. Many factors influence communication. Examples of these factors include environment, territoriality, values, personal space, attitudes, and time. The nurse must be aware of these and other factors and not let them block effective communication. It is difficult to carry out effective critical thinking when communication is breaking down.

## *Predicting and Managing Potential Complications*

Predicting and managing potential complications requires critical thinking. Nurses must look at the big picture in order to predict potential complications that may exist for individual clients. The starting point is to know common complications related to a client's condition, then consider individual differences that may address additional concerns.

For example, all surgical clients are at risk for atelectasis and pneumonia. Interventions such as deep breathing and coughing exercises, early ambulation, and the use of an incentive spirometer are planned. However, an 18-year-old athlete in excellent physical condition who has undergone a laparoscopic appendectomy is at much less risk for these complications than a 60-year-old obese client with a history of cigarette smoking who has undergone a colon resection.

## *Resolving Conflicts*

Conflict cannot be avoided. Conflict happens on a daily basis. Nurses are often in a rapidly paced climate, full of urgency and serious consequences if errors are made. In this kind of environment, conflict is inevitable.

Nurses in all areas of client care must be able to maintain calm, avoid conflict, and if conflict should occur, handle it in a constructive manner. These characteristics serve to promote an atmosphere that is optimal for critical thinking to take place.

## *Resolving Ethical Dilemmas*

Because ethical dilemmas are typically extremely complex issues, they require professionals to use critical thinking skills. A code of ethics provides a point of reference for nurses to use when faced with ethical dilemmas. The American Nurses' Association, the International Council of Nurses, and the Canadian Nurses' Association have all adopted a code of ethics. Nurses can use these to help guide their thinking processes when faced with an ethical dilemma.

## *Setting Priorities*

Setting priorities or prioritizing is a thinking skill constantly used by nurses in all client care environments. Prioritizing can be a simple task or a complex task that involves comparing and contrasting data and sorting relevant from irrelevant information.

Nurses prioritize:

- When caring for a group of clients and deciding which clients to see first and which clients can wait.
- When caring for a specific client to determine which assessments and interventions are most important and must be carried out first.

In some settings, protocols are in place to help with prioritizing. For example, triage nurses in the emergency department typically follow a procedure in which clients with chest pain or eye injuries take priority. For other client problems, these nurses use their established knowledge base and experience to determine which clients must be seen first.

## *Delegating*

When delegating care, nurses engage in many critical thinking skills and strategies. According to the National Council of State Boards of Nursing (1997), delegating refers to "transferring to a competent individual the authority to perform a selected nursing task in a selected situation" (p. 2). Delegating requires nurses to engage in assessing, planning, assigning, supervising, and evaluating. Each of these roles requires a high degree of critical thinking and decision making. When engaged in delegation activities, nurses are accountable that the delegation process is accurately and responsibility carried out in all client care situations.

## *Teaching Others*

In all aspects of life, teaching is empowering. Nurses empower clients through teaching. Teaching can occur informally any time a nurse interacts with a client. Teaching is also formalized through the written plan of care. One example is discharge teaching, which typically addresses specific areas such as medications, diet, activity restrictions, and follow-up visits. Another example of formalized teaching is diabetic teaching, which often involves written guidelines with a checklist to ensure all areas are covered.

Critical thinking skills are used in teaching. Nurses consider all factors, looking at the big picture, in order to individualize the teaching plan. For example, discharge teaching has a different focus if the client is going home alone, discharged home with a caregiver, or transferred to an extended-care facility.

### *Evaluating Responses*

The thinking skills in this category include:
- Evaluating and correcting thinking.
- Evaluating data.

- Supporting conclusions with evidence.

## *Evaluating and Correcting Thinking*

After using critical thinking to resolve a problem, make a decision, or plan client care, it is important to evaluate the thinking that occurred. Evaluating thinking means reflecting on what just happened, how the situation was handled, and what lessons can be learned for use in similar situations in the future.

This type of self-evaluation promotes professional development, enhances self-esteem, and fosters insight into one's own thinking. Thinking about one's thinking is part of the total critical thinking process. The following questions may be used to evaluate thinking:

- What thinking skills were used? Were they effective?
- Were the outcomes what was expected? If not, were the outcomes acceptable or perhaps better than expected? If the outcomes were not acceptable, what might be done differently in the future?
- How did the thinking impact all the people affected, such as the client, significant others, and other healthcare providers? Was the impact positive or negative?

It is helpful to discuss with co-workers the thinking skills used in a situation. Ask how they might have handled the situation and be ready to change if change is needed.

## *Evaluating Data*

Evaluating data is the basis for several steps of the nursing process. Data collection is part of the assessment step. Accurate and complete data collection provides a database on which to formulate diagnoses and interventions. Data collection is carried out again during the evaluation step to determine if the interventions were effective.

Because data collection is such an important part of the nursing process, it is necessary for nurses to evaluate the data for accuracy. Many times, nurses must question the data collected, collect additional data, or take further steps to verify accuracy. Inadequate data collection can have a detrimental effect on client outcomes.

## *Supporting Conclusions with Evidence*

Nurses often have intuitive feelings about what is happening with clients. Intuition can be quite helpful as a starting point but should not be the sole means for identifying problems. It is important for nurses to collect data that support suspected problems and formulate nursing diagnoses based on evidence rather than jumping to conclusions and focusing in the wrong direction. Applying the steps of the nursing process helps ensure a systematic, scientific approach to data collection and analysis.

It is important for students to be aware of just what critical thinking is and have the opportunity to discuss examples of the skills and strategies such as those reviewed above. This provides a foundation of knowledge to use in the application of critical thinking to client care.

## Critical Thinking Learning Activities for Nursing Students

This section provides a sampling of critical thinking activities. Most of the activities can be modified for beginning students, and all can be used for intermediate and advanced students. Feel free to use these or to modify them for use with a specific group of students. Use these examples to stimulate creativity within yourself to develop many more of your own critical thinking activities for your nursing students.

The critical thinking activities described in this section include:

- Delegating and Prioritizing Exercise.
- Client-Care Critical Thinking Activity.
- Nursing Abilities Critical Thinking Tool.
- Three Approaches to Planning Client Care.
- Critical Thinking Activity: "Putting It All Together."

### *Delegating and Prioritizing Exercise*

See Figures 32.1 and 32.2 for the Delegating and Prioritizing Exercise. The purpose of this exercise is to help students develop the skills of delegating and prioritizing, two highly important skills in all areas of nursing. This particular exercise addresses the medical/surgical client but can be modified to fit any nursing situation. This tool is included on the CD-ROM accompanying this book for easy access.

### *Client-Care Critical Thinking Activity*

See Figures 32.3 and 32.4 for the Client-Care Critical Thinking Activity. This activity focuses the students' attention on gathering pertinent information about a client and conducting an initial client assessment, then using that information to determine the most important aspects of care. This tool is included on the CD-ROM accompanying this book for easy access.

### *Nursing Abilities Critical Thinking Tool*

In the chapter of this book titled *Approval: National Council of State Boards of Nursing*

Nancy Spector points out that some states have specific curricular regulations that educators should follow. One such regulation in Minnesota is called the *Nursing Abilities to be Evaluated*. This prompted me to develop this tool titled *Nursing Abilities Critical-Thinking Tool* (see Figure 32.5). The purpose of this tool is to focus students' attention on important nursing abilities. Directions for three educational levels are included. This tool is included on the CD-ROM accompanying this book for easy access.

Figure 32.1 - Delegating and Prioritizing Exercise, Page 1

---

### Delegating and Prioritizing Exercise
### Medical/Surgical Client

**Today you have the following team members working with you:** an LPN/LVN and a CNA.

**Step 1:**
Obtain the following information on three clients. You might use information from the shift report, cardex, and medication administration record.

Name:
Medical Diagnosis:
Nursing care for today:
      Activity:                     Assistance needed with activity:
      Diet:                         Assistance or special needs related to diet:
      Pain rating:
            Medications ordered for pain:
            Side effects of analgesics:
      Safety issues:
      IV fluids:
      Medications: Fill out the information on the attached sheet for each medication (see Figure 32.2).
      State of fluid balance:
      Labs scheduled for today:
            How the labs relate to nursing care:
      Diagnostics studies scheduled for today:
            How the studies relate to nursing care:
      Dressing changes:
      Suctioning:
      Enema:
      Other treatments:

**Step 2:**
Visit each client and perform a quick, two-minute assessment of both the client and the client's environment.

---

Figure 32.1 - Delegating and Prioritizing Exercise, Page 1 cont.

---

**Step 3:**
1. Prioritize which client you should care for first, second, and third. Why?
2. What are the primary assessments that should be completed first for each client? Why?
3. What nursing interventions need to be carried out for each client?
4. What interventions will you do first?
5. Which of the above interventions will you delegate and to whom? Why?
6. What information will you give to the person to whom you are delegating the task and what information will you collect after the task is finished?

---

Figure 32.2 - Delegating and Prioritizing Exercise, Page 2

---

### Medication Information

On another sheet of paper, fill in the following information for each medication to be administered while you are caring for this client.

**Name of medication:**
1. Classification of the medication.
2. Reason why the medication was ordered.
3. When it will be administered.
4. Teaching that needs to be done relative to the medication.
5. Any special instructions regarding administration of this medication.

Which medication for each client is most important to give on time?
Which medication can be given toward the end of the window of time and still be given "at the right time" without adverse effects?

**Medications administered at other times:**
What other medications are prescribed for the client that were administered on the previous shift or will be administered on the next shift?
How will those medications affect the client assessments and the care you will be giving this shift?

---

Figure 32.3 - Client-Care Critical Thinking Activity, Page 1

---

### Client-Care Critical Thinking Activity

On a separate sheet of paper, answer the following:

1. Client information:
   Age:
   Reason for admission:
   Date of admission:
   Diagnostic procedures:
   Surgical procedure:
   Diet:
   Activity:

2. Medications:
   Drug:
   Reason why it was prescribed:
   Therapeutic effects expected:
   Adverse effects to monitor:
(Complete for all medications prescribed.)

3. Client history:
   Important information from history:
   From the history, the most important data impacting this
   hospitalization is:

4. Diagnostic tests:
   Name of test:
   Why was this test ordered?
   (Complete for each test ordered.)

5. Problems occurring for this client during the preceding 24 hours:

   How were the above problems handled?

6. Was the physician called for any reason? If so, why?
   What information was gathered prior to notifying the physician?
   What actions were taken?

7. Potential problems that could occur for this client:

   Interventions to prevent the potential problems:

---

Figure 32.4 - Client-Care Critical Thinking Activity, Page 2

8. Look at the client's nursing care plan:
    List the nursing diagnoses:

    Prioritize the nursing diagnoses:

    How did you determine the order of prioritization of the nursing diagnoses?

    What are the interventions for the top two nursing diagnoses?

    Prioritize those interventions:

    Which of these interventions can you delegate to an unlicensed person?

9. Look at the shift report sheets for the past 24 hours. Based on those report sheets, what is the MOST IMPORTANT nursing intervention for you to carry out this shift?

10. If the physician came in at this moment and discharged this client, what are the most important teaching instructions for this client?

11. What if……………………….

(Ask me to complete this question for you to answer.)
Here the teacher poses a "What if" question based on the information the student collected.

Figure 32.5 - Nursing Abilities Critical Thinking Tool

---

**Nursing Abilities Critical Thinking Tool**

**Beginning Students:** For each of the nursing abilities listed below, write a brief statement of how you addressed each one for each client you cared for today.

**Intermediate Students:** For each of the nursing abilities listed below, write a nursing diagnosis–if applicable–for each client. Write a brief statement of how you addressed each nursing ability for each client you cared for today.

**Advanced Students:** For each of the nursing abilities listed below, write a nursing diagnosis–if applicable–for each client, then write a goal statement, outcome criteria, and interventions for each diagnosis. For items that do not require a nursing diagnosis, write a brief statement of how you addressed each one for each client you cared for today.

1. Provide for physical safety
2. Prevent spread of pathogens
3. Determine when necessary to use sterile technique
4. Maintain sterility
5. Maintain skin and mucous membrane integrity
6. Promote respiratory function
7. Promote circulatory function
8. Promote fluid and nutrition balance
9. Promote elimination
10. Promote physical activity
11. Promote restoration/maintenance of physical independence
12. Provide for physical comfort
13. Provide for rest and sleep
14. Provide for personal hygiene

---

## *Three Approaches to Planning Client Care*

The purpose of this activity is for students to compare and contrast three approaches to planning client care. For the same client, students should:
- Complete a traditional care plan.
- Construct a concept map (use the guidelines provided in the chapter in this book titled *Using Concept Maps to Foster Critical Thinking* by Deanne Couey).
- Develop a clinical pathway or care map (guidelines for this are presented in Figures 32.6, 32.7, and 32.8.). These guidelines are included on the CD-ROM accompanying this book.

After completing the above, students are asked to address a variety of questions that compare and contrast these three approaches. Following are examples of questions that can be used:
- How does each approach organize client care?
- How does each approach foster collaboration among healthcare disciplines?
- How does each format help evaluate the client's response to care and in revising the plan of care?

Figure 32.6 - Instructions for Completing the Care Map

---

**Guidelines for Completing the Care Map**

1. Read through the client's chart and fill out the Care Map form.

2. If this was an elective admission, such as for surgery, include preoperative testing, etc., in the Prior To Admission (PTA) column.

3. Record the care given on each day. For most categories you will include a nursing diagnosis and desired outcome. The columns in that category labeled PTA, Day 1, Day 2, and Day 3 will include both nursing interventions documented in the chart related to that category as well as care provided by other disciplines. For example, under respiratory you will include nursing interventions such as deep breathing and coughing as well as any respiratory therapy treatments administered.

4. Complete a medication sheet for each medication prescribed.

5. Using your textbook, study the typical care provided for a client with that particular diagnosis. Compare this with the care provided as documented on the care map.

6. On the Care Map Variance Record, note:

---

Figure 32.6 - Instructions for Completing the Care Map cont.

(a) any differences from the typical treatment due to a pre-existing condition (such as a chronic illness), and

(b) any differences from the expected care due to a problem that arose during the client's stay (unexpected happenings), such as a postoperative temperature or adverse reaction to an antibiotic. Explain the action taken to treat or care for any of the unexpected happenings.

Figure 32.7 - Care Map

| Care Map | | | | |
|---|---|---|---|---|
| **Medical Diagnosis** | **PTA** | **Day 1** | **Day 2** | **Day 3** |
| **Consults** | | | | |
| **Activity & Safety**<br>  Nursing Diagnosis:<br>  Desired Outcome: | | | | |
| **Circulatory/Neurovascular**<br>  Nursing Diagnosis:<br>  Desired Outcome: | | | | |
| **Comfort/Pain Mgmt.**<br>  Nursing Diagnosis:<br>  Desired Outcome: | | | | |
| **Elimination**<br>  Nursing Diagnosis:<br>  Desired Outcome: | | | | |
| **Fluids/IV**<br>  Nursing Diagnosis:<br>  Desired Outcome: | | | | |
| **Hygiene**<br>  Nursing Diagnosis:<br>  Desired Outcome: | | | | |
| **Infection**<br>  Nursing Diagnosis:<br>  Desired Outcome: | | | | |
| **Integument**<br>  Nursing Diagnosis:<br>  Desired Outcome: | | | | |
| **Neurological**<br>  Nursing Diagnosis:<br>  Desired Outcome: | | | | |
| **Nutrition**<br>  Nursing Diagnosis:<br>  Desired Outcome: | | | | |
| **Respiratory**<br>  Nursing Diagnosis:<br>  Desired Outcome: | | | | |
| **Sleep/Rest**<br>  Nursing Diagnosis:<br>  Desired Outcome: | | | | |
| **Psychosocial**<br>  Nursing Diagnosis:<br>  Desired Outcome: | | | | |
| **Teaching**<br>  Required for care during<br>  hospitalization | | | | |
| **Discharge Planning**<br>**Discharge Teaching** | | | | |

Figure 32.8 - Care Map Variance Record

| Care Map Variance Record | |
|---|---|
| **Variance** | **Action Taken** |
| | |
| | |
| | |

### *Critical Thinking Activity: "Putting It All Together"*

This final critical thinking activity involves role playing. The purpose of the activity is to provide students an opportunity to use observational skills, gather complete and accurate data, and then act on that data. In this skit, students are put into an action-filled, simulated emergency that is challenging and exciting. Given a particular scenario, several students perform assigned roles as the remaining students observe and critique the actor's response to the emergency situation. Everyone is drawn into the action, which students love, as they become **real** nurses. This activity, designed by Lynn Engelmann, may be used with advanced students, who have a working knowledge of the basic principles of emergency nursing and anaphylactic shock. See Figure 32.9 for details of this activity. The ideas for this activity were drawn from Laskowski-Jones (1995) *First-Line Emergency Care: What Every Nurse Should Know.*

Figure 32.9 - Critical Thinking Activity: Putting It All Together

---

Putting It All Together

Directions: Three students perform the following roles:
- Victim
- Rescue nurse: Neighbor next door
- Victim's spouse

Props:
- Blanket for victim to lay on
- Rake
- Red dot (to simulate bee sting and erythema)
- Medi-alert bracelet, stating, "allergic to bee stings"

Instructions:

One student plays the victim, who is stung by a bee. This event is not witnessed by the rescue nurse. The rescue nurse is instructed to respond to the emergency, doing what the nurse deems appropriate. The victim's spouse does not know what happened, only that her spouse collapsed while raking leaves. Audience is not given information on the problem.

Action:
- Victim is outside raking leaves.
- Victim suddenly grabs his leg, falls to the ground, and stridor ensues.
- Spouse finds victim and calls for the nurse who lives next door.
- Nurse implements emergency actions. Ideally, action by nurse would include:
  - Securing the area for safety, throwing rake out of way so there is safe access to victim.
  - Performing a primary assessment, assessing ABCs, opening airway, and directing spouse to call 9-1-1.
  - Performing secondary assessment, finding bee sting site, asking spouse about allergies..
  - Noting medi-alert bracelet, asking spouse about epi-pen.
  - Administering epinephrine, placing victim in rescue position, covering victim with blanket.

At the end of the performance, students evaluate any actions that were missing in the process, and discuss what actions are taken when responding to emergency situations.

---

# Conclusion

Developing critical thinking is an ongoing process in relation to the nursing content under study. As nursing knowledge increases, so should students' ability to use critical thinking skills to handle increasingly complex nursing situations. Working through a variety of these activities provides a venue for this ongoing process with the end goal that critical thinking will become intuitive and routine.

# Learning Activities

1. Pick three critical thinking skills and develop a one-minute assignment® in your area of practice for students to apply these skills.
2. Choose one of the five critical thinking activities presented in this chapter. Assign the activity. Discuss with a colleague the learning outcomes achieved by the students completing this activity.
3. Review the works of three critical thinking theorists. Develop a personal definition of critical thinking. Compare that definition with one used in the nursing program in which you teach or from which you graduated.
4. For each of the critical thinking activities presented in this chapter, determine which of the critical thinking skills and strategies are used as the student works through each activity.

# References

Alfaro-LeFevre, R. (1999). *Critical thinking in nursing: A practical approach.* Philadelphia, PA: Saunders.

Alfaro-LeFevre, R. (2001). *Evaluating critical thinking: How do you read minds?* [online]. Available: http://nsweb.nursingspectrum.com/cfforms/GuestLecture/

Caputi, L. (2003a). *The critical thinking tutorial.* Glen Ellyn, IL: College of DuPage.

Ennis, R. (1992, March 27-30). *Critical thinking: What is it?* Proceedings of the 48th Annual Meeting of the Philosophy of Education Society, Denver, CO.

Hatcher, D. (1995). *Critical thinking and epistemic obligations* [online]. Available: http://www.shss.montclair.edu/inquiry/spr95/hatcher2.html

Kozier, B., Erb, G., Berman, A. J., & Burke, K. (2000). *Fundamentals of nursing: Concepts, process, and practice.* Upper Saddle River, NJ: Prentice-Hall.

Laskowski-Jones, L. (1995). First-line emergency care: What every nurse should know. *Nursing 95, 25*(1), 34-45.

McDonald, M. (2002). *Systematic assessment of learning outcomes: Developing multiple-choice exams.* Boston, MA: Jones & Bartlett.

McPeck, J. E. (1990). *The meaning of critical thinking: Critical thinking and education.* New York: St. Martin Press.

National Council of State Boards of Nursing. (1997). *Role development: Critical components of delegation curriculum outline.* Chicago: Author.

Paul, R., & Elder, L. (2001). *Critical thinking: Tools for taking charge of learning and your life.* Upper Saddle River, NJ: Prentice Hall.

# Accreditation, Approval, and Certification

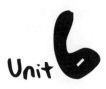

Unit 6

# Chapter 33: AN OVERVIEW OF NURSING PROGRAM ACCREDITATION

Susan Abbe, MS, PhD, RN

*It is our opinion that nursing faculty are dedicated professionals who work hard to educate nurses at the highest possible level of competence. These faculty are typically proud of their programs and proud of their graduates. One way to publicly proclaim their fine programs is to seek accreditation. By obtaining accreditation, the world knows the program has met standards established by an outside body – a form of external evaluation. This chapter explains what accreditation is all about, its history, and its current status. – Linda Caputi and Lynn Engelmann*

## Introduction

Nursing regulates the profession in three ways: licensure, certification, and accreditation. The nursing profession called for professional regulation in the early 1900s as a means of protecting the public from incompetent practitioners. Licensure is the process by which a governmental agency gives affirmation to the public that individuals engaged in an occupation or profession have minimal education, qualifications, and competencies necessary to practice in a safe manner. Upon graduation from a nursing education program, a person is eligible to write the National Council Licensure Examination (NCLEX®-RN or NCLEX®-PN), qualifying the candidate to practice nursing. This exam validates that the individual has acquired basic knowledge required for minimal safe practice; it does not recognize exceptional performance. Currently, each state board of nursing licenses and sanctions registered nurses and practical nurses as authorized by the State Nurse Practice Act and accompanying regulations.

Educational Philosophy

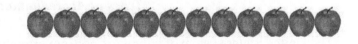

To facilitate student learning; to encourage inquiry and creativity; and to be a resource. – Susan Abbe

Certification is the process by which an organization, association, voluntary agency, or state licensing board grants recognition that an individual has met predetermined criteria specified for practice in an area of specialization. There are over 20 recognized nursing certification organizations representing various nursing specialties. Examples of entities that grant certification include:

- American Nurses Credentialing Center (ANCC).
- Board of Certification for Emergency Nursing.
- National Association of School Nurses.
- National Certification Board of Pediatric Nurse Practitioners/Nurses (NCBPNP/N).
- Wound, Ostomy, and Continence Nurses Society.

Nurse certification involves an individual passing an examination in a specialty area of nursing to testify that the nurse has achieved a certain level of competence in the particular area. The individual initiates the certification process, and although many jobs may require certification, it is a voluntary process. See the chapter in this book titled *Certification in Nursing* by Andrea Tacchi for more information on certification.

## Accreditation

Accreditation in nursing education is a system for recognizing educational institutions and programs that have been found to meet established standards. The status of recognition conveys to the educational community and the public confidence that a certain level of performance, integrity, and quality has been met. In the United States, accreditation is a voluntary, nongovernmental process that uses peer review to determine if academic programs meet public confidence. Accreditation indicates that the institution or program has accepted the responsibility of continuous self-evaluation. The accreditation process requires a rigorous self-evaluation, an appraisal by respected and competent peers, and a subsequent review and decision by an external agency. Accreditation is ideally grounded in collegiality and the voluntary search for quality improvement. Accreditation applies to institutions or programs, distinguishing it from licensure and certification, which apply to individuals.

### *Types of Accreditation*

The United States system of voluntary, non-governmental evaluation promotes education quality either through institutional (regional or national) accreditation or programmatic (specialized or professional) accreditation. Regional accrediting bodies accredit public and private, nonprofit and for-profit, and two- and four-year institutions. National accrediting bodies accredit public and private institutions; nonprofit and for-profit institutions; frequently single-purposed institutions, including distance learning colleges and universities; private career institutions; and faith-based colleges and universities. Programmatic accrediting bodies accredit specific units, schools, or programs within institutions.

Institutional and programmatic accreditations are complementary. The focus of a regional accrediting agency considers the characteristics of the whole institution as a total operating unit. The accrediting agency provides assurance that the general characteristics of the college, university, or school have been examined and found to be satisfactory. The standards established by institutional accrediting agencies are broad in nature to reflect the components of the entire institution as well as the wide range of purposes and scopes of post-secondary and higher education. There are six regional accrediting bodies:

- Middle States Association of Colleges and Schools.
- New England Association of Schools and Colleges.
- North Central Association of Colleges and Schools.
- Northwest Association of Schools and Colleges.
- Southern Association of Colleges and Schools.
- Western Association of Schools and Colleges.

In contrast, a specialized accrediting agency focuses its attention on an individual program within a post-secondary or higher education institution. The focus on a specific program provides assurance that the particular program has met the external accreditation standards. The accrediting agency conducting the evaluation of a program preparing students for a profession or occupation is often associated with the professional association(s) for the field. Thus, specialized accreditation is recognized as providing an essential assurance of the scope and quality of professional or occupational preparation.

Nursing has two agencies offering specialized accreditation for nursing education programs: National League for Nursing Accrediting Commission (NLNAC) – an independent subsidiary of the National League for Nursing (NLN) – and the Commission on Collegiate Nursing Education (CCNE) – an autonomous arm of the American Association of Colleges of Nursing (AACN). NLNAC is responsible for the specialized accreditation of all types of nursing education programs: master's, baccalaureate, associate, diploma, and practical nursing. CCNE is responsible for the specialized accreditation of baccalaureate and higher degree programs in nursing.

### *History of Nursing Accreditation*

Nursing has a long history of voluntary efforts to raise its educational standards, and accreditation has played an essential role in these efforts. As early as 1894, the American Society of Superintendents of Training Schools for Nursing, the first national nursing organization in the United States, was founded to assure the public that schools were preparing nurses who were adequately educated to serve the community. The Society's Constitution and By-laws, Article II, stated, "The objectives of the Society shall be to further the best interests of the nursing profession by establishing and maintaining a universal standard of training, and by promoting fellowship among its members by meetings, papers, and discussions on nursing subjects, and by interchange of options" (Deforge, n.d.). Linda Richards served as its first president.

In 1912, the Society changed its name to the National League for Nursing Education and, in 1917, published the *Standard Curriculum for Schools of Nursing*. Between 1912 and 1948, four additional organizations, primarily concerned with the quality of nursing education, came into existence:

- The Association of Collegiate Schools of Nursing (ACSN).
- The National Association for Practical Nurse Education (NAPNE).
- The National Organization for Public Health Nursing (NOPHN).
- The American Association of Industrial Nurses (AAIN).

The Conference of Catholic Schools of Nursing of the Catholic Hospital Association, a national group, also was active in the field of nursing education. During this time, these national nursing organizations recognized that accreditation was imperative for the improvement of nursing education. Four of the organizations instituted accreditation services for the educational programs with which they were concerned:

- NOPHN in 1920 for colleges and university programs in public health nursing.
- ACSN in 1932 for college and university nursing education programs.
- Council on Nursing Education of the Catholic Hospital Association in 1938 for schools of nursing conducted under Catholic auspices.
- National League for Nursing Education (NLNE) in 1939 for programs in basic professional nursing, both hospital and college controlled.

The existence of several accrediting groups led to confusion and overlapping of services.

Prior to a formal reorganization, the four organizations worked together through the Joint Committee on Unification of Accrediting Activities (JCUAA) to provide accreditation services. In 1948, the National Nursing Accrediting Service (NNAS) was formed, under the auspice of the JCUAA, to unify accreditation activities offered by the four organizations. The NNAS was discontinued in 1952 when the NLN was formed. The NLN represented the merging of three nursing groups with common goals for advancing nursing service and nursing education. The NLN became the first nursing education organization to gain recognition by the U.S. Department of Education (then part of the U.S. Department of Health, Education and Welfare) as nursing education's official accrediting body. Accreditation of nursing education programs became the function of NLN Division of Nursing Education. See the chapter in this book titled *Accreditation: National League for Nursing Accrediting Commission (NLNAC)* by Susan Abbe for more information on NLNAC.

In 1996 a second organization was created as an accrediting body for nursing education programs at the baccalaureate and graduate education level. This organization is the Commission on Collegiate Nursing Education (CCNE), an autonomous arm of the American Association of Colleges of Nursing (AACN). See the chapter in this book titled *Accreditation: Commission on Collegiate Nursing Education (CCNE)* by Mary Collins for more information on CCNE.

## Purpose, Benefits/Value, and Role of Accreditation

Accreditation has two fundamental purposes:
- Assure the quality of the nursing program.
- Assist in the improvement of the program.

These two purposes encompass responsibilities such as:
- Upholding agreed-upon standards for educational quality and public accountability.
- Evaluating nursing education programs in relation to their stated purpose(s) and the agreed-upon standards for accreditation.
- Involving institutional and nursing administration, faculty, and students in the process of continuous self-assessment.
- Bringing together practitioners, administrators, faculty, and students to improve the preparation of graduates to meet their responsibilities to society.
- Providing for external peer review.

In fulfilling its two purposes – quality assurance and program improvement – the value of specialized accreditation of nursing education programs benefits four primary constituencies:
- The public.
- Students.
- Educational institutions.
- The profession.

### *The Public*

The public is given assurance that the program in nursing has been reviewed by a qualified, independent group of peers and found to be in conformity to the general expectations of post-secondary and higher education and the profession. The public is also assured that accredited programs will continue to implement improvements that reflect changes in knowledge and practice generally accepted in the nursing and education community. Programs are publicly identified that have successfully undergone the voluntary activities directly linked to the accreditation process for the quality of the nursing program.

### The Student

The second constituency, the student, is given assurance that the educational activities of a nursing program that has satisfactorily undergone the accreditation process will be at the level of quality necessary to meet the needs of the student. Accreditation provides assistance in the smooth transfer of credits and courses between institutions and programs or the admission of students to advanced degrees. Accreditation status of the program may be noted by employers when evaluating potential candidates for employment. Specialized accreditation is a "stamp of approval" and confers the status accreditation brings on its programs.

### Educational Institutions

Post-secondary and higher education institutions – the third constituency – benefit from specialized accreditation through the stimulus provided for self-evaluation and self-directed improvement. In addition, the reputation of the institution is enhanced when programs offered by the institution are accredited. Another benefit is that the institution can gain eligibility for the participation of itself and its students in certain government and private funding or grant programs as accreditation is considered an indicator of the quality of education offered at the institution. Accreditation can aid in student and faculty recruitment.

### The Profession

The profession benefits from accreditation as it provides a means for the profession to set the requirements for the preparation of its practitioners. Accreditation contributes to the unity of the profession as it brings together administrators, faculty, and students in an effort directed at improvement.

Bellack, Gelmon, O'Neil, and Thomsen (1999) cited seven perceived benefits of accreditation for nursing education programs:

1. A hallmark of program excellence, adherence to high standards, and prestige and recognition.
2. Professional marketability and educational mobility of graduates.

3. The opportunity to engage in periodic self-study as a basis for improvement.
4. Demonstrated accountability to funders, consumers, and the public.
5. Peer review and consultation.
6. Leverage for an equitable share of institutional resources.
7. Entitlement to federal funds.

The top three benefits of accreditation identified by survey respondents were program excellence, prestige, and recognition (71%, n = 342), marketability and mobility of graduates (67%, n = 323), and self-evaluation for program improvement (56%, n = 268).

Accreditation has played an important role in the success of the American higher education system because of its voluntary nature and its status as a nongovernmental process. The primary role of accreditation is to promote high standards. Accreditation serves as the agent that encourages nursing programs to "push the outside of the envelope," to not accept the status quo, and to be the vision for the future of where nursing education needs to go.

## Challenges/Issues Facing Accreditation

Five challenges/issues facing faculty when making the decision to seek accreditation include:

- The necessity of accreditation.
- The duplication and cost of accreditation.
- The opinion of some that accreditation is a barrier to innovation in education.
- The need to implement an integrated, automated, electronic information system.
- The incorporation of distance education.

### *The Necessity of Accreditation*

The value of accreditation is generally believed to be worthwhile by participants and the public. It is through accreditation that continuous improvement is encouraged, professional excellence is demonstrated, and peer review and collaboration are hallmarks. Currency of content and quality of instruction are critical aspects of the institution maintaining its market share. Accreditation contributes to demonstrating this quality.

### *The Duplication and Cost of Accreditation*

Questions that arise are: What research has been done to show there is "value added"? and does the valued added outweigh the various costs of achieving and maintaining accreditation? Currently, college and university presidents are questioning whether it is necessary to maintain specialized accreditation if the institution has regional accreditation. Each specialized accrediting body has its own accreditation standards and its own set of policies and procedures, often overlapping but still distinct, that need to be followed. The interchange of information and material among various accrediting agencies is infrequent. With the proliferation of specialized accrediting bodies, institutions often find numerous agencies on campus during any one year. A tremendous amount of time is involved, for the institution and specific programs, in the preparation required prior to the site visit as well as at the time allotted for the review. Inherent in the issue of duplication is the matter of cost. Some costs to the institution are direct, such as the site visit fees, but other costs are indirect, such as faculty time.

### *Barriers to Innovation in Education*

For years, critics of accreditation have said that accreditation sets up barriers that inhibit innovation and creativity in education. Accreditation is based on agreed-upon standards that when implemented may be seen as barriers to faculties trying new teaching methodologies or curriculum designs. Standards are not always viewed as reflecting current educational trends or having been developed with the profession or public's input. Faculty concerns center on not being in compliance with a particular standard, thus jeopardizing the accreditation status.

### *The Need to Implement an Integrated, Automated, Electronic Information System*

Accreditation standards often incorporate language that addresses how an institution or program uses information technology. However, these same accrediting agencies are not always able to follow their own expectations. It is not uncommon for accrediting agencies to require self-study reports and supporting information to be submitted in hard copy. Even when the institution has the ability to support electronic submission of information the accrediting agency itself does not have the ability to receive it.

### *The Incorporation of Distance Education*

An educational trend affecting accreditation is the introduction of new educational methodologies, such as distance education. Accreditation provides assurance to the public of the quality of an institution or specific program, not necessarily the delivery system. Guidelines need to address distance learning to ensure continued quality in those education programs that use technology. The question that is asked is, "How can the quality of distance education be assured?" The American Association of Colleges of Nursing (AACN,

1999) has available a white paper on distance technology. This may be helpful for schools using this methodology for delivering education.

## Conclusion

Accreditation is still one of the primary guarantees of academic quality. When academic quality is recognized to exist in a particular program, nurses prepared in those programs enter the workforce prepared to provide quality care. When facing the current healthcare issues, the need for responsive accreditation measures to guarantee quality of the preparation of future nursing practitioners is imperative. Quality is and will remain an issue of concern to all healthcare professionals in facing the challenges to come.

## Learning Activities

1. Consider the five challenges/issues facing accreditation, select one, take either the pro or con platform, and examine the area in more depth, supporting your position.
2. Compare the accreditation standards for NLNAC and the Commission on Collegiate Nursing Education (CCNE). Identify areas of strength and areas of concern for each. Propose potential solutions for areas of concern.

## References

American Association of Colleges of Nursing (1999). *White Paper: Distance technology in Nursing Education*. Washington, DC: Author.

Bellack, J. P., Gelmon, S. B., O'Neil, E. H., & Thomsen, C. L. (1999). Responses of baccalaureate and graduate programs to the emergence of choice in nursing accreditation. *Journal of Nursing Education, 38*, 53-61.

Deforge, V. M. (n.d.). *A century of leadership in nursing*. Boston, MA: Department of Nursing Massachusetts College of Pharmacy and Allied Health Sciences.

## Bibliography

Barnum, B. S. (1997). Licensure, certification, and accreditation. *Online Journal of Issues in Nursing* [online]. Available: www.nursingworld.org/ojin/tpc4/tpc42.htm

Gelmon, S. B., O'Neil, E. H., Kimmey, J. R., & the Task Force on Accreditation of Health Professions Education. (1999). *Strategies for change and improvement: The report of the task force on accreditation of health professions' education*. San Francisco, CA: Center for the Health Professions, University of California at San Francisco.

National League for Nursing [NLN]. (1963). *The school improvement program of the National League for Nursing, 1951-1960.* New York: Author.

# Chapter 34: ACCREDITATION: NATIONAL LEAGUE FOR NURSING ACCREDITING COMMISSION (NLNAC)

Susan Abbe, MS, PhD, RN

*This chapter provides a clear overview of the inception, mission, structure, and role of the National League for Nursing Accrediting Commission (NLNAC). Dr. Abbe details the evaluation process, highlighting the three steps involved when seeking accreditation. Nursing faculty may find themselves returning to this chapter, again and again, to gain a full appreciation of the self-regulatory guidelines and expectations inherent to the NLNAC.*
*– Lynn Engelmann and Linda Caputi*

## Introduction

The National League for Nursing (NLN) Board of Governors approved the establishment of an independent entity within the organization to be known as the National League for Nursing Accrediting Commission (NLNAC). NLNAC began operations in January, 1997, with sole authority and accountability for carrying out the responsibilities of accreditation of nursing programs. NLNAC accredits 1,456 nursing education programs including master's, baccalaureate, associate degree, diploma, and practical nursing.

## Inception of NLNAC

The NLN Board of Governors' action to establish the NLNAC was necessary to comply with the U.S. Department of Education regulations concerned with conflict of interest

## Educational Philosophy

To facilitate student learning; to encourage inquiry and creativity; and to be a resource. – Susan Abbe

interest when membership organizations are also involved with recognizing educational programs for accreditation. In 1992, Higher Education Amendments to the Higher Education Act (HEA) required greater governmental oversight and an increase in the gate-keeping responsibilities of the federal government, states, and accrediting agencies. The regulations required accrediting bodies to increase monitoring activities. This was a shift away from voluntary accreditation and a move toward regulatory activities. NLNAC, through its standards, had to address such oversight activities as monitoring of student loan default rates, conducting unannounced site visits, submitting business plans when branch campuses are established, and reporting of substantive changes. Unannounced site visits were removed from monitoring following future amendments to the HEA.

The U.S. Department of Education has recognized the NLNAC/NLN since 1952 and has included the organization on its initial list of recognized accrediting agencies. NLNAC/NLN has been continually recognized by the Department of Education since that time. The NLN was also recognized by the Council on Postsecondary Accreditation (COPA), 1977-1993, and the Commission on Recognition of Postsecondary Accreditation (CORPA), 1993-1996. In 2000, the NLNAC was accredited by the Council for Higher Education Accreditation (CHEA). NLNAC maintains accountability to the programs and schools it accredits as well as to the public it serves by undergoing periodic external reviews by the U.S. Department of Education and the Council of Higher Education Accreditation.

## Mission and Goals of NLNAC

The NLNAC is the entity that is responsible for the specialized accreditation of all types of nursing education programs: master's, baccalaureate, associate degree, diploma, and practical nursing. The **mission** is as follows:

NLNAC supports the interests of nursing education, nursing practice, and the public by the functions of accreditation. Accreditation is a voluntary, self-regulatory process by which nongovernmental associations recognize educational institutions or programs that have been found to meet or exceed standards and criteria for educational quality. Accreditation also assists in the further improvement of the institutions or programs as related to resources invested, processes followed, and results achieved. The monitoring of certificate, diploma, and degree offerings is tied closely to state examination and licensing rules and to the oversight of preparation for work in the profession. The **goals** are to:
- Promulgate a common core of standards and criteria for the accreditation of nursing programs found to meet those standards and criteria.
- Strengthen educational quality through assistance to associated programs and schools

and evaluation processes, functions, publications, and research.

- Advocate self-regulation in nursing education.
- Promote peer review.
- Foster education equity, access, opportunity, and mobility, and preparation for employment based upon type of nursing education.
- Serve as gatekeeper to Title IV-HEA programs for which NLNAC is the accrediting agency. These include some practical nursing and all hospital diploma programs eligible to participate in programs administered by the Department of Education or other federal agencies. (NLNAC, 2002, p. 1)

The NLNAC accreditation program is founded on the belief that specialized accreditation provides assurance that schools and programs meet or exceed agreed-upon standards and criteria. The accreditation process requires a rigorous self-evaluation by the program, an appraisal by peers, and review and decision by the NLNAC governing body. Achievement of accreditation indicates to the general public and to the educational community that a nursing program has clear and appropriate educational objectives and is providing the conditions under which its objectives can be fulfilled. Emphasis is placed upon the total nursing program and its compliance with established standards and criteria in the context of current practice and anticipated future direction.

NLNAC believes that the approach to accreditation is that of an enabling process rather than a rigid or prescriptive process. Accreditation is expected to reflect each individual nursing program's goals and roles within its particular community. Accreditation is based on consensus building that is informed by the collective wisdom of administrators, faculty, students, peer reviewers, commissioners, and the public. At the same time, NLNAC cannot accept the status quo and must "push the envelop" in order to advance the profession of nursing.

## The Commission

NLNAC is governed by a committee of 15 members elected by the NLN membership. Nine commissioners are nurse educators, three commissioners are nursing service representatives, and three commissioners are public members.

The Commission has the sole authority to determine accreditation status or withhold accreditation status from applicant programs. The Commission, composed of experts in education, nursing education, administration, nursing service, health care, and business, applies the standards and criteria of accreditation within and across program types within the context of a global perspective. In addition, the Commission has the responsibility for the management, financial decisions, policy making, and general administration of the NLNAC.

# Standards and Criteria

The importance of standards to assuring quality of the accreditation process has been mentioned previously. Standards are the substance of accreditation, emphasizing learning, community, responsibility, integrity, and quality. Standards are agreed-upon rules set forth to provide quality assurance concerning educational preparation of members of the profession. Criteria are board statements that frame the issues that need to be examined in evaluation of the individual standards. In 1996, the NLN Board of Directors adopted a common core of standards and criteria across all five program types to which NLNAC has continued to subscribe. For more information on the NLN see the chapter in this book titled *National League for Nursing (NLN)* by Susan Abbe.

The NLNAC has seven accreditation standards in the areas of mission and governance, faculty, students, curriculum and instruction, resources, integrity, and educational effectiveness.  In addition there are 23 criteria.

# NLNAC Accreditation Standards for Academic Quality

1. Mission and governance.  There are clear and publicly stated mission and/or philosophy and purposes appropriate to post-secondary or higher education in nursing.
2. Faculty. There are qualified and credentialed faculty appropriate to accomplish the nursing education unit purposes and strengthen its educational effectiveness.
3. Students. The teaching and learning environment is conducive to student academic achievement.
4. Curriculum and instruction. The curriculum is designed to accomplish its educational and related purposes.
5. Resources.  Resources are sufficient to accomplish the nursing education unit purposes.
6. Integrity. Integrity is evident in the practices and relationships of the nursing education unit.
7. Educational effectiveness. There is an identified plan for systematic evaluation including assessment of student academic achievement.

The educational program has a responsibility to demonstrate that there is a comprehensive, systematic evaluation plan of all program components in place. The findings from the evaluation are then used for development, maintenance, and revision of the program as based on aggregate, trended data. The core activity of a systematic evaluation and assessment should be the process of determining whether the various parts and the entire program are, in fact, achieving the mission, goals, objectives, and outcomes. A central concern of accreditation is with the degree to which the evaluation and assessment processes are directed toward and result in program improvement.

## Evaluation Process

The NLNAC's procedure for evaluation of nursing education programs is a comprehensive three-step process. The first step is the self-study and site visit. The second step is the review by a peer evaluation review panel of the reports written about the program. The final step is a review of the process and the decision on accreditation status by the NLNAC Commissioners.

### *The First Step*

The first step of the process is the self-study and site visit. In preparation for the site visit, the program conducts a self-study to determine to what extent it is meeting the accreditation standards and criteria. The self-assessment process precedes the writing of the self-study report and includes the following activities:

- Review of the philosophy and beliefs of voluntary, specialized accreditation and the philosophy and beliefs of the NLNAC accreditation specifically.
- Thorough exploration of the beliefs and the objectives of the program and the services of the nursing unit.
- Assessment of the philosophy and the objectives of the nursing unit in terms of current trends and needs in nursing education.
- Evaluation of the extent to which the nursing unit is achieving its objectives, based on an analysis of all its activities.
- Careful consideration of various ways and means by which the objectives may be more fully attained. (NLNAC, 2002, p. 24)

The conclusions derived from the data accumulated as a result of the self-study process serve as a basis for continuing development and improvement of the program and as a basis for evidence of how both the accreditation standards and criteria and the nursing unit's stated objectives are being met. These conclusions should be clearly set forth in the self-study report.

The self-study report is the primary document used by the program evaluators (site visitors), the evaluation review panel members, and the Commissioners to understand the nursing education program. The self-study report is written by the faculty and administration of the nursing education unit using the accreditation standards and criteria in effect at the time of the scheduled visit. There are four sections to the report:

1. Executive summary which provides a brief overview of the program.
2. Standards and criteria which demonstrates the extent to which the nursing education program is meeting the standards – mission and governance, faculty, student, curriculum and instruction, resources, integrity.
3. Standard and criterion – educational effectiveness which provides an opportunity to present and discuss the comprehensive plan for program evaluation and to identify what decisions were made for program improvement based on analysis of data.
4. Appendix which offers supporting information.

Faculty play both a leadership and dynamic role in the self-study process and the preparation of the self-study report. It is their unique story that is being told and no one can tell it as well as the faculty themselves. Ownership and belief in the value of accreditation must be felt by the faculty. There are many ways faculty can be involved in the writing of the self-study report. One suggestion is to form a Steering Committee/Self-Study Committee with subcommittees composed of faculty responsible for each of the seven standards. All faculty (or as many as appropriate for large faculties) need to be assigned to a standard based on interest or expertise. As each standard is prepared it needs to be shared with the entire faculty for comment and editing. As faculty are writing the self-study report, NLNAC professional staff are available to provide guidance through such avenues as conducting telephone conference calls, answering e-mail questions, and reading draft copies of the report. Yearly, NLNAC offers a Self-Study Forum in two locations around the country where nursing faculty and administrators receive current information regarding the writing of the self-study report and an update of current policies and program evaluation.

A minimum time frame for preparing for the site visit is approximately one year. A timeline should be developed that takes into consideration the writing of each standard and criteria, editing of the report at established intervals, and conducting the final edit of the entire document, printing and binding of the report, and mailing of the report and catalog to the program evaluators and NLNAC six weeks prior to the visit date. Faculty determine a timeline for accreditation activities taking into account other on-going program activities that are anticipated but not related to accreditation, such as, submission of a grant proposal, faculty workload, faculty retirement, or involvement in special institutional activities.

The site visit gives the school an avenue to demonstrate and highlight information presented in the self-study report. The site visit provides an opportunity for interaction among all concerned: administrators, faculty, students, staff, and program-specific peer evaluators. It also affords an opportunity for the site visitors to see firsthand what is being presented by the nursing program and allows for clarifying, verifying, and amplifying of program materials. At the conclusion of the visit, the site visitors prepare a report that includes verification of data, documentary statements, and additional descriptive material essential to a clear and concise picture of all aspects of the nursing program. The team makes a recommendation for accreditation status to the Commission.

Accreditation visits are usually scheduled for three days – Tuesday, Wednesday, and Thursday with the team arriving mid-afternoon on Monday. During the three days the team meets with the nurse administrator, chief executive officer of the governing organization, other institutional administrator persons (such as the financial officer), nursing faculty, students, general education faculty, student support personnel, learning resource personnel, clinical agency personnel, and the public. The team also tours clinical agencies, the library, learning resource center, and nursing program facilities, such as classrooms and faculty offices.

At the conclusion of the visit the team, as content experts, prepares a report of the visit entitled *The Program Evaluator Report*. The program evaluators document the extent that the nursing program is in compliance with the standards. The report clarifies, amplifies, and verifies the self-study report, as necessary, to give a concise picture of all aspects of the program. The team also identifies areas needing development and makes a recommendation to the NLNAC Commissioners regarding accreditation status.

The team chairperson is responsible for submitting the program evaluator report to NLNAC where a professional staff member reviews the report for completeness and appropriateness of information. The team chairperson is contacted for clarification if the staff person has any questions about the content of the report. Following this review the program evaluator report is sent to the nurse administrator for review for "error of fact." Substantive comments received from the nurse administrator are shared with the team chairperson for determination of inclusion into the report. The final report is mailed to the nurse administrator and the evaluation review panel members with a copy placed in the school file.

### The Second Step

The second step of the accreditation process is the review of the findings of the site visitors by program-specific evaluation review panels. There are four panels: master's and baccalaureate, associate degree, diploma, and practical nursing. The role of the evaluation review panels is to assure that the process of peer evaluation is carried out according to the accreditation standards and criteria. The panel members review the findings and make a recommendation for accreditation status to the NLNAC Commissioners. Evaluation review panel members bring to the discussion specific program expertise as designated by the panel's program type. They apply the accreditation standards and criteria within the program type from the context of a national perspective.

An NLNAC Commissioner serves as chairperson for each evaluation review panel. Three panel members are assigned to present the program to the entire evaluation review panel for discussion. The Commissioners at the next regularly scheduled meeting make the final accreditation decision.

The goal of the first and second steps of the evaluation process is to promote a seamless review that has integrity and that does justice to the program under review. The role of NLNAC professional staff is to facilitate the work of both review groups.

## *The Third Step*

The final step in the accreditation process is for the NLNAC Commissioners to consider the recommendations of the peer evaluators, review the materials provided by the specific program, and take action. Accreditation of the nursing education program will be granted or withheld. The Commission has the sole authority to determine the accreditation status or withhold accreditation from the applicant program.

Accreditation status granted by NLNAC Commissioners for initial or continuing accreditation is:

Initial Accreditation
- Grant accreditation for five (5) years when the nursing program is in compliance with all accreditation standards.
- Deny accreditation when the nursing program does not present evidence of being in compliance with all accreditation standards.

Continuing Accreditation
- Grant accreditation for eight (8) years when the nursing program is in compliance with all accreditation standards.
- Grant accreditation for two years when the nursing program is in non-compliance with one or two accreditation standards.
- Require a focused report and/or a focused visit to discuss the areas of non-compliance; if areas are found in compliance, the program will receive an additional six years for an eight year accreditation.
- Grant accreditation for two years, place on warning, when the nursing program is in non-compliance with more than two accreditation standards.
- Require a full self-study and site visit to address all accreditation standards.

## Products and Services

NLNAC provides its accredited nursing programs and interested constituencies with the following products and services:
- Initial accreditation and continuing accreditation of nursing programs yearly.
- Continuous monitoring of all accredited nursing programs.
- *Accreditation Manual.*

- *Interpretive Guidelines for Standards and Criteria* for:
  - Master's degree programs in nursing.
  - Baccalaureate degree programs in nursing.
  - Associate degree programs in nursing.
  - Diploma programs in nursing.
  - Practical nursing programs.
- *Directory of Accredited Nursing Programs.*
- Educational forums:
  - Self-study forum.
  - Program evaluator forum.
- Consultation.
- Annual report.
- NLNAC website.

## Headquarters

The NLNAC is located at 61 Broadway, New York, New York, 10006; telephone: 212-363-5555/ext 153.

Please visit the NLNAC website at www.nlnac.org. For easy launching, this website address is located on the CD accompanying this book. Simply launch your internet browser, put the CD-ROM in the drive, go to Chapter 34 on the CD, and then click on the website address.

## Learning Activities

1. Read a nursing program's most recent self-study report, evaluate how the program of nursing applied the NLNAC standards and criteria, and identify areas of program improvement.
2. Identify any changes the program would need to implement to meet NLNAC accreditation standards.

## References

National League for Nursing Accrediting Commission [NLNAC]. (2002). *Accreditation manual and interpretative guidelines by program type.* New York: Author.

# Chapter 35: ACCREDITATION: COMMISSION ON COLLEGIATE NURSING EDUCATION (CCNE)

Mary S. Collins, MS, PhD, RN, FAAN

*Dr. Collins walks us down the path the American Association of Colleges of Nursing (AACN) took to establish a task force in nursing education to examine the need for, and role of, the Commission on Collegiate Nursing Education (CCNE). The CCNE's evolution, purpose, mission, governance, and values are described herein. The process of accreditation involves self-study and an on-site evaluation to validate how well the self-study reflects compliance with CCNE standards. Dr. Collins offers suggestions as to what schools of nursing can do to prepare for and maintain CCNE accreditation, including continuous academic improvement activities. – Lynn Engelmann and Linda Caputi*

## Introduction

For anyone who is a faculty member in an institution of higher education in the United States, the term **accreditation** is a familiar one. However, it is a term that is often misunderstood or ignored until a program or institution becomes a part of the activities that lead to accreditation. Accreditation for the majority of nursing programs is an important one and is an important factor in the development of high-quality nursing education. The public is the ultimate benefactor of such activities as quality nursing education produces quality graduates and practitioners of nursing.

### Educational Philosophy

I believe that the role of teaching for students of nursing is to help them grow and develop as professionals. Within the classroom I try to create a course where the student will grow not only in content but also in awareness of the profession and how he/she can contribute. Students grow and develop differently and within differing time sequences. It is my challenge to create a learning environment where each student can meet objectives in his/her own time and way. It is also important to have students understand the context of learning, practice, and professional behavior within a changing knowledge-based practice, evolving healthcare system, and a rigorous professional environment. – Mary S. Collins

# Role of Accreditation

According to the Council for Higher Education Accreditation (CHEA) (2002), accreditation is the primary means by which the quality of higher education institutions and programs is assured in the United States. Additionally, accreditation is a form of self-regulation in which colleges, universities, and programs have come together to develop standards, policies, and procedures for self-examination and judgment by peers. Accreditation is a widely practiced activity in higher education and is pervasive at both the program and institutional level. CHEA (2002) stated that in 2001, approximately 6,300 institutions and 17, 500 programs held accredited status.

Accreditation is carried out by private, nonprofit agencies that accredit entire institutions such as **regional** accrediting agencies or that focus on programs such as law, nursing, public health, and medicine by **specialty** accrediting agencies. All agencies require programs or institutions to participate in activities such as the production of a self-study, review by peers, and a judgment about their accreditation status. The judgments are based on standards that have been developed by the accrediting agency with consultation from their constituents.

There are approximately 80 accrediting organizations in the United States. In order to assure quality decisions on accreditation, these agencies also undergo scrutiny by the CHEA, by the federal government through the United States Department of Education, or both. Those that are approved receive **recognition** status.

The Association of Specialized and Professional Accreditors (ASPA) represents specialty programs. ASPA focuses on the needs of specialty programs within institutions of higher education. In an effort to meet the needs of program accreditation, ASPA created a framework for accreditation activities performed by its member organizations. The ethical framework is called the *Code of Good Practice* (ASPA, 1995) and offers an objective view of accreditation and the ethical practices necessary for accreditors.

# Historical Development of CCNE

## *Task Force on Nursing Accreditation*

Following several years of requests by constituent members of the American Associated of Colleges of Nursing (AACN), the AACN Task Force on Nursing Accreditation (TFNA) was created by the Board of Directors. AACN members asked the Board of Directors to investigate both general accreditation and nursing accreditation. In October 1995, the AACN TFNA was created. Dr. Linda Amos, dean of nursing at the University of Utah, was appointed chair of the eight-member TFNA. The purpose of the TFNA was derived from the strategic planning put in place by AACN. With input from its constituent members and the Board of Directors of AACN, the TFNA was asked to focus on "assessing AACN's role in the accreditation of nursing education and in assuring quality through the development and implementation of standards for nursing education"(AACN, 1996, p.1 ). The Board of Directors of AACN asked the newly appointed task force to explore the fiscal, professional, regulatory, and statutory aspects of conducting specialized accreditation and to present a report to the membership regarding the feasibility of AACN assuming the responsibility for baccalaureate and graduate nursing accreditation.

Over the next year, the TFNA completed an extensive list of activities aimed at understanding the issues surrounding accreditation, issues regarding accreditation, and the constituent members of AACN. The activities completed by the TFNA included:

- Monitored activities of accreditation in higher education.
- Conducted interviews with 25 specialized accrediting agencies.
- Developed a matrix to analyze costs, membership, purposes, and processes utilized by these specialized accrediting agencies.
- Reviewed literature on credentialing, certification, licensure, and accreditation in nursing and higher education.
- Analyzed the results of a comprehensive questionnaire/survey of membership, identifying issues, costs, and recommended directions for accreditation in nursing.
- Met with a member of the Department of Education to review the criteria and process for becoming a Department of Education-recognized accreditation agency.
- Analyzed several reports and consulted with individuals in a variety of other higher education organizations.
- Held open forums with the membership to discuss issues, listen to questions and concerns, and advise about the future direction of accreditation.
- Remained apprised of the status of other accrediting agencies in nursing.
- Met with other professional nursing organizations to explore possible collaborative activities in the future accreditation of baccalaureate and graduate programs in nursing.

## *Report of the TFNA*

The TFNA prepared a report that incorporated all of the materials gathered during its year of fact finding. The report stated the conclusion that with the many changes occurring in nursing education, higher education, and general and specialty accreditation, there is a need for:

- A new conceptualization of nursing education.
- Collaboration with specialty groups in the review process.
- A role in the development of standards of accreditation for specialty certifying agencies.

The TFNA also recommended that AACN take the lead role in creating a new entity, a nonprofit organization that would serve the sole purpose of accreditation services to baccalaureate and graduate programs in nursing. Further, AACN would not change its structure or organization. To that end, the focus of accreditation for the new organization would be for baccalaureate and graduate nursing only. AACN would also take a lead role in bringing other relevant groups to this new alliance of nursing organizations interested in accreditation.

> The TFNA recommends that the AACN assume the leadership in accreditation, which will create a new future for the advancement of baccalaureate and graduate education and resultant accountability to the public. The Task Force believes a plan for accreditation of baccalaureate and graduate programs that includes the creation of a new and separate organization, with new processes and criteria, and which is based on a sound and reasonable financial plan that is feasible, appropriate, and timely. This plan should include baccalaureate and graduate entry preparation as well as preparation for advanced practice nursing, and it should address the roles of specialty organizations in accreditation of programs. The Task Force on Accreditation makes this recommendation because it is consistent with the AACN's mission and vision for the future (AACN, 1996, p. 8).

## *Action to Create An Organization*

The report of the TFNA was sent to the Board of Directors of AACN in the summer of 1996. The Board approved the report on August 31, 1996. It was distributed to its members for action at the fall semiannual meeting of AACN held in Washington, DC, in October, 1996. During the fall semiannual meeting, the organization voted overwhelming to take the lead in developing an alliance of organizations to streamline and coordinate activities around accreditation and to establish a new entity that would have the sole purpose of providing accreditation services to baccalaureate and graduate nursing programs (Syllabus, 1996).

The Commission on Collegiate Nursing Education (CCNE) was created as an outcome of that Fall Semiannual Meeting of AACN. An Accreditation Steering Committee was formed to organize the governing structure, finance the agency, and create the accreditation process using recommendations from member schools.

The mission of CCNE defines its distinctive purpose, its relationship with AACN, and its focus on nursing education.

> The Commission on Collegiate Nursing Education (CCNE) is a specialized

accrediting agency contributing to the improvement of the public's health. An autonomous arm of the American Association of Colleges of Nursing, CCNE ensures the quality and integrity of baccalaureate and graduate degree nursing education programs. As a voluntary and self-regulatory process, CCNE accreditation serves the public interest by assessing and identifying programs that engage in effective educational practices (CCNE, 2001a, p. 1).

In order to transition to the new accrediting agency, programs were offered a process whereby schools of nursing would be recognized for achieving accreditation by another agency. Schools were encouraged to apply for this transitional status. Careful consideration was given to applicants, and those approved were given preliminary approval status with the identification of the date for the first site visit and accreditation action. Three hundred and eighteen programs received preliminary approval.

## Organization of the Commission on Collegiate Nursing Education

CCNE has identified five general purposes for which the organization is established. These purpose are:
1. To hold nursing education programs accountable to the community of interest – the nursing profession, consumers, employers, higher education, students, and their families – and to one another by ensuring that these programs have mission statements, goals, and outcomes that are appropriate for programs preparing individuals to enter the field of nursing.
2. To evaluate the success of a nursing education program in achieving its mission, goals, and outcomes.
3. To assess the extent to which a nursing education program meets accreditation standards.
4. To inform the public of the purposes and values of accreditation and to identify nursing education programs that meet accreditation standards.
5. To foster continuing improvement in nursing education programs – and thereby in professional practice (CCNE ,1998, p. 3).

The governance of CCNE is composed of a Board of Commissioners, committees, and the CCNE staff. A 13-member Board of Commissioners that represents the organization's community of interest governs CCNE. The Board includes faculty and deans/directors of nursing education programs, professional nurses, professional consumers, and public consumers.

In addition, there are five standing committees, which include the:
- Accreditation Review Committee.
- Budget Committee.
- Nominating Committee.
- Report Review Committee.
- Hearing Committee.

The staff, under the direction of the executive director and associate director, administers all aspects of the accreditation process and all activities of the Board and standing committees.

CCNE is autonomous in all aspects of its evaluation and accreditation activities, including but not limited to the establishment of bylaws, standards, policies, and procedures; control of its financial affairs; implementation of its operating rules; selection of its members, evaluators, and consultants; and the administration of its own affairs (CCNE, 2001a, p. 3).

CCNE is a values-driven organization. These core values permeate all of the activities and actions of the organization and are agreed upon by the Board of Commissioners, staff, standing committees, and site evaluators. All constituents review the values frequently. The following is a list of the values of CCNE:
- Fostering **trust** in the process, in CCNE, and in the professional community.
- Focusing on stimulating and supporting **continuous quality improvement** in nursing education programs and their outcomes.
- Being **inclusive** in the implementation of its activities and maintain openness to the **diverse institutional and individual opinions** of the interested community.
- Relying on **review and oversight by peers** from the community of interest.
- Maintaining **integrity** through a consistent, fair, and honest accreditation process.
- Valuing and fostering **innovation** in both the accreditation process and the programs to be accredited.
- Facilitating and engaging in **self-assessment**.
- Fostering an educational climate that supports program students, graduates, and faculty in their pursuit of **life-long learning**.
- Maintaining a high level of **accountability** to the public served by the process, including consumers, students, employers, programs, and institutions of higher education.
- Maintaining a process that is both **cost-effective and cost-accountable**.
- Encouraging programs to develop graduates who are **effective professionals and socially responsible citizens.**
- Assuring **autonomy and due process** in its deliberations and decision-making

processes (CCNE, 2001b, p. 2-3).

## An Overview of Accreditation

For nursing faculty, accreditation has several perspectives. Accreditation can be seen as:

- A time consuming activity.
- A set of activities not usual to the typical faculty member's actions.
- An exercise in writing a self-study, then visitors evaluating their courses, committee work, and program.

Accreditation is an ongoing process that has several highlights but no beginning or end. Faculty may focus on the highlights such as the production of the self-study report document or the site evaluation. However, accreditation is also a set of on-going activities which enables the program to continue to meet high standards of quality in nursing education.

The length of time of accreditation by CCNE is variable. For programs seeking initial accreditation, the maximum term is 5 years. For programs who have received preliminary approval, the maximum term is ten years.

In keeping with its value of continuous quality improvement, CCNE also requires periodic reports. Each accredited program submits an annual report as well as a Continuous Improvement Progress Report at the mid point of the term of accreditation. The purpose of these reports is to provide information on the progress of the program's development and to help faculty assess their plans and programs.

## Process of Accreditation

Ideally, the process of accreditation would be seamless. It would not have a beginning or an end. Faculty members and administrators would put into place a set of processes that produce total quality improvement. There comes a point when a program requests accreditation by CCNE. That point can be related to:

- The fact that the time period designated for preliminary approval is expiring and the program needs to be considered for continuing accreditation.
- The nursing program did not apply for preliminary approval and is requesting initial approval by CCNE.
- The nursing program has added additional programs that it is requesting to be evaluated for accreditation.

The chief administrator of the nursing program requesting accreditation review by CCNE sends a formal letter to CCNE. A date is set by CCNE for the site evaluation.

As the nursing program prepares for the process of self-study, a series of documents, prepared by CCNE, are helpful and provide guidance in the development of the self-study report. These documents include:

- *Standards for Accreditation of Baccalaureate and Graduate Nursing Education Programs.*
- *Procedures for Accreditation of Baccalaureate and Graduate Nursing Education Programs.*
- *General Advice for Programs Hosting an On-Site Evaluation by CCNE.*
- *Checklist of Activities in a CCNE Accreditation Review.*

### *Elements of the Accreditation Process*

For many faculty, the activities of accreditation begin with the self-study. However, the self-study can be successful only if it has the appropriate materials and data ready to analyze. Many activities within the nursing program need to be implemented as they are developed and not wait until it is time for accreditation activities. Familiarity with requirements of the self-study activity is critical. Because there is a fundamental value and purpose of CCNE of continuous quality improvement, it is important to view courses, committee work, program development, and evaluation, as well as all activities of the nursing program, with a focus on improvement. Questions need to be posed about how to improve all aspects of the program. Then methods of improvement need to be sought. Finally, a way of measuring whether the solutions are successful and have contributed to the overall improvement of the program are critical to the analysis of the identified issues/problems.

### *Self-Study Preparation*

The focus of the self-study is to determine program quality and program effectiveness. The process of self-assessment and self-analysis should result in an analytical document that reflects all accreditation standards. The self-study document must reflect the use of data, its analysis, and its use to continuously improve the program. Again, CCNE can provide documents which can aid in the self-study preparation and planning for the on-site evaluation.

Plans, activities, and responsibility for self-study preparation vary with each program. Some programs begin with strategic plans, others with self-study groups, and others begin by assigning one or more faculty the responsibility of writing the self-study document (which has a maximum limit of 75 pages). Preparation time varies, but it usually takes an academic year to view, describe, and analyze all activities in which the school participates. Programs can also view examples of completed studies at the CCNE offices in Washington, DC.

## On-Site Evaluation

The on-site evaluation is conducted after all required materials, including the self-study, are submitted to CCNE. The evaluation is conducted to assess the program's compliance with CCNE standards. The on-site evaluation team has three objectives:

1. To validate the findings and conclusions of the self-study document.
2. To collect information to be used by the Accreditation Review Committee (ARC) and the CCNE Board of Commissioners to assess compliance with the CCNE accreditation standards.
3. To gain insight into the plans of program officials and faculty to engage in continued self-improvement for the educational program.

The site evaluators are selected from a group of nursing faculty, nursing education administrators, and practicing nurses who have all received evaluator training. A team of three or four members usually conducts a three-day, on-site evaluation. During this time, the team reviews a variety of supporting documents prepared by the nursing program, which helps to demonstrate the program's compliance with the CCNE standards. This body of evidence is placed in a resource room for easy access by the site evaluators. At the end of the visit, the evaluation team summarizes their evaluation. The school is informed verbally of the findings of the team in regard to whether their program(s) have met the key elements and standards. The site evaluation team does not formulate a recommendation regarding accreditation. After the visit, the completed team report is sent to both CCNE and the program.

The written report of the site evaluation team is submitted to the program several weeks after the visit. An institutional response to the report is invited. The program can offer corrections and comments regarding opinions and conclusions in the Site Evaluators' Report. Programs can also offer any new information or materials it has developed since the site evaluation until the Board of Commissioners makes their final decision for accreditation.

## Accreditation Review Committee (ARC)

The ARC is provided copies of the program self-study, the evaluation team's report, and the response to the team's report submitted by the chief nursing administrator. The ARC considers all materials carefully and formulates a recommendation regarding the proposed action to be taken by the CCNE Board of commissioners. The action by the Board of Commissioners includes:

- The accreditation status and the period of accreditation.
- The identification of any areas where the program is not in compliance with CCNE standards.
- A schedule for progress or special reports to be submitted, and for the conduct of subsequent comprehensive or focused evaluations, if needed (CCNE, 2001b).

## *Board of Commissioners*

At the next Board of Commissioners meeting following the ARC meeting, the Board considers the recommendation of the ARC. They may accept that recommendation or choose to take alternative actions that the Board considers appropriate.

## *Potential Outcomes*

The outcomes that the Board determines include:

- Accreditation.
- Reaffirmation of accreditation.
- Accreditation denied.
- Accreditation withdrawn.
- Termination of accreditation: closed programs and voluntary withdrawal from accreditation.

The Board of Commissioners has the final decision-making authority to grant, deny, reaffirm, or withdraw accreditation (CCNE, 2002b, p. 12-13). By the spring of 2003, CCNE had accredited 305 institutions. An additional 85 programs continue to hold preliminary approval while awaiting their first accreditation activities with CCNE. With only 5 years of accreditation activity, 68% of all baccalaureate and graduate nursing programs in the United States have either preliminary approval or accreditation status with CCNE.

## Costs

The costs for accreditation activities vary widely in relation to the size and complexity of the program, faculty and staff time, self-study and manuscript preparation, and organizational activities. CCNE assess programs a flat fee for hosting the on-site evaluation. The fee is intended to cover team travel, lodging, and other expenses of the site evaluators. Typical programs have three to four site evaluators. For academic year 2004 the fee is

$1,400 per site evaluator. The typical team of three site evaluators would produce a fee of $4,200 and a team of four site evaluators would produce a fee of $5,600.

## Roles and Responsibilities of the Nursing Program

The chief nursing administrator takes responsibility for the leadership of all program related accreditation activities. Components of the activities may be delegated to individual administrators, faculty, or program committees. The chief nursing administrator is the individual with whom CCNE communicates regarding the scheduling of the on-site evaluation, the site evaluators, comments regarding the evaluation team report, and the person who submits any additional information relevant to the final decision of accreditation.

Faculty have a responsibility to become familiar with the accreditation process, the *CCNE Standards for Accreditation of Baccalaureate and Graduate Nursing Education Programs*, and materials for which they are responsible that will be helpful in the analysis of the program. Faculty need to be familiar with their role in accreditation. The information can be reviewed during orientation of new faculty or during a faculty workshop. Faculty need to be aware of the key elements for each standard so that, when appropriate, they may submit examples of evidence in support of each key element and standard. Data about each course, its outcome, and recommendations for changes can offer direction for continuous quality improvement. Faculty need to be current regarding professional practice and professional standards, which have been selected to improve program quality. Faculty also need to familiarize themselves with the new terminology of CCNE accreditation, including terms such as **a community of interest**. CCNE resources are available to assist programs with these requirements.

Standing committees of the nursing program are often charged with the responsibility of curriculum development, student performance, and program evaluation and effectiveness. Committees need to keep accurate records of their meetings and activities, including the identification of issues brought forward, their rationale for action, the action taken, and the analysis of whether the action was effective in producing continuous quality improvement for the program. Records need to reflect the data used to make recommendations for action and measurement of expected results.

Students have the opportunity to participate in several activities related to accreditation. Individually or within student organizations, they have responsibility to give input into course and faculty evaluation, program improvement, clinical experiences, and support services within both the program and the college or university. Participation on committees may be another way for students to become involved. During the on-site evaluation, students are given the opportunity to meet with evaluators to give feedback on the self-study document and how well the program is meeting the CCNE standards.

Many university constituents, as well as members of the community of interest, can offer comments, data, and input into the program's self-assessment and self-analysis. These same constituents are also important to on-site evaluation in validating the program's compliance with the CCNE standards.

## Continuous Quality Improvement Activities

Continuous quality improvement is a hallmark of CCNE accreditation. Yet for many programs, it is a new framework in which to view program assessment, evaluation, and improvement. Accreditation activities, including continuous quality improvement, must become an integral part of the daily functioning of a program. All nursing faculty, administration, and staff need to incorporate quality standards into ongoing activities and ask critical questions, such as:

- What are the issues/concerns presented by courses, students, clinical agencies, etc?
- What do the data indicate?
- What are the solutions?
- Did the data indicate that the solutions were appropriate?

Faculty, administrators, and staff can then measure effective changes in the program.

The key to effective analysis is the development of appropriate measurement systems. Faculty members have long used anecdotal and informal information to produce change. When measurement systems using data are put in place, outcomes can be compared among students, courses, time intervals, program changes, and ultimately, program outcomes. Focusing on outcomes rather than processes produces information that can inform change.

Faculty members can build into courses the measurements needed to have information regarding how well the coursework is meeting the program goals and objectives. Identifying the contributions of the course through objectives, evaluations, and outcomes can clearly delineate how the course meets program outcomes. Although CCNE does not prescribe a specific course of action regarding how the program meets quality expectations, it is important to have a method or methods whereby all aspects of the program can be improved.

Selecting methods of consensus or what manner of data collection is appropriate to the program is a matter of choice for each program. It is imperative that all personnel involved in the nursing program be responsible for measurement of expected results within their faculty/administrative roles. When data indicate that actual results and expected results are inconsistent, analysis of the differences can suggest changes to improve actual results and outcomes. After the implementation of the changes, it is critical to determine if these changes have been effective and ultimately improve the quality of the nursing program.

Accreditation is an important function of nursing education. Accreditation must become an integral part of the daily functioning of the program, not an episodic event. By incorporating quality standards of nursing education into ongoing activities, seamless development of the program is assured (Collins, 1997).

## Websites

Following is a list of websites that may be helpful in learning more about accreditation and the CCNE. For easy launching, these are also located on the CD accompanying this book. Simply launch your internet browser, put the CD-ROM in the drive, go to Chapter 35 on the CD, and then click on the website address.

- Association of Specialized and Professional Accreditors (ASPA): www.aspa-usa.org
- Commission on Collegiate Nursing Education (CCNE): www.aacn.nche.edu
- Council for Higher Education (CHEA): www.chea.org

## Learning Activities

1. Identify four outcomes currently in place in the baccalaureate or graduate program in which you teach. Discuss how the outcomes could be used to demonstrate compliance with CCNE standards.
2. Analyze course data guided by expected results of program outcomes. If the expected results are less than projected, identify strategies and activities which can be put in place to improve expected results. How will the results be measured?
3. Identify one issue that you would like to resolve within your nursing program. Analyze two program outcomes that do not meet expected results and suggest continuous quality improvement activities related to the resolution of this issue.

# References

American Association of Colleges of Nursing [AACN]. (1996). *Report of the task force on nursing accreditation*. Washington, DC: Author.

Association of Specialty and Professional Accreditors [ASPA]. (1995). *Code of good practice*. Washington, DC: Author.

Collins, M.S. (1997, August 13) Issues of accreditation: A dean's perspective. *Online Journal of Issues in Nursing*. Retrieved from http://www.nursingworld.org/ojin/tcp4/4cp4_1.htm.

Commission on Collegiate Nursing Education [CCNE] (1998). *Standards for accreditation of baccalaureate and graduate nursing education programs.* Washington, DC: Author

Commission on Collegiate Nursing Education [CCNE]. (2001a). A *new model for changing times: Annual report, 2001*. Washington, DC: Author.

Commission on Collegiate Nursing Education [CCNE]. (2001b). *Procedures for accreditation of baccalaureate and graduate nursing education programs* (amended May, 2001). Washington, DC: Author.

Commission on Collegiate Nursing Education [CCNE]. (2002). *Directory of accredited baccalaureate and master's degree programs in nursing.* Washington, DC: Author.

Council for Higher Education. (2002). *Accrediting organizations in the U.S.: How do they operate to assure quality* (Fact sheet #5). Washington, DC: Author.

Syllabus. (1996). AACN members overwhelming endorse action to establish alliance to accredit nursing higher education. *American Association of Colleges of Nursing. 22*(6), 1.

# Chapter 36: APPROVAL: NATIONAL COUNCIL OF STATE BOARDS OF NURSING (NCSBN)

Nancy Spector, MSN, DNSc, RN

*Dr. Spector takes us through the inception and process of professional regulation, highlighting distinctions and overlap between accreditation and approval. As we look at approval issues as designated by the National Council of State Boards of Nursing (NCSBN), we discover a compelling history. Rationale and preparation for site visits are detailed, along with the recently written Model Nursing Practice Act. We found this chapter a unique contribution for the clarity it brings to the approval process. – Lynn Engelmann and Linda Caputi*

## Introduction

Professional regulation in nursing is defined as the process whereby governmental agencies grant legal authority for an individual who has met specified qualifications and demonstrated a minimum entry-level competence to practice a chosen profession (Sheets, 1996). This definition is used to provide the framework for this chapter. Although this definition implies that regulation is mandated by governments, a developing body of literature asserts that professions are regulated by licensure, certification (as opposed to state-issued certification), and accreditation (Barnum, 1997). However, this chapter makes a distinction between regulation and licensure versus accreditation and certification because the former are governmental mandates.

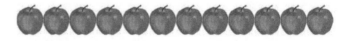

### Educational Philosophy

I believe more of our resources should be used to teach undergraduate nursing students. These are our nurses of the future. Too often in nursing education our best and brightest teach in graduate programs. I also believe that all nursing students should have outstanding clinical experiences and teachers because that is where much of the learning takes place. – Nancy Spector

Regulation can be on four levels (National Council Position Paper, 1993):
- Designation/recognition.
- Registration.
- State-issued certification.
- Licensure.

The least restrictive level is designation/recognition, and regulation at this level does not limit the right of the nurse to practice; neither can the state inquire about incompetence. It merely provides the public with information about nurses with special credentials. Likewise, registration does not involve state inquiry into the scope of practice, or competence; it merely involves providing information to an official roster. This is the most elementary level of regulation.

The next level is state-issued certification, which allows for the legal authority to practice. A few states issue state certification to advanced practice nurses, though state-issued certification does not include a defined scope of practice. The federal government has used the term **certification** to define credentialing by a nongovernmental agency, and a few boards of nursing have used the term to authorize advanced practice. The most restrictive type of regulation is licensure, in which the professional must demonstrate minimal competency to practice and the state has the authority to take disciplinary action should licensees violate the law or rules under which they are regulated (Sheets, 2002).

## Brief History of State Approval of Nursing Schools

The approval of nursing programs is part of the regulatory process carried out by the state boards of nursing in the 61 states and territories of the United States. The approval process can be defined as "official recognition of nursing education programs which meet standards established by the board of nursing" (NCSBN, 1994, p. 2). See Figure 36.1 for relevant definitions.

The early struggle for nursing regulation began in England with what has been termed the Thirty Years' War. The debate was one of self-regulation versus legal regulation. Some nurses viewed legal regulation as an opportunity to establish uniform qualifications, thus safeguarding the profession and the public. However, others, including Florence Nightingale, believed the focus should be on social and moral standards of the nurse rather than the abilities of the nurse. The physicians and hospital administrators feared that legal registration would lessen their control over nurses and grant nurses "undeserved" professional status (International Council of Nurses, 1985; Weisenbeck & Calico, 1991). While this debate was raging, New Zealand enacted the first international regulation law on August 12, 1901. Ellen Dougherty of New Zealand was the first nurse – worldwide – to

Figure 36.1 – Relevant Definitions

**Accreditation** – a voluntary process by private agencies which is an external quality review by peers to assure that an educational program meets established standards for structure, function, and performance (Sheets, 2002).

**Approval** – official recognition of nursing education programs which meet standards established by the board of nursing.

**APRN** – advanced practice registered nurses, including certified nurse midwives (CNMs), clinical nurse specialists (CNSs), certified registered nurse anesthetists (CRNAs), and nurse practitioners (NPs) (NCSBN, 2002).

**Certification** – either state-issued or voluntary; if state issued, it allows for the legal authority to practice; if voluntary, it is a professional credential that recognizes that a practitioner has passed a professional certification exam given by a private agency, and it does not grant a legally defined scope of practice (Sheets, 2002).

**Designation/Recognition** – provides the public with information about nurses with special credentials. It is the least restrictive type of regulation, and it does not limit the right of the nurse to practice, nor can the state inquire about incompetence.

**Licensure** – the most restrictive form of professional regulation where regulated activities are complex, requiring specialized knowledge and skill and independent decision-making. In the licensure process, predetermination of qualifications is made (for example, passing the NCLEX® in nursing), monitoring of qualifications is often ongoing, and licensure provides authority to take disciplinary action if the law or rules are not followed (Sheets, 2002).

**Nurse Practice Act** – the statutes that authorize the board of nursing to promulgate rules that are necessary for the implementation of the nurse practice act (Weisenbeck & Calico, 1991).

**Registration** – does not involve state inquiry into the scope of practice or competence; it merely involves providing information to an official roster.

**Regulation** – the process whereby governmental agencies grant legal authority for an individual who has met specified qualifications and demonstrated a minimum entry-level competence to practice a chosen profession.

**Rules** – regulations that are consistent with the nurse practice act. These rules cannot go beyond the law, and once enacted, they have the force of the law. Some states refer to these as the regulations, though this chapter will refer to them as the rules.

**State Boards of Nursing** – exist for the purpose of protecting health, safety, and welfare of the public. They license nurses, discipline nurses for unsafe practice, and develop rules and approve nursing education programs.

be registered ("Nurse Dougherty," 2001; Weisenbeck & Calico, 1991).

Although the first reference to the employment of nurses in the United States was in 1777, it was not until 1903 that North Carolina enacted the first registration law for nursing, followed by New York, New Jersey, and Virginia (Flanagan, 1976; Weisenbeck & Calico, 1991). Soon thereafter, state boards of nursing began to emerge for the purpose of regulating nurses. By 1906, inspectors of schools or hospitals with nurse training programs began making program visits for approval. One of the first nurse inspectors was Annie Damer in New York (American Nurses Association [ANA], 2001; N. Birnbach, personal communication, July 29, 2002).

The early regulation of nurses protected the title of those who met a minimum set of criteria for registration. Those requirements included:

- Completion of an educational program that met standards set by the board of nursing.
- Successful completion of a written and performance examination.
- Evaluation of moral and character fitness. (Weisenbeck & Calico, 1991)

However, these early registration acts did not define the scope of practice for nursing; it took 35 years for the first state, New York (in 1938), to become the first state to define the scope of practice and to adopt a mandatory licensure law.

Safriet (2002) asserted that nursing was "relegated to a scope of practice that was by definition 'carved out' of medicine's universal domain" (p. 308). Because physicians were the first to secure licensure, Safriet stated, the rest of the healthcare fields had to defer to physicians, whose scope of practice is extremely pervasive. According to Safriet a physician could practice gynecology, oncology, orthopedics, pediatrics, retinal surgery, or psychiatry using outdated treatment modalities--all with the same license that the physician obtained years ago. Realistically, physicians do not do this, though Safriet contended that it is not the law that constrains them. Safriet reminded nurses that only three decades ago, nurses needed orders for starting IVs or taking a blood pressure. Until the 1970s, only physicians had the authority to pierce ears.

Resistance to mandatory licensure came from hospital administrators who realized there would be an economic effect from adopting a compulsory law. Therefore, it was not until the mid-1960s that all states had adopted definitions of nursing, delineating the scope of practice along with mandatory licensure.

The mission of state boards of nursing includes developing rules and approving nursing education programs for the purpose of protecting the health, safety, and welfare of the public. Boards also have the legal authority to license nurses and to discipline nurses for unsafe practice (NCSBN, 1998).

## Accreditation Versus Approval

Although approval is mandated by the state boards of nursing for the purpose of protecting the health, safety, and welfare of the public, accreditation is a voluntary, nongovernmental, peer-review process to assure that programs are meeting standards of structure, function, and performance. The first nursing accreditation program began in 1916, and currently, two private agencies accredit nursing programs. The National League for Nursing Accrediting Commission (NLNAC) accredits practical, associate-degree, diploma, baccalaureate, and master's nursing programs, and the Commission on Collegiate Nursing Education (CCNE) accredits baccalaureate and master's nursing programs. Historically, professions have had only one accrediting agency, so the competitive model is a new concept and bears watching (Sheets, 2002). Boards of nursing approve practical, associate-degree, diploma, and baccalaureate nurses, and some boards approve advanced practice nurses. Although there is some redundancy in the process, NCSBN and accrediting agencies are working together to make the process more seamless for schools of nursing.

However, there are some major differences between approval and accreditation:

- State boards of nursing approve nursing programs for minimal standards of practice and from the point of view of public protection. Because of this, the criteria from state boards of nursing must be met, rather than being met at different levels, as is the case with accreditation.
- State boards of nursing monitor and sanction nursing programs through statutory authority. The professional accreditation process, however, focuses on the quality and integrity of nursing programs (CCNE, 1998).
- With the accrediting process, schools can lose their accreditation status, but they cannot be shut down. The boards of nursing, through legal authority, can close programs that do not meet their criteria, after the programs have been given a reasonable opportunity to comply with the standards.
- Accreditation is voluntary, while approval is mandatory.
- State boards of nursing approve practical, associate-degree, diploma, baccalaureate, and sometimes advanced practice nursing programs, but NLNAC and CCNE only accredit certain nursing programs.
- By law, the state boards of nursing monitor the licensure exams so they align with current practice. To do this, they conduct comprehensive studies and job analyses. Although private accreditors often conduct their own research, the law does not mandate that they do so.
- State boards of nursing may make emergency visits to the nursing program if problems are reported to them.
- State boards of nursing are in the unique position of being able to demonstrate great awareness of statewide nursing education needs, but accreditation is a national pro-

cess.
- State boards of nursing do all of this at little cost to nursing programs, but private accreditation can be quite costly (Gloor, 2001).

In addition to approval and accreditation, schools must also meet standards of other agencies. For example, they must meet the standards of the Occupational Safety and Health Administration (OSHA), as well as be in compliance with the Americans with Disabilities Act (ADA). The parent institutions may be required to meet standards set by various state or regional agencies, e.g., North Central Association of Colleges and Schools. Practice settings also must follow regulations set by state agencies, and most of them seek voluntary accreditation from the Joint Commission on Accreditation of Health Care Organizations (JCAHO).

## Rationale for Regulation of Nursing Education Programs

State boards of nursing exist to protect public health and the safety and welfare of individuals. State approval of nursing programs ensures that nursing is practiced by minimally competent licensed nurses within an authorized scope of practice. The preparation of nurses who practice safely is closely linked to the provision of safe patient care (Gloor, 2001). This is especially important currently because there is a national focus on unsafe nursing and medical practices.

Effective communication with the many stakeholders in regulation, such as schools of nursing, nurse educators, accrediting entities, nursing organizations, and the community, is necessary for effective regulation. Yet approval can also present unique opportunities to nursing because it can provide databases and information-sharing to individual boards as well as to the nursing educational community and nursing organizations (Gloor, 2001).

The regulation process is carried out somewhat differently by each of the 61 boards of nursing, with the underlying assumption that there are many different ways to effectively regulate education. Creative and visionary ways of regulating nursing programs are, however, shared among the various boards of nursing (Gloor, 2001). Sharing of information occurs in a variety of ways, including during monthly education network conference calls coordinated by NCSBN and at the NCSBN annual and midyear meetings. The Nursing Practice and Education Committee of NCSBN found that most of the 61 state boards of nursing have the following roles in common (Gloor, 2001):
- Granting approval to basic nursing education programs.
- Monitoring and sanctioning programs at risk, according to the statutes.
- Demonstrating awareness of state nursing education needs.
- Participating in standard setting in basic nursing education programs.

In 1997-1998, the Nursing Practice and Education Committee of NCSBN reviewed current educational standards. This committee found that all state boards were working on public protection by assuring consumers that they would receive safe student-provided and professional-provided nursing care. Further, the state boards of nursing all mandated that students be given educational opportunities that prepared them for entry to practice and licensure within that state (Gloor, 2001). This same committee developed 10 indicators of quality nursing education programs (see Appendix 36.1).

## Legal Basis of the Board of Nursing's Authority to Regulate Nursing

Although laws generally state that boards of nursing have the responsibility to establish criteria for licensure, thereby protecting public health and safety, the states vary in their statutes and regulations regarding approval of nursing programs. Of the 61 state boards of nursing (see Appendix 36.2 for a list of the 61 state boards of nursing), the majority of boards has the responsibility of licensure (57), licensure renewal (56), establishing practice standards (57), making definitive practice decisions (48), and regulating advanced practice (51) (NCSBN, 2000). Further, the majority of boards has statutory authority to approve nursing education programs (see Table 36.1).

Table 36.1 - State Boards' Responsibilities for Approval of Five Types of Educational Programs

|        | Basic | RN-BSN | RN Certificate | Graduate | CEU |
|--------|-------|--------|----------------|----------|-----|
| Yes    | 57    | 18     | 15             | 14       | 18  |
| No     | 3     | 37     | 39             | 41       | 39  |
| Other  | 1     |        | 2              |          | 2   |

Licensure and the state-based regulatory system in the United States are founded in the 10th Amendment of the U.S. Constitution, often referred to as the states' rights amendment (Hutcherson & Williamson, 1999). Each state and territory enacts nurse practice acts that describe the scope of practice for nurses. The statutory language is written in broad terms to allow for evolution of practice. Boards of nursing then develop administrative rules that are consistent with the nurse practice act. These rules can not go beyond the law, and once enacted, they have the force of the law. During the development of the rules, public comment periods are allowed so practitioners can attend hearings and participate in rule making (Sheets, 2002). Please see Appendix 36.3 for the 2002 Model Administrative Educational Rules and Appendix 36.4 for the 2002 Model Practice Act, which were approved in August, 2002, at the annual meeting of NCSBN. These models, developed by the Practice, Regulation, and Education Committee of NCSBN, provide direction for the various state boards of nursing when enacting laws or developing the rules and regulations.

## Purpose and Process of the Site Visit

The site visit, sometimes termed the **survey visit**, is conducted by representatives of a state board of nursing. The primary goal of the site visit is to gather information to determine if the school is meeting the criteria set in the board of nursing's rules (see Appendix 36.3 for Model Administrative Education Rules). Site visits are routinely made for initial approval of a new school. After initial approvals, visits are ordinarily made at regular intervals, which may differ from state to state (see Table 36.2).

Table 36.2 - Length of Time Approval is Granted in Individual States

|  | # of Programs |
|---|---|
| **1 Year** | 11 |
| **2 Years** | 3 |
| **3 Years** | 3 |
| **4 Years** | 9 |
| **5 Years** | 2 |
| **6 Years** | 2 |
| **7 Years** | 0 |
| **8 years** | 5 |
| **Other** | 7 = Variable<br>5 = up to 5 years<br>3 = up to 8 years<br>2 = Indefinite<br>1 = 4 – 8  years<br>1 = Variable, maximun 8 years<br>1 = Not specified |

- RN, PN, CEU programs are reported together
- Source: NCSBN, 2000 Profiles of Member Boards

Boards may also schedule a visit if the program is initiating a satellite program or off-campus offering or if the nursing program is about to initiate a major curriculum change. Further, an emergency visit may be made if there are reports of noncompliance of the administrative education rules. The site visits ordinarily take from a few hours to three days, depending on the nature of the visit (NCSBN, 1995).

Some boards of nursing are recognized as accrediting agencies by the U.S. Department of Education, and in 10 of those states, approval is granted if the program meets national accreditation standards. Further, if the nursing program seeks national accreditation, nearly half the state boards of nursing coordinate their visits with accrediting agencies in an attempt to avoid duplication of efforts, as well as to streamline the process for nursing programs (see Table 36.3).

Most state boards of nursing have education consultants who make these visits, and often, two visitors survey the schools. When there are two site visitors, tasks can be divided, thus shortening the length of the visit. Moreover, if there are conflicts during a survey, a second perspective can be invaluable. In the case of two visitors, a "lead visitor" is usually designated, and the responsibilities of each are clarified before the visit.

The site visitors are usually prepared at least at the master's degree level, and often they are doctorally prepared. Although the site visitor may have had experience in academia, it is imperative for the visitor to have the ability to evaluate nursing curricula.

Communication skills, such as writing, interviewing, and listening, are all important when conducting a site visit. The site visitor must create an environment in which a candid exchange can take place. When a milieu of objectivity, adaptability, and openness is achieved, the process becomes positive for the nursing program as well as for the visitors (NCSBN, 1995).

Although site visitors take on various roles when visiting nursing programs, their major role is that of a **regulator** for the purpose of safeguarding the public. In this role, visitors provide information about compliance and noncompliance of the administrative education rules. In the **consultant** role, the visitor can make clarifications and provide new information. As a **facilitator**, the site visitor can encourage the participants to share information in an open environment. Site visitors are **fact finders** because they comprehensively gather information from a variety of sources. Last, site visitors take on the role of **problem solver**, thus assisting programs to identify ways to meet the requirements of the state boards of nursing (NCSBN, 1995).

Table 36.3 - Summary for Criteria for Board Approval

| | Yes (# of Boards) | No (# of Boards) | Other (# of Boards) |
|---|---|---|---|
| **% of first-time writers on NCLEX®** | 44 | 15 | 2 |
| **NCLEX®passing rate** | 85-95% of national pass rate- 3<br>75-80% of national pass rate- 19<br>Other – 16 | 23 | |
| **Minimum Theory Hours:**<br>**PN/VN**<br>**LPN/VN – AD**<br>**RN Diploma**<br>**RN AD**<br>**RN-Baccalaureate** | 17<br>6<br>6<br>9<br>9 | 33<br>31<br>34<br>40<br>41 | 11<br>24<br>21<br>12<br>11 |
| **Minimum Clinical Hours:**<br>**LPN/VN**<br>**LPN/VN – AD**<br>**RN Diploma**<br>**RN AD**<br>**RN-Baccalaureate** | 13<br>3<br>3<br>4<br>3 | 36<br>36<br>40<br>46<br>47 | 12<br>22<br>18<br>11<br>11 |
| **Board is recognized as An accrediting agency by the US Dept. of Ed.** | 5 | 52 | 4 |
| **Approval/accreditation granted to nursing programs that meet national accreditation standards** | 10 | 43 | 8 |
| **Approval/accreditation visits are coordinated** | 28 | 25 | 8 |

# Preparation for the Site Visitors

Initial contact with program directors should provide nursing programs with adequate time to submit requested materials and to prepare for the site visit. The nursing program should know the reason for the visit and have a clear idea of the agenda, including identification of documents to review, which individuals are to be interviewed, and which facilities are to be toured. If possible, the nursing program should participate in setting the schedule. The site visitor may alert the administrator of the parent institution of the purpose and dates of the visit.

## *Submission of Documents*

Most boards of nursing require a self-study or self-evaluation document prior to the approval process. When boards and accrediting bodies collaborate on the approval visit, sometimes the board accepts the self-study written for accreditation, perhaps with an addendum addressing where the document addresses the boards' rules (L. Shores, personal communication, October 11, 2002). The Model Education Rules (see Appendix 36.3) give an overview of the documentation that is generally required. This document was developed at NCSBN by the Practice, Regulation, and Education Committee to be used as guidelines for state boards to use when establishing their education rules. Each board of nursing differs as to when the program should submit written materials. One jurisdiction may ask for submission of the self-study prior to the visit, although others may ask for documentation at the time of the site visit. Other boards may ask for a combination of pre-visit and on-site document review (NCSBN, 1995).

Boards may request materials pertaining to the organization and administration of the nursing program (NCSBN, 1995). Many states require documentation that the institution is regionally accredited within their jurisdiction. Organizational charts of the nursing school as well as the parent organization are often requested. Careful review of these charts can clarify the administrative authority of the head of the program. Job descriptions of faculty/ staff are often reviewed for consistency with current practice and appropriateness to the nursing program. Review of the nursing program's budget is important for ascertaining the adequacy of resources to meet the goals and objectives of the school. Often, this review includes state allocation, subsidized salaries, tuition, grants, special initiative funds, endowments, aggregate faculty and staff salaries, and operating costs of the program. There is a careful review of funds allocated for professional development and travel as well as the library and learning resources. Contracts with each practice setting should delineate each party's responsibilities as well as the time frame and termination clause. Contracts with non-practice settings may also be reviewed; for example, there may be contracts with off-campus offices or simulated practice settings. Boards may also require a total program evaluation plan to review all aspects of the nursing program from recruitment to graduate evaluation. This plan is a tool, and validation of its implementation should be found in faculty minutes, course materials, NCLEX® results, etc.

Boards of nursing may ask for documentation regarding the curriculum and course materials. Although the Model Education Rules (see Appendix 36.3) are broadly stated, many state rules are extremely specific for curricular requirements. For example, the Minnesota Rules (Minnesota Rules, 2002), section 6301.1800, *Nursing Abilities to be Evaluated*, include the ability to provide for physical safety; prevent spread of pathogens; determine when necessary to use sterile technique; maintain sterility; maintain skin and mucous membrane integrity; promote respiratory and circulatory function; promote fluid and nutrition balance; promote elimination; promote physical activity; promote restoration/maintenance of physical independence; provide for physical comfort; provide for rest and sleep; and provide for personal hygiene.

Some of the materials that may be reviewed are the philosophy and mission of the program and the overall curricular plan. Individual syllabi with accompanying course goals, content, and learning activities may be evaluated. Evaluation tools, examples of students' work, and course evaluations often are requested. Courses are reviewed for relevancy, and the reference lists are evaluated for being up-to-date. The same criteria are used for evaluating distance-learning courses and for reviewing other courses. Some state boards of nursing have requirements for minimum theory or clinical hours (see Table 36.3).

The program is evaluated for internal consistency, meaning that the individual components of the curriculum relate to each other and to the theoretical framework of the program. Internal consistency suggests that a curriculum progresses logically within the program's framework. For example, the program's philosophy may describe the students as mature, responsible, and self-directed, whereas its policies may contain inflexible student requirements or its curriculum may not provide for self-direction (NCSBN, 1995). A combination of reviewing written documents and interviewing faculty and students is often the best method of evaluating the curriculum.

Faculty qualifications are also reviewed, in terms of licensure status, educational degrees, employment history, teaching responsibilities, and professional development. Teaching and non-teaching responsibilities of the faculty are carefully considered. See Tables 36.4 and 36.5 for a breakdown of the state boards of nursing degree requirements for nursing program administrators and faculty in various nursing programs.

The Model Education Rules (see Appendix 36.3) also provide suggestions for the qualifications of faculty and program administrators. Faculty/student ratios are often reviewed, as is the ratio of full-time to part-time faculty. The process of faculty evaluation and promotion is reviewed, and the visitors look for evidence of student input into faculty evaluations. The faculty handbook and bylaws are often excellent sources of faculty data.

Table 36.4 - Program Administrator Requirements

|  | LPN Programs | RN—Diploma* | RN—AD* | RN—BSN* |
|---|---|---|---|---|
| BSN | 11 | 3 | 4 | 0 |
| MSN | 17 | 20 | 39 | 29 |
| Doctorate | 1 | 4 | 5 | 19 |
| Other | 32 | 35 | 16 | 17 |

* Programs are listed under MSN, as well as "Doctorate preferred"

Table 36.5 - Requirements for Faculty Qualifications

|  | LPN | RN--Diploma | RN--AD | RN—BSN* |
|---|---|---|---|---|
| BSN | 21 | 3 | 2 | 1 |
| MSN | 8 | 12 | 26 | 34 |
| Doctorate | 0 | 0 | 0 | 0 |
| Other | 32 | 34 | 33 | 33 |

*Some state boards were listed twice

Reviewers may request documentation about current preceptors, including licensure status, educational qualifications, employment, and relevancy of student placements

State boards of nursing request information about the nursing student body. Policies regarding admission, progression, graduation, and health requirements are investigated, and it is important that these policies be published in the appropriate catalogues and handbooks. The state boards vary widely in their requirements for reviewing student records, though confidentiality always must be maintained.

Documentation of the students' NCLEX® scores may be requested. Forty-four state boards of nursing have required NCLEX® pass rates (see Table 36.3) for first-time writers of the exam. If a program's pass rate falls below the mandated level, the board usually requests a plan from the program for improving its scores within a reasonable timeframe to regain compliance with this rule.

Visitors tour the facilities and carefully evaluate the resources of nursing programs. Classrooms, learning resource centers, and equipment should be adequate in number, size, and quality so the program's goals can be met. Offices and meeting space should be adequate for the number of faculty. Library and audiovisual resources should be comprehensive and current, and they should be accessible to all students. This is especially important when students take distance-learning courses. There should be adequate support services for faculty and students alike. Documentation regarding clinical agencies may include accrediting status, opportunities for learning experiences, facilities, and resources.

## *Planned Meetings and Tours*

In preparation for site visitors, a schedule of meetings and tours is usually planned. Meetings are intended to clarify and/or verify the documents submitted. Separate meetings with the program administrator, faculty, and students allow for an objective exchange of information. Agendas of the meetings should be carefully planned, and the length should be between 30 and 60 minutes. Site visitors usually want to meet with the administrator of the parent institution as well. Tours of the campus, classrooms, faculty offices, libraries, conference rooms, and resource centers should also be planned. Site visitors often tour the clinical agency, although this depends on the individual jurisdiction.

The initial site visit is with the program dean or director, and this sets the tone for the visit. This meeting covers changes in the program since the last visit, any upcoming changes, a general description of the facilities and financial resources, and issues to be raised with the administrator of the parent institution. The visitors meet with the faculty members and adjunct faculty to discuss the curriculum, the program's strengths and weaknesses, the clinical agencies, and the faculty workload. Site visitors may take the opportunity to discuss any trends of regulation in that particular jurisdiction (NCSBN, 1995).

Meetings are scheduled with students – or consumers – of the program. These meetings may take place in the classroom or in the clinical agency. The site visitors may discuss the students' perceptions of the program and its strengths and weaknesses, faculty-student interactions, learning activities, clinical practice settings, and regulatory issues. If students raise internal issues that are not within the jurisdiction of the state board of nursing, the visitors should direct them to the appropriate resources, always remaining objective and nonjudgmental (NCSBN, 1995).

Not all jurisdictions visit the practice setting, although several do. If the state board of nursing collaborates with NLNAC or CCNE when making site visits, representatives typically survey the clinical agency with the accreditors. If the visitors do tour the practice arena, they evaluate the learning experiences offered in these facilities, the client population, and the communication process between faculty and nurses in the setting.

When meeting with the administrator of the parent institution, visitors review the purpose of the visit and discuss possible outcomes. The dean or director of the program should be present at this meeting, and the discussion may include nursing shortage information, future plans of the nursing program, financial support of the nursing program, and the patterns of present and future enrollment of the college as well as the nursing program. Please see Figure 36.2 for a template of a recent approval report from a site visit by the

Iowa State Board of Nursing.

Figure 36.2 – Template of a Site Visit Report*

1) Accrediting agencies and dates of last accreditation
2) Demographic data of nursing program (student enrollment & faculty numbers)
3) NCLEX® pass rates for past 5 years
4) Advanced practice certification examination pass rates for past 5 years
5) Agencies with contracts, addresses, date of contract, last review date
6) Faculty:  name, license # & expiration, status, position, teaching responsibility, education, enrollment, hire date, faculty with ARNP certification
7) Organization & administration of the program
8) Resources of the controlling organization
9) Curriculum
10) Faculty (i.e., faculty development, teaching load, faculty/student ratios, etc.)
11) Program responsibilities (i.e., student policies)
12) Clinical facilities
13) Preceptors
14) The program will notify the state board of nursing when NCLEX® scores fall lower than 95% of the national passing percentage for two consecutive calendar years.

*Each of these headings has numerous subheadings
Source: E. Gloor, personal communication, September, 2002.

The last meeting during the site visit is usually termed the exit interview. All findings and recommendations are shared at this time, and they must be documented and referenced to the board's rules. At this time, the date at which the report is to be presented to the board of nursing is specified. Some jurisdictions require that the dean or director of the nursing program be present at this meeting. Site visitors should remind the nursing program that their findings are only recommendations and that the board of nursing will make the final decision on approval status.

## Board of Nursing's Report

It is the responsibility of the site visitors to complete an accurate report of the visit, based on the program's compliance with the education rules of that jurisdiction. Some boards require documentation on how the program is in compliance with each rule, although others may require documentation only in the areas of noncompliance. If the program is in noncompliance of the rules, it is important that clear recommendations are made to bring the program in compliance.

Some boards of nursing send the school a copy of the initial report of the site visit to allow faculty an opportunity to respond, and others send the initial report to the board of the state boards. Most reports are discussed with the board within four to eight weeks after the visit has been conducted. The presence of the dean or director of the program is sometimes required at the board meeting, depending on the jurisdiction. The board acts upon the recommendations presented in the report of the site visit.

See Appendix 36.3 for the terminology for approval status, as defined in the Model Education Rules. This document states that **initial approval** is given to a school in order to be able to admit students. Once students are admitted, they are often given (depending on the state board) **provisional approval**. **Ongoing approval** is the approval of nursing programs that go through a satisfactory site visit. Ongoing approval is reevaluated anywhere from one year (11 state boards) to an indefinite number of years (Wisconsin) (see Table 36.2). **Conditional approval** is given when a school has not met all of the board's criteria. In most cases, the nursing program is given a reasonable time to meet the rules of the board of nursing. Often the program is required to submit a plan outlining, in detail, its plans for bringing the program into compliance with the board's rules. **Denial of approval** is given when a program has been given time to comply with the rules and has failed to do so or when a program fails substantially to meet the standards for nursing education.

However, boards of nursing are highly variant in the terms they use for approval status. For example, the North Carolina State Board of Nursing uses the following terms: **approval with stipulations**; **provisional approval**; **probational approval**; **discontinuance of program** (K. Apply, personal communication, September 26, 2002). Alternatively, the approval status terms at the Minnesota Board of Nursing are **initial approval**, **continuing approval**, **loss of approval**, **and reinstatement of approval** (Minnesota Rules, 2002). Although the terms are often different, the definitions are similar.

## Regulation in Advanced Practice Nursing

In the 1960s, several events led to the development of the advanced practice role in nursing. Medicare and Medicaid increased the number of people who received federal funds for health care, and at the same time, the federal government forecasted a shortage of physicians. The emerging women's movement in the U.S. led to an increased demand for personal and professional autonomy of women. Thus, more women were seeking nurse midwives for care rather than the traditional male obstetrician. Specialized care units, such as ICUs and neonatal care units, were being established in hospitals with the resultant need for better prepared nurses (Safriet, 1992). Nurse practitioner programs were established. In 1971, Idaho became the first state to legislate diagnosis and treatment as a part of the scope of practice of advanced practice nurses. Although it was pathbreaking at the time, it was somewhat restrictive. Since then, most states have statutorily recognized advanced practice roles of nurses to various degrees.

Please see Table 36.6 for the number of states that regulate specific types of advanced practice nursing with a certificate or a license. Currently, 54 boards of nursing specifically regulate advanced practice nursing as a separate group within their jurisdictions. In 2002, NCSBN (2002b) published a position paper regarding regulation of advanced practice nursing, which incorporated a review of the background of regulation of advanced practice nursing as well as a review of education, certification, and accreditation as a basis for regulation. In this paper, NCSBN recommended that **advanced practice registered nurse** (APRN) be used as an umbrella term to designate appropriately credentialed and educated nurses, such as nurse anesthetists, nurse midwives, nurse practitioners, and clinical nurse specialists, who have primary responsibility in the direct care of patients. NCSBN further suggested that licensure be granted only when the APRN education program and the area of the certification exam are congruent. To improve public protection and promote informed healthcare decisions, NCSBN believes that future movement should be toward consistency with regard to education, titles, and the use of terminology. The NCSBN position paper recommends broad, rather than specific, preparation; for example, adult nurse practitioner would be preferred to diabetes educator.

The NCSBN (2002b) position paper recommends that APRNs be educated at the graduate level. The specialty should be consistent with the certification that the individual is seeking. The nursing curriculum should be broad and include biological, behavioral, medical, and nursing sciences relevant to the specialty, and there should be a minimum of 500 supervised clinical hours. Clinical experience should be directly related to the specialty, and the preceptor should be appropriately educated and licensed for that role. For licensure, the position paper also recommended that the APRN graduate from an accredited educational program. It is critical that the APRN program meet established standards such as those set by the *Essentials of Master's Preparation for Advanced Practice Nursing* (American Association of Colleges of Nursing [AACN], 1996), the *National Task Force Criteria for Evaluation of Nurse Practitioner Programs* (National Task Force on Quality Nurse Practitioner Education, 1997, 2002), or the *Standards for Accreditation of Nurse Anesthesia Educational Programs* (American Association of Nurse Anesthetists[AANA], 1999).

It is imperative for boards to have criteria for evaluating APRN programs for regulatory purposes, so NCSBN (2002a) developed *APRN Certification Examination Review Program: Requirements for Accrediting Agencies and Criteria for APRN Certification Programs*. See Figure 36.3 for recommended educational criteria for APRNs.

Table 36.6 - Types of Advanced Practice that were Regulated in 2000

| Type of Program | Regulated by State Boards? |
|---|---|
| Certified Nurse Midwife | Yes: 50;  No: 4 |
| Certified Registered Nurse Anesthetist | Yes: 50;  No: 5 |
| Clinical Nurse Specialist (psych/mental health) | Yes: 34;  No: 20 |
| Clinical Nurse Specialist – other types | Yes: 28;  No: 18 |
| Clinical  Nurse Specialist – No specialty | Yes: 31;  No: 24 |
| Acute Care Nurse Practitioner | Yes: 33;  No: 21 |
| Adult Health Nurse Practitioner | Yes: 35;  No: 20 |
| Child Health/Pediatric Nurse Practitioner | Yes: 34;  No: 21 |
| College Health Nurse Practitioner | Yes: 14;  No: 41 |
| Emergency Nurse Practitioner | Yes: 19;  No: 36 |
| Family Nurse Practitioner | Yes: 35;  No: 20 |
| Family Planning Nurse Practitioner | Yes: 22;  No: 33 |
| Geriatric Nurse Practitioner | Yes: 33;  No: 22 |
| Neonatal Nurse Practitioner | Yes: 33;  No: 22 |
| Nurse Practitioner (no designation) | Yes: 28;  No: 27 |
| OB/GYN or Women's Health Nurse Practitioner | Yes: 34;  No: 21 |
| Psychiatric/Mental Health Nurse Practitioner | Yes: 28;  No: 27 |
| School Health Nurse Practitioner | Yes: 31;  No: 24 |

Source:  National Council of State Boards of Nursing (2000).
*Note:  Information was not available for all state boards of nursing so the numbers do not add up to 61 boards of nursing.*

Figure 36.3 - Recommended Educational Requirements for APRN Programs

---

- Current licensure in the United States.
- Graduation from an APRN program, meeting the following requirements:
  - Education program offered by an accredited college or university offers a degree with a concentration in the advanced nursing practice specialty the individual is seeking.
  - If post-master's certificate programs are offered, they must be offered through the above institutions.
  - Both direct and indirect clinical supervision must be congruent with current national specialty organizations and nursing accrediting guidelines.
- The curriculum includes, but is not limited to:
  - Biological, behavioral, medical and nursing sciences relevant to practice as an APRN in the specified category.
  - Legal, ethical, and professional responsibilities of the APRN.
  - Supervised clinical practice relevant to the specialty of the APRN.
- The curriculum meets the following criteria:
  - Curriculum is consistent with competencies of the specific areas of practice.
  - Instructional track/major has a minimum of 500 supervised clinical hours overall.
  - The supervised clinical experience is directly related to the knowledge and role of the specialty and category.

All individuals, without exception, seeking a national certification must complete a formal didactic and clinical advanced practice program meeting the above criteria.

---

Source:  (National Council of State Boards of Nursing, 2002a)

# Conclusion

Approval in prelicensure nursing programs is similar to accreditation, although there are some distinct differences. Although approval is for the purpose of ongoing safe practice and protection of the public, accreditation sets standards for quality education programs. In order to limit redundancy for nursing programs, site visits for accreditation and approval often are collaborative, and this is the trend for the future. In the regulation of APRN programs, educational consistency across programs and a broad education are important for public protection and are thus important in approvals. Approval of prelicensure and APRN nursing programs is an integral part of nursing regulation.

Please visit the National Council of State Board of Nursing at www.ncsbn.org. For easy launching, this address is located on the CD accompanying this book. Simply launch your internet browser, put the CD-ROM in the drive, go to Chapter 36 on the CD, and then click on the website address.

## Learning Activities

1. You are the education consultant for a state board of nursing and are to visit a private university's baccalaureate nursing program for ongoing approval. It has a baccalaureate program that admits students as freshman and also as transfer students. Using the NCSBN (2002) Model Education Rules and the information in this chapter, discuss which documents, such as syllabi, data, instruments, etc., you will ask the school to submit to help you to decide if the school is in compliance with the state's rules. Be creative.

2. As the Director of Education at NCSBN, you are asked to develop evidence-based criteria for the state boards of nursing to use when approving schools. Outline a proposal for this project. What will be your timeline? What are some of the criteria that you will use? How will you support these criteria with evidence?

3. You are scheduled to visit a large ADN program in a community college. What meetings will you schedule to achieve the goals of your visit?

### References

American Association of Colleges of Nursing [AACN]. (1996). *Essentials of master's education for advanced practice nursing.* Washington, DC: Author.

American Association of Nurse Anesthetists [AANA]. (1999). *Standards for accreditation of nurse anesthesia educational programs.* Park Ridge, IL: Author.

American Nurses Association [ANA]. (2001). *ANA hall of fame: Annie Damer* [online]. Retrieved October 20, 2002, from http://www.nursingworld.org/hof/ damera.htm

Barnum, B. S. (1997). Licensure, certification, and accreditation. *Online Journal of Issues in Nursing* [online]. Retrieved August 20, 2002, from http://www.nursingworld. org/ojin/tpc4/tpc4_2.htm.

Commission on Collegiate Nursing Education [CCNE]. (1998). *Standards for accreditation of baccalaureate and graduate nursing education programs.* New York: Author.

Flanagan, L. (1976*). One strong voice.* Kansas City, MO: ANA.

Gloor, E. (2001). *The essential link between nursing education and public protection.* NCSBN Summit of States, August 6, 2001.

Hutcherson, C., & Williamson, S. H. (1999). Nursing regulation for the new millennium: The mutual recognition model. *Online Journal of Issues in Nursing* [online]. Retrieved August 20, 2002, from http://www.nursingworld.org/ojin/topic9/ topic9_2.htm

International Council of Nurses. (1985). *Report on the regulation of nursing: A report of the present, a position for the future.* Geneva, Switzerland: Author.

*Minnesota rules.* (2002). Retrieved October 3, 2002, from http://www.revisor.leg.state. mnus/arule/6301/0100.html

National Council of State Boards of Nursing [NCSBN]. (1993). *Regulation of advanced nursing practice* (position paper). Chicago: Author.

National Council of State Boards of Nursing [NCSBN]. (1994). *Model administrative rules.* Chicago: Author.

National Council of State Boards of Nursing [NCSBN]. (1995). *Guidelines for education program surveyors: A series of learning modules.* Chicago: Author.

National Council of State Boards of Nursing [NCSBN]. (1998). *Position paper related to approval of nursing education programs by boards of nursing.* Chicago: Author.

National Council of State Boards of Nursing [NCSBN}. (2000). *Profiles of member boards.* Chicago: Author.

National Council of State Boards of Nursing [NCSBN]. (2002a). *APRN certification examination review program: Requirements for accrediting agencies and criteria for APRN certification programs.* Chicago: Author.

National Council of State Boards of Nursing [NCSBN]. (2002b). *Regulation of advanced practice nursing: 2002 National Council of State Boards of Nursing position paper.* Chicago: Author.

National Task Force on Quality Nurse Practitioner Education. (1997, 2002). *National task force guidelines for evaluation of nurse practitioner programs.* Washington, DC: American College of Nurse Practitioners.

*Nurse Dougherty was first: Nursing regulation in New Zealand 1901-2001* [online]. (2001). Retrieved August 23, 2002, from http://www.vuw.ac.nz/nsemid/ndwf/

Safriet, B. (1992). Healthcare dollars and regulatory sense: The role of advanced practice nursing. *Yale Journal on Regulation, 9,* 417-488.

Safriet, B. (2002). Closing the gap between *can* and *may* in healthcare providers' scopes of practice: A primer for policymakers. *Yale Journal on Regulation, 19*(2), 301-334.

Sheets, V. (1996). *Public protection or professional self-preservation*? Unpublished manuscript, National Council of State Boards of Nursing.

Sheets, V. (2002). *An overview of the accreditation of healthcare education and the regulation of healthcare practitioners.* (Unpublished paper: National Council of State Boards of Nursing).

Weisenbeck S. M., & Calico, P. A. (1991). Licensure and related issues in nursing. In Delaughery (Ed.), *Issues and trends in nursing.* St. Louis, MO: CV Mosby.

Appendix 36.1 - Indicators of Quality Nursing Education Programs that Relate to Public Protection

1. Consistency of program outcomes with state laws and administrative rules.
2. Consistency of program outcomes with general standard of practice.
3. Consistency of program outcomes with needs and expectations of consumers.
4. Consistency of program outcomes with a comprehensive systematic evaluation plan that incorporates continuous quality improvement.
5. Evidence of faculty and student participation in program planning, implementation, evaluation, and improvement.
6. Consistency of program outcomes with a curriculum that provides diverse learning experiences.
7. Fiscal, human, physical, and learning resources that support program outcomes and quality improvement.
8. Program administrator who is a professionally and academically qualified registered nurse with institutional authority and administrative responsibility.
9. Professionally and academically qualified nurse faculty sufficient in number and expertise to accomplish program outcomes and quality improvement.
10. Evidence that information communicated by the nursing program is fair, accurate, inclusive, and consistent.

(Gloor, 2001)

Appendix 36.2 - The 61 State Boards of Nursing

| Area I | Area II | Area III | Area IV |
|---|---|---|---|
| Alaska | Illinois | Alabama | Connecticut |
| American Samoa | Indiana | Arkansas | Delaware |
| Arizona | Iowa | Florida | District of Columbia |
| California RN & PN | Kansas | Georgia RN & PN | Maine |
| Colorado | Michigan | Kentucky | Maryland |
| Guam | Minnesota | Louisiana RN & PN | Massachusetts |
| Hawaii | Missouri | Mississippi | New Hampshire |
| Idaho | Nebraska | North Carolina | New Jersey |
| Montana | North Dakota | Oklahoma | New York |
| Nevada | Ohio | South Carolina | Pennsylvania |
| New Mexico | South Dakota | Tennessee | Puerto Rico |
| N. Mariana Islands | West Virginia RN & PN | Texas RN & PN | Rhode Island |
| Oregon | Wisconsin | Virginia | Vermont |
| Utah | | | U.S. Virgin Islands |
| Washington | | | |
| Wyoming | | | |

* Please note:  California, West Virginia, Georgia, Louisiana, & Texas all have separate RN and PN Boards of Nursing.

Appendix 36.3 - National Council of State Boards of Nursing 2002 Model Nursing Administrative Rules for Nursing Education

---

Following is the *Nursing Education* section of the *Model Nursing Administrative Rules*:

**A. Purpose of Standards**
1.  To ensure that graduates of nursing education programs are prepared for safe and effective nursing practice.
2.  To provide criteria for the development, evaluation, and improvement of new and established nursing education programs.
3.  To assure candidates are educationally prepared for licensure and recognition at the appropriate level.

**B. Standards of Nursing Education**
1.  The purpose and outcomes of the nursing program shall be consistent with the Nursing Practice Act and board-promulgated administrative rules, regulations, and other relevant state statutes.
2.  The purpose and outcomes of the nursing program shall be consistent with generally accepted standards of nursing practice appropriate for graduates of the type of nursing program offered.
3.  The input of consumers shall be considered in developing and evaluating the purpose and outcomes of the program.
4.  The nursing program shall implement a comprehensive, systematic plan for ongoing evaluation that is based on program outcomes and incorporates continuous improvement.
5.  Faculty and students shall participate in program planning, implementation, evaluation, and continuous improvement.
6.  The curriculum shall provide diverse learning experiences consistent with program outcomes.
7.  The fiscal, human, physical, and learning resources are adequate to support program processes and outcomes.
8.  The nursing program administrator shall be a professionally and academically qualified registered nurse with institutional authority and administrative responsibility for the program.
9.  Professionally and academically qualified nurse faculty is sufficient in number and expertise to accomplish program outcomes and quality improvement.
10. Program information communicated by the nursing program shall be fair, accurate, inclusive, consistent, and readily available to the public.

**C. Models for Implementing Standards**
The evaluation model for achievement of these standards is determined by each individual jurisdiction, and may be met by state approval and/or through accreditation by a recognized national, regional, or state accreditation body.

**D. Required Components for Nursing Education Programs**
The organization and administration of the nursing education program shall be consistent with the law governing the practice of nursing by:
1.  **Administrator Qualifications**
    a. The administrator of the nursing education program shall be a registered nurse, licensed or privileged to practice in this state, with the additional education and experience necessary to direct the program preparing graduates for the safe and effective practice of nursing. The

Appendix 36.3 - National Council of State Boards of Nursing 2002 Model Nursing Administrative Rules for Nursing Education cont.

administrator is accountable for the administration, planning, implementation, and evaluation of the nursing education program.

b. In a program preparing for practical/vocational nurse licensure:
   (1) minimum of a master's degree with a major in nursing;
   (2) educational preparation or experience in teaching, curriculum development, and administration, including at least two years of clinical experience; and
   (3) a current knowledge of nursing practice at the practical/vocational level.

c. In a program preparing for registered nurse licensure:
   (1) a doctoral degree in nursing or a master's degree with a major in nursing and a doctoral degree;
   (2) educational preparation or experience in teaching, curriculum development, and administration, including at least two years of clinical experience; and
   (3) a current knowledge of professional nursing practice.

2. **Faculty**
   a. There shall be sufficient a number of qualified faculty to meet the objectives and purposes of the nursing education program.
   b. Qualifications:
      (1) Nursing faculty who teach in a program leading to licensure as a practical/vocational nurse shall:
         (a) be currently licensed or privileged to practice as a registered nurse in this state;
         (b) have a minimum of a master's degree with a major in nursing; and
         (c) have < > years of clinical experience.
      (2) Nursing faculty who teach in programs leading to licensure as a registered nurse shall:
         (a) be currently licensed or privileged to practice as a registered nurse in this state;
         (b) have a minimum of a master's degree in nursing with a major in nursing; and
         (c) have < > years of clinical experience.

3. **Adjunct Clinical Faculty**
   Faculty employed solely to supervise clinical nursing experiences of students shall meet all the qualifications above.

4. **Interdisciplinary Faculty**
   Faculty who teach nonclinical nursing courses, e.g., issues and trends, nursing law and ethics, pharmacology, nutrition, research, management, and statistics, shall have advanced preparation appropriate to these areas of content.

5. **Preceptors**
   Clinical preceptors may be used to enhance clinical learning experiences after a student has received clinical and didactic instruction in all basic areas, for that course or specific learning experience. Clinical preceptors should be licensed at or above the level for which the student is

Appendix 36.3 - National Council of State Boards of Nursing 2002 Model Nursing Administrative Rules for Nursing Education cont.

preparing.

6. **Students**
   a. Students shall be provided the opportunity to acquire and demonstrate the knowledge, skills, and abilities for safe and effective nursing practice.
   b. All policies relevant to applicants and students shall be available in writing.
   c. Students shall be required to meet the health standards and criminal background checks as required in the state.

7. **Curriculum**
   a. The curriculum of the nursing education program shall enable the student to develop the nursing knowledge, skills, and competencies necessary for the level and scope of nursing practice.
   b. The curriculum shall include:
      (1) Content regarding legal and ethical issues, history and trends in nursing, and professional responsibilities;
      (2) Experiences which promote the development of leadership and management skills and professional socialization consistent with the level of licensure;
      (3) Learning experiences and methods of instruction consistent with the written curriculum plan; and
      (4) Courses including, but not limited to:
         (a) content in the biological, physical, social, and behavioral sciences to provide a foundation for safe and effective nursing practice;
         (b) the nursing process; and
         (c) didactic content and clinical experience in the promotion, prevention, restoration, and maintenance of health in clients across the life span and in a variety of clinical settings.
   c. Delivery of instruction by distance-education methods must be congruent with the program curriculum plan and enable students to meet the goals, competencies, and objectives of the educational program and standards of the board.

E. **Initial Approval of Nursing Education Programs**
   Before a nursing education program is permitted to admit students, the program shall submit evidence of the ability to meet the Standards for Nursing Education (Section B above).

F. **Provisional Approval of New Nursing Education Programs**
   The board may grant provisional approval when it determines that a program is not fully meeting approval standards. This type of approval is usually granted until graduation of the first class from a nursing program.

G. **Ongoing Approval of Nursing Education Programs**
   All nursing education programs shall be reevaluated every < > years, upon request of the nursing education program or at the discretion of the board to ensure continuing compliance with the

Appendix 36.3 - National Council of State Boards of Nursing 2002 Model Nursing Administrative Rules for Nursing Education cont.

Standards for Nursing Education (Section B above).

**H.  Conditional Approval of Nursing Education Programs**
   1.  If the board determines that an approved nursing education program is not meeting the criteria set forth in these regulations, the governing institution shall be given a reasonable period of time to submit an action plan and to correct the identified program deficiencies.
   2.  The Board may grant conditional approval when it determines that a program is not fully meeting approval standards.

**I.   Denial or Withdrawal of Approval**
   1.  The board may deny provisional (initial) approval when it determines that a new nursing education program will be unable to meet the standards for nursing education.
   2.  The board may withdraw approval if:
       a.  It determines that a nursing education program fails substantially to meet the standards for nursing education.
       b.  The nursing education program fails to correct the identified deficiencies within the time specified, the board may withdraw approval.

**J.   Appeal**
   A program denied approval or given less than full approval may appeal that decision within a < > month period.

   All such actions shall be effected in accordance with due process rights and the <NAME OF STATE> Administrative Procedures Act and/or Administrative Rules of the Board.

**K.  Reinstatement of Approval**
   The board may reinstate approval if the program submits evidence of compliance with the plan within the specified time frame.

**L.   Closure of Nursing Education Program and Storage of Records**
   A nursing education program may close voluntarily or may be closed due to withdrawal of board approval.  Provision must be made for maintenance of the standards for nursing education during the transition to closure; for placement for students who have not completed the nursing program; and for the storage of academic records and transcripts.

Appendix 36.4 - National Council of State Boards of Nursing Model Nursing Practice Act

# Article I. Title and Purpose

**Section 1.** *Title of Act.* This Act shall be known and may be cited as The <NAME OF STATE> Nursing Practice Act.

**Section 2.** *Description of Act.* An Act concerning the regulation of the practice of nursing that creates and empowers the State Board of Nursing to regulate the practice of nursing and to enforce the provisions of this act.

**Section 3.** *Purpose.* The legislature finds that the practice of nursing is directly related to the public welfare of the citizens of the state and is subject to regulations and control in the public interest to assure that practitioners are qualified and competent. It is further declared that the practice of nursing, as defined in the Act, merits and deserves the confidence of the public and that only qualified persons be permitted to engage in the practice of nursing. The legislature recognizes that the practice of nursing is continually evolving and responding to changes within healthcare patterns and systems.

# Article II. Definitions and Scope

**Section 1.** *Practice of Nursing.* The *practice of nursing* means assisting clients or groups to attain or maintain optimal health, implementing a strategy of care to accomplish defined goals, and evaluating responses to nursing care and treatment. Nursing practice includes (1) basic health care that helps both clients and groups of people cope with difficulties in daily living associated with their actual or potential health or illness status, and (2) those nursing activities that require a substantial amount of scientific knowledge or technical skill. Nursing practice includes, but is not limited to:

a. Providing comfort and caring.
b. Providing attentive surveillance to monitor client conditions and needs.
c. Promoting an environment conducive to well being.
d. Planning and implementing independent nursing strategies and prescribed treatment in the prevention and management of illness, injury, disability, or achievement of a dignified death.
e. Promoting and supporting human functions and responses.
f. Providing health counseling and teaching.
g. Collaborating on aspects of the health regimen.
h. Advocating for the client.

Nursing is both an art and a scientific process founded on a professional body of knowledge; it is a learned profession based on an understanding of the human condition across the lifespan and the relationship of a client with others and within the environment. Nursing is a dynamic discipline that is continually evolving to include more sophisticated knowledge, technologies, and client care activities.

**Section 2.** *Registered Nurse.* Practice as a registered nurse means the full scope of nursing, with or without compensation or personal profit, that incorporates caring for all clients in all settings; and

Appendix 36.4 - National Council of State Boards of Nursing Model Nursing Practice Act cont.

includes, but is not limited to:

a. Providing comprehensive assessment of the health status of clients, families, groups, and communities.
b. Developing a comprehensive nursing plan that establishes nursing diagnoses; sets goals to meet identified healthcare needs; and prescribes nursing interventions.
c. Implementing nursing care through the execution of independent nursing strategies and prescribed medical regimen.
d. Managing nursing care through cohesive, coordinated care management within and across care settings.
e. Delegating and assigning nursing interventions to implement the plan of care.
f. Providing for the maintenance of safe and effective nursing care rendered directly or indirectly.
g. Promoting a safe and therapeutic environment.
h. Providing health teaching and counseling to promote, attain, and maintain the optimum health level of clients, families, groups, and communities.
i. Advocating for clients, families, groups, and communities by attaining and maintaining what is in the best interest of the client or group.
j. Evaluating responses to interventions and the effectiveness of the plan of care.
k. Communicating and collaborating with other healthcare professionals in the management of health care and the implementation of the total healthcare regimen.
l. Acquiring and applying critical new knowledge and technologies to practice domain.
m. Managing, supervising, and evaluating the practice of nursing.
n. Teaching the theory and practice of nursing.
o. Participating in development of policies, procedures, and systems to support the client.
p. Other acts that require education and training as prescribed by the board. Additional nursing services shall be commensurate with the registered nurse's experience, continuing education, and demonstrated competencies.

Each registered nurse is accountable to clients, the nursing profession, and the board for complying with the requirements of this Act and the quality of nursing care rendered; and for recognizing limits of knowledge and experience and planning for management of situations beyond the nurse's expertise.

**Section 3.** *Licensed Practical/Vocational Nurse.* Practice as a licensed practical/vocational nurse means a directed scope of nursing practice, with or without compensation or personal profit, under the supervision of the registered nurse, advanced practice registered nurse, licensed physician, or other healthcare provider authorized by the state to delegate healthcare activities and functions; and includes, but is not limited to:

a. Collecting data and conducting focused assessments of the health status of clients.
b. Planning nursing care during care episode for clients with stable conditions.
c. Participating in the development and modification of the comprehensive plan of care for all types of clients.
d. Implementing the appropriate aspects of the strategy of care within the LPN/VN scope of practice.
e. Participating in nursing care management through delegating, assigning, and directing nursing

Appendix 36.4 - National Council of State Boards of Nursing Model Nursing Practice Act cont.

interventions that may be performed by others, including other LPN/VNs, that do not conflict with the act.

f. Maintaining safe and effective nursing care rendered directly or indirectly.

g. Promoting a safe and therapeutic environment.

h. Participating in health teaching and counseling to promote, attain, and maintain the optimum health level of clients.

i. Serving as an advocate for the client by communicating and collaborating with other health service personnel.

j. Participating in the evaluation of client responses to interventions.

k. Communicating and collaborating with other healthcare professionals in the nursing practice management.

l. Providing input into the development of policies and procedures.

m. Other acts that require education and training as prescribed by the board. Additional nursing services shall be commensurate with the licensed practical nurse's experience, continuing education, and demonstrated competencies.

Each nurse is accountable to clients, the nursing profession, and the board for complying with the requirements of this Act and the quality of nursing care rendered; and for recognizing limits of knowledge and experience and planning for management of situations beyond the nurse's expertise.

**Section 4.** *Advanced Practice Registered Nurse.* Advanced practice registered nursing by nurse practitioners, registered nurse anesthetists, nurse midwives, or clinical nurse specialists is based on knowledge and skills acquired in basic nursing education; licensure as a registered nurse; graduation from or completion of a graduate level APRN program accredited by a national accrediting body and current certification by a national certifying body in the appropriate APRN specialty. Practice as an advanced practice registered nurse means an expanded scope of nursing, with or without compensation or personal profit, and includes but is not limited to:

a. Assessing clients, synthesizing and analyzing data, and understanding and applying nursing principles at an advanced level.

b. Analyzing multiple sources of data, identifying alternative possibilities as to the nature of a healthcare problem and selecting appropriate treatment.

c. Making independent decisions in solving complex client care problems.

d. Developing a plan that establishes diagnoses, sets goals to meet identified healthcare needs, and prescribes a regimen of health care.

e. Performing acts of diagnosing, prescribing, administering, and dispensing therapeutic measures, including legend drugs and controlled substances, within the advanced practice registered nurse's focus of practice.

f. Managing clients' physical and psychosocial health-illness status.

g. Providing for the maintenance of safe and effective nursing care rendered directly or indirectly.

h. Promoting a safe and therapeutic environment.

i. Providing expert guidance and teaching.

j. Participating in client and health systems management.

k. Advocating for clients, groups, and communities by attaining and maintaining what is in the best .

Appendix 36.4 - National Council of State Boards of Nursing Model Nursing Practice Act cont.

interest of the client or group.

l.   Evaluating responses to interventions, the effectiveness of the plan of care, and the health regimen.

m.   Communicating and working effectively with clients, families, and other members of the healthcare team.

n.   Utilizing research skills and acquiring and applying critical new knowledge and technologies to practice domain.

o.   Teaching the theory and practice of advanced practice nursing.

Each advanced practice registered nurse is accountable to clients, the nursing profession, and the board for complying with the requirements of this Act and the quality of nursing care rendered; for recognizing limits of knowledge and experience, planning for management of situations beyond the nurse's expertise; and for consulting with or referring clients to other healthcare providers as appropriate. This act shall supersede all prior inconsistent statutes, rules or regulations regarding this subject.

**Section 5. *Board.*** "Board" means the <NAME OF STATE> Board of Nursing.

**Section 6. *Other Board.*** "Other Board" means the comparable regulatory agency in any U.S. state, territory, or the District of Columbia.

**Section 7. *License.*** "License" means a current document permitting the practice of nursing as a registered nurse, licensed practical nurse, or advanced practice registered nurse.

**Section 8. *Other Definitions.***

a.   **Absolute discharge from sentence** – completion of any court-imposed sentence, including imprisonment, probation, parole, community supervision, or any form of court supervision.

b.   **Assignment** – designating nursing activities to be performed by another nurse or assistive personnel that are consistent with his/her scope of practice (licensed person) or role description (unlicensed person).

c.   **Chief Administrative Nurse** – the registered nurse who oversees the provision of nursing services in an organization, regardless of title.

d.   **Client** – the client as the recipient of care may be an individual, family, group, or community.

e.   **Compact** – an interstate compact is an agreement between two or more states established for the purpose of remedying a particular problem of interstate concern.

f.   **Comprehensive assessment by the RN** – an extensive data collection (initial and ongoing) for clients, families, groups, and communities addressing anticipated changes in client conditions as well as emergent changes in a client's health status; recognizing alterations to previous client conditions; synthesizing the biological, psychological, and social aspects of the client's condition; evaluating the impact of nursing care and using this broad and complete analysis to make independent decisions and nursing diagnoses; planning nursing interventions; and evaluating need for different interventions and the need to communicate and consult with other health team members.

g.   **Cooperation** – a joint effort of cooperating, assisting, and working together for a common benefit.

h.   **Delegation** – transferring to a competent individual the authority to perform a selected nursing task in a selected situation.

Appendix 36.4 - National Council of State Boards of Nursing Model Nursing Practice Act cont.

i. **Emergency** – a sudden state of danger, conflict, or crisis requiring immediate action.

j. **Focused assessment by the LPN/VN** – an appraisal of the client's status and situation at hand, contributing to ongoing data collection, and deciding who needs to be informed of the information and when to inform.

k. **Healthcare Provider** – an individual authorized (e.g., licensed or certified) to prescribe and/or administer various aspects of health care.

l. **Licensure by Endorsement** – the granting of authority to practice based on an individual's licensure (having met comparable requirements) in another jurisdiction.

m. **Licensure by Examination** – the authority to practice nursing based on an assessment of minimum competency by such means as the boards shall determine.

n. **Nurse Licensure Compact (NLC)** – a compact between participating states to facilitate the regulation of nurses. The compact is adopted by each state legislature and allows a nurse licensed in a compact state to practice under a multistate privilege in all other compact states.

o. **Nurse Licensure Compact Administrators (NLCA)** – the administrators of each compact state who are responsible for implementing and coordinating the NLC.

p. **Person** – an individual, corporation, partnership, association, unit of government, or other legal entity.

q. **Prescriptive Authority** – the power to determine the need for drugs, immunizing agents, or devices; selecting the remedy; and writing a prescription to be filled by a licensed pharmacist.

r. **Standards of Nursing Practice** – those standards adopted by the board that interpret legal definitions of practice.

s. **Nursing Student** – a person who is studying in an approved education program.

t. **Unauthorized practice** – practice of licensed practical/vocational nursing, registered nursing, or advanced practice registered nursing by any person who has not been authorized to practice nursing under the provision of this Act.

# Article III. The Board of Nursing

**Section 1.** *Membership; Appointment; Nominations; Term of Office; Removal; Vacancies; Qualifications; Immunity.*

a. The board of nursing shall consist of < > members to be appointed by the Governor < > days prior to the expiration of the term of office of a current member. Nominations for appointment may be made to the Governor by any interested individual, association, or any other entity, provided that such nominations be supported by a petition executed by no less than < > qualified voters in this state. These nominations shall not be binding upon the Governor.

b. The membership of the board shall be at least < > members of registered nurses; at least < > members of licensed practical/vocational nurses; at least < > members of advanced practice registered nurses; and at least < > members representing the public.

   1. Each registered nurse member shall be an eligible voting resident in this state, licensed in good standing under the provisions of this chapter, currently engaged in the practice of nursing as a registered nurse, and shall have no less than five (5) years of experience as a registered nurse, at least three (3) of which immediately preceded appointment.

Appendix 36.4 - National Council of State Boards of Nursing Model Nursing Practice Act cont.

    2.      Each licensed practical/vocational nurse member shall be an eligible voting resident in this state, licensed in good standing under the provisions of this chapter, currently engaged in the practice of nursing as a licensed practical/vocational nurse, and shall have no less than five (5) years of experience as a licensed practical/vocational nurse, at least three (3) of which immediately preceded appointment.

    3.      Each advanced practice registered nurse member shall be an eligible voting resident in this state, licensed in good standing under the provisions of this chapter, currently engaged in the practice of nursing as an advanced practice registered nurse, and shall have no less than five (5) years of experience as an advanced practice registered nurse, at least three (3) of which immediately preceded appointment.

    4.      The representatives of the public shall be eligible voting residents of this state who are knowledgeable in consumer health concerns, and shall not be associated with the provision of health care or be enrolled in any health-related education program.

    5.      Membership shall be restricted to no more than one (1) person who is associated with a particular agency, corporation, other enterprise or subsidiary at one time.

c.    Members of the board shall be appointed for a term of < > years.

    1.      The present members of the board holding office under the provisions of the <NAME OF ACT BEING AMENDED OR REPEALED> shall serve as members for their respective terms.

    2.      No member shall serve more than two (2) consecutive full terms. The completion of an un-expired portion of a full term shall not constitute a full term for purposes of this section. Any board member initially appointed for less than a full term shall be eligible to serve two (2) additional terms.

    3.      An appointee to a full term on the board shall be appointed by the Governor before the expiration of the term of the member being succeeded and shall become a member of the board on the first day following the appointment expiration date. Appointees to unexpired terms shall become members of the board on the day following such appointment.

    4.      Each term of office shall expire at midnight on the last day of the term of the appointment or at midnight on the date on which any vacancy occurs. If a replacement appointment has not been made, the term of the Member shall be extended until a replacement is made.

d.    Any vacancy that occurs for any reason in the membership of the board shall be filled by the Governor in the manner prescribed in the provisions of this article regarding appointments. Vacancies created by reason other than the expiration of a term shall be filled within < > days after such vacancy occurs. A person appointed to fill a vacancy shall serve for the unexpired portion of the term.

e.    The governor may remove any member from the board for neglect of any duty required by law or for incompetence or for unprofessional or dishonorable conduct. The general laws of this state controlling the removal of public officials from office shall be followed in dismissing board members.

f.    All members of the board shall have immunity from individual civil liability while acting within the scope of the duties as board members.

g.    In the event that the entire board, an individual member, or staff is sued, the Attorney General shall appoint an attorney to represent the involved party.

h.    Board meetings and hearings shall be open to the public. In accordance with the law, the board may in its discretion conduct part of the meeting in executive session closed to the public.

Appendix 36.4 - National Council of State Boards of Nursing Model Nursing Practice Act cont.

**Section 2.** *Powers and Duties.* The Board shall:

a. Be responsible for interpretation and enforcement of the provisions of this Act. The board shall have all of the duties, powers, and authority specifically granted by and necessary to the enforcement of this Act, as well as other duties, powers, and authority as it may be granted by appropriate status.

b. Be authorized to make, adopt, amend, repeal, and enforce such administrative rules consistent with law as it deems necessary for the proper administration and enforcement of this Act and to protect the public health, safety, and welfare.

c. Be authorized to make, adopt, amend, repeal, and enforce such administrative rules consistent with the law, as it deems necessary for the regulation of advanced nursing practice.

d. Further be authorized to do the following without limiting the foregoing:

   1. Develop standards for nursing education.
   2. Enforce educational standards and rules set forth by the board.
   3. Require criminal background checks on applicants and licensees.
   4. License qualified applicants for RN and LPN/VN licensure by examination or endorsement, and renew and reinstate licenses.
   5. Regulate the advanced practice of nursing by advanced practice registered nurses.
   6. Regulate the clinical support of nursing services by unlicensed assistive personnel regardless of title.
   7. Maintain a record of all persons regulated by the board.
   8. Develop and enforce standards for nursing practice.
   9. Develop rules to govern delegation by and to nurses.
   10. Develop standards for maintaining competence of licensees continuing in or returning to practice.
   11. Collect and analyze data regarding nursing education, nursing practice, and nursing resources.
   12. Issue subpoenas in connection with investigations, inspections, and hearings.
   13. Access to records as reasonably requested by the board to assist the board in its investigation; the board shall maintain any records obtained pursuant to this paragraph as confidential data.
   14. Order licensees to submit to physical, mental health, or chemical dependency evaluations for cause.
   15. Cause prosecution of allegations of violations of this Act.
   16. Conduct hearings, compel attendance of witnesses, and administer oaths to persons giving testimony at hearings.
   17. Close discipline sessions and hearings to the public.
   18. Discipline licensees as needed.
   19. Maintain membership in national organizations that develop and regulate the national licensure examinations and exclusively promote the improvement of the legal standards of the practice of nursing for the protection of the public health, safety, and welfare.
   20. Establish alternative programs for monitoring of nurses who voluntarily seek treatment for chemical dependency, mental health, or physical health conditions that could lead to disciplinary action by the board.
   21. Regulate the manner in which nurses announce their practice to the public.
   22. Issue a modified license to practice nursing to an individual to practice within a limited scope of practice or with accommodations or both, as specified by the board.

Appendix 36.4 - National Council of State Boards of Nursing Model Nursing Practice Act cont.

23. Inform licensees on an established basis about changes in law and rules regarding nursing practice.
24. Maintain records of proceedings as required by the laws of this state.
25. Provide consultation, conduct conferences, forums, studies and research on nursing education and practice.
26. Appoint and employ a qualified registered nurse to serve as Executive Officer and approve such additional staff positions as may be necessary, in the opinion of the board, to administer and enforce the provisions of the Act.
27. Delegate to the Executive Officer those activities that expedite the functions of the board.
28. Develop disaster preparedness plan.
29. Employ professional and support staff, investigators, and legal counsel and other personnel necessary for the board to carry out its functions.
30. Require such surety bonds as are deemed necessary.
31. Determine and collect reasonable fees.
32. Receive and expend funds in addition to appropriations from this state, provided such funds are received and expended for the pursuit of the authorized objectives of the board of Nursing; such funds are maintained in a separate account; and periodic reports of the receipt and expenditures of such funds are submitted to the Governor.
33. Adopt a seal that shall be in the care of the Executive Officer and shall be affixed only in such a manner as prescribed by the board.

This Act shall not be construed to require the board of nursing to report violations of the provisions of the Act whenever, in the board's opinion, the public interest will be served adequately by a suitable written notice of warning.

**Section 3.** *Executive Officer.* The Executive Officer shall be responsible for:
a. The performance of administrative responsibilities of the board.
b. Employment of personnel needed to carry out the functions of the board.
c. The performance of any other duties as the board may direct.

**Section 4.** *Compensation.* Each member of the board shall receive, as compensation, a reasonable sum for each day the member is engaged in performance of official duties of the board and reimbursement for all expenses incurred in connection with the discharge of such official duties.

## Article IV.  Administrative Procedures Act – Application

The <NAME OF STATE> State Administrative Procedures Act is hereby expressly adopted and incorporated herein as if all the provisions of such Act were included in this Act.

## Article V.  Licensure

**Section 1.** *Requirements.* Each applicant who successfully meets the requirements of this section shall be entitled to licensure as a registered nurse or licensed practice/vocational nurse, whichever is applicable,

Appendix 36.4 - National Council of State Boards of Nursing Model Nursing Practice Act cont.

---

as follows:

a. Licensure by Examination. An applicant for licensure by examination to practice as a registered nurse or licensed practical/vocational nurse shall:
1. Submit a completed application and fees as established by the board.
2. Be a graduate of a board-approved nursing education program or a program that meets criteria comparable to those established by the board in its rules.
3. Be proficient in English language as set forth in the board rules.
4. Pass an examination authorized by the board.
5. Have committed no acts or omissions which are grounds for disciplinary action as set forth in Article IX, Section 2, of this Act, or, if such acts have been committed and would be grounds for disciplinary action, the board has found after investigation that sufficient restitution has been made.
6. If convicted or pled *nolo contendre* to one or more felonies, has received an absolute discharge from the sentences for all felony convictions < > years prior to the date of filing an application pursuant to this chapter.
7. Meet other criteria established by the board.
b. Licensure by Endorsement. An applicant for licensure by endorsement to practice as a registered nurse or licensed practical/vocational nurse shall:
1. Submit a completed application and fees as established by the board.
2. Have committed no acts or omissions which are grounds for disciplinary action in another jurisdiction or, if such acts have been committed and would be grounds for disciplinary action as set forth in Article IX, Section 2, of this Act, the board has found after investigation that sufficient restitution has been made.
3. Be a graduate of a board-approved nursing education program which meets criteria comparable to those established by this board and which prepares for the level of licensure being sought.
4. Pass an examination authorized by the board.
5. Be proficient in English language as set forth in the board rules.
6. Submit verification of licensure status directly from the U.S. jurisdiction of licensure by examination, Nur*sys* (or the Coordinated Licensure Information System).
7. Meet continued competency requirements as stated in Article V, Section 3 and as set forth in board rules.
8. If convicted or pled *nolo contendre* to one or more felonies, has received an absolute discharge from the sentences for all felony convictions five or more years prior to the date of filing an application pursuant to this chapter.
9. Meet other criteria established by the board.
c. Initial Licensure for Advanced Practice Registered Nurse. An application for initial licensure as an advanced practice registered nurse shall:
1. Be licensed as a registered nurse (unencumbered).
2. Be a graduate from or have completed a graduate level APRN program accredited by a national accrediting body.
3. Be currently certified by a national certifying body in the APRN specialty appropriate to educational preparation.

Appendix 36.4 - National Council of State Boards of Nursing Model Nursing Practice Act cont.

4. Submit a completed written application and appropriate fees as established by the board.

5. Provide evidence as required by the board in its rules.

6. Have committed no acts or omissions which are grounds for disciplinary action in another jurisdiction or, if such acts have been committed and would be grounds for discipline under Article IX, Section 2, of this Act, the board has found after investigation that sufficient restitution has been made.

d. The board may issue a license by endorsement to practice as an advanced practice registered nurse under the laws of another state and, in the opinion of the board, the applicant meets the qualifications for licensure in this jurisdiction.

e. Temporary Permits

1. Applicants for Endorsement. The board may issue, upon the request of an applicant, a temporary permit to practice nursing at the same level of licensure to an individual currently licensed in another jurisdiction of the United States who submits an application in accord with the rules of the board.

2. Individuals Previously Licensed to Practice Nursing Enrolled in Refresher Courses. The board may issue a temporary permit to provide direct client care as part of a nursing refresher course, as permitted in board rules.

3. APRN Temporary Permits. The board may issue, upon request of the applicant, a temporary permit to practice advanced practice nursing to an applicant authorized to practice at that level in a U.S. jurisdiction who submits an application in accord with the rules of the board.

## Section 2. *Examinations.*

a. The board shall authorize the administration of the examination to applicants for licensure as registered nurses or licensed practical/vocational nurses.

b. The board may employ, contract, and cooperate with any entity in the preparation and process for determining results of a uniform licensure examination. When such an examination is utilized, access to questions and answers shall be restricted by the board.

c. The board shall determine whether a licensure examination may be repeated, the frequency of reexamination, and any requisite education prior to reexamination.

## Section 3. *Renewal of Licenses.*

a. Licenses issued under this Act shall be renewed every < > years according to a schedule established by the board.

b. An applicant for licensure renewal shall submit a verified statement that indicates whether the applicant has been convicted of a felony, and if convicted of one or more felonies, indicates the date of absolute discharge from the sentences for all felony convictions.

c. 1. A renewal license shall be issued to a registered nurse or licensed practical/vocational nurse who remits the required fee and satisfactorily completes any other requirements established by the board as set forth in rules.

2. A renewal license shall be issued to an advanced practice registered nurse who maintains national certification in the appropriate APRN specialty through an ongoing certification maintenance program of a nationally recognized certifying body [or applicants for whom no recognized certification is available must participate in a competence maintenance program], remits the required fee, and

Appendix 36.4 - National Council of State Boards of Nursing Model Nursing Practice Act cont.

satisfactorily completes any other requirements established by the board as set forth in rules.

d. Failure to renew the license shall result in forfeiture of the right to practice nursing in this state.

### Section 4. *Reinstatement of Licenses.*

a. A licensee whose license has lapsed by failure to renew may apply for reinstatement according to the rules established by the board. Upon satisfaction of the requirements for reinstatement, the board shall issue a renewal of license.

a. A licensee whose license has been suspended, revoked, or otherwise removed shall comply with all requirements set forth in the board's discipline order.

### Section 5. *Modified License.* The board may consider issuing a modified license to an individual who has successfully completed a board approved nursing program and who is able to practice without compromise to the public safety within a modified scope of practice or with accommodations or both as specified by the board.

### Section 6. *Duties of Licensees.* The nurse shall comply with the provisions of this act. The burden of responsibility is on the licensee to know and practice according to the laws and regulations of the state.

a. In response to board inquiries, provide relevant and truthful personal, professional, or demographic information requested by the board to perform its duties in regulating and controlling nursing practice in order to protect the public health, safety, and welfare. Failure to provide the requested information may result in nonrenewal of the license to practice nursing and/or licensure disciplinary action.

b. Submit to a physical or mental evaluation by a designated < > when directed in writing by the board for cause. If requested by the licensee, the licensee may also designate a < > for an independent medical examination. Refusal or failure of a licensee to complete such examinations shall constitute an admission of any allegations relating to such condition. All objections shall be waived as to the admissibility of the examining < > testimony or examination reports on the grounds that they constitute privileged communication. The medical testimony or examinations reports shall not be used against a registered nurse, licensed practical nurse, or advanced practice registered nurse in another proceeding and shall be confidential. At reasonable intervals, a registered nurse, licensed practical nurse or advanced practice registered nurse shall be afforded the opportunity to demonstrate competence to resume the practice of nursing with reasonable skill and safety to clients.

c. Report to the board those acts or omissions which are violations of the Act or grounds for disciplinary action as set forth in Articles VIII and IX of this Act.

## Article VI. Titles and Abbreviations

### Section 1. *Titles and Abbreviations for Licensed Nurses.*

a. Only those persons who hold a license to practice nursing in this state shall have the right to use the following title abbreviations:
   1. Title: "Registered Nurse" and the abbreviation "RN."
   2. Title: "Licensed Practical/Vocational Nurse" and the abbreviation "LPN/VN."
   3. Title: "Advanced Practice Registered Nurse" and the abbreviation "APRN."

b. It shall be unlawful for any person to use the title "Nurse," "Registered Nurse," "Licensed

Appendix 36.4 - National Council of State Boards of Nursing Model Nursing Practice Act cont.

Practical/Vocational Nurse," "Advanced Practice Registered Nurse," or their authorized abbreviations unless permitted by this Act.

**Section 2.** *Titles and abbreviations for Temporary Permits.* Any person who has been approved as an applicant for licensure by endorsement and has been granted a temporary permit shall have the right to use the titles < > and abbreviations < > designated by the state.

## Article VII. Approval of Nursing Education Programs

**Section 1.** *Approval Standards.* The board shall, by administrative rules, set standards for the establishment and outcomes of nursing education programs, including clinical learning experiences, and approve such programs that meet the requirements of the Act and the board administrative rules.

**Section 2.** *Initial Approval Required.* An educational institution that seeks to provide a diploma, degree, or certificate in nursing to students in this jurisdiction shall apply to the board and submit evidence that its nursing program(s) meets or will meet the standards established by the board. If, upon review, the board determines that the program(s) meets established standards, it shall grant approval.

**Section 3.** *Provisional or Interim Approval of New Programs.* Provisional approval of new programs may be granted contingent upon conditions set forth by the board in administrative rules.

**Section 4.** *Continuing Approval of Nursing Programs.* The board shall periodically review educational nursing programs and require nursing education programs to submit evidence of compliance with standards and administrative rules. If, upon review of such evidence, the board determines that the program(s) meets the established standards, it shall grant continuing approval. The board will publish a list of approved programs.

**Section 5.** *Denial or Withdrawal of Approval.* The board may deny or withdraw approval or take such action as deemed necessary when nursing education programs fail to meet the standards established by the board, provided that all such actions shall be in accordance with this state's Administrative Procedures Act and/or the Administrative Rules of the board. A process of appeal and reinstatement shall be delineated in board rules.

**Section 6.** *Reinstatement of Approval.* The board shall reinstate approval of a nursing education program upon submission of satisfactory evidence that its program meets the standards established by the board.

## Article VIII. Violations and Penalties

**Section 1.** *Violations.*
Every employer of a licensed nurse and every person acting as an agent for such a nurse in obtaining employment shall verify the current status of the licensee's authorization to practice within the provisions of this chapter. As used in this section, the term "agent" includes, but is not limited to, a nurses' registry.

Appendix 36.4 - National Council of State Boards of Nursing Model Nursing Practice Act cont.

No person shall:

a. Engage in the practice of nursing as defined in the Act without a valid, current license, except as otherwise permitted under this Act.
b. Practice nursing under cover of any diploma, license, or record illegally or fraudulently obtained, signed, or issued unlawfully or under fraudulent representation.
c. Practice nursing during the time a license is suspended, revoked, surrendered, inactive, or lapsed.
d. Use any words, abbreviations, figures, letters, title, sign, card, or device tending to imply that he or she is a registered nurse, licensed practical nurse, or advanced practice registered nurse unless such person is duly licensed so to practice under the provisions of this Act.
e. Fraudulently obtain or furnish a license by or for money or any other thing of value.
f. Knowingly employ unlicensed persons in the practice of nursing.
g. Fail to report information relating to violations of this Act.
h. Conduct a program for the preparation for licensure under this chapter unless the program has been approved by the board.
i. Conduct courses or providing consultation that conflict with the scope and standards of practice set forth in this Act and in rules of the board.
j. Otherwise violate or aid or abet another person to violate any provision of this Act.
k. Engage in irregular behavior in connection with the licensure examination, including, but not limited to, the giving or receiving of aid in the examination or the unauthorized possession, reproduction, or disclosure of examination questions or answers.

**Section 2.** *Penalties.*  Violation of any provision of this article shall constitute a misdemeanor or felony as defined by rule.

**Section 3.** *Criminal Prosecution.*  Nothing in this Act shall be construed as a bar to criminal prosecution for violation of the provisions of this Act.

**Section 4.** *Civil Penalties.*  The board may, in addition to any other sanctions herein provided, impose on any person violating a provision of this Act, or Administrative Rules of the board, a civil penalty not to exceed <$> for each count or separate offense.

## Article IX.  Discipline and Proceedings

**Section 1.** *Authority.*  For any one or combination of the grounds set forth below, the board of nursing shall have the power to:

a. Refuse to issue or renew a license.
b. Limit a license.
c. Suspend a license.
d. Revoke a license.
e. Place a license on probation.
f. Reprimand or otherwise discipline a licensee.
g. Impose a civil penalty not exceeding $10,000 for each separate violation.
h. Impose fines of up to ($).

Appendix 36.4 - National Council of State Boards of Nursing Model Nursing Practice Act cont.

i.   Take any other action justified by the facts in the case.

**Section 2.** *Grounds for Discipline.* The board may discipline a licensee or applicant for any or a combination of the following grounds [as defined by regulations adopted by the board]:

a.   **Failure to Meet Requirements** – the failure to demonstrate the qualifications or satisfy the requirements for licensure contained in Article V. In the case of a person applying for a license, the burden of proof is upon the applicant to demonstrate the qualifications or satisfactions of the requirements.

b.   **Criminal Convictions** – convictions by a court or entry of a plea of *nolo contendere* to a crime in any jurisdiction that relates adversely to the practice of nursing or to the ability to practice nursing.

c.   **Fraud and/or Deceit** – employment of fraud or deceit in procuring or attempting to procure a license to practice nursing, in filing any reports or completing client records, in signing any report or records in the nurse's capacity as a registered nurse, licensed practical/vocational nurse, or advanced practice registered nurse or in submitting any information or record to the board.

d.   **Action in Another Jurisdiction** – a nurse's license practice nursing or another healthcare profession or a multistate practice privilege has been denied, revoked, suspended, restricted or otherwise disciplined in this or any other state.

e.   **Unsafe Practice/Unprofessional Practice** – actions or conduct including, but not limited to:
   1.   Failure or inability to perform registered nursing, practical nursing, or advanced practice nursing, as defined in Article II, with reasonable skill and safety.
   2.   Unprofessional conduct, including a departure from or failure to conform to board standards of registered nursing, practical nursing, or advanced practice nursing.
   3.   Failure to supervise the performance of acts by any individual working at the nurse's direction.
   4.   Failure of a chief administrative nurse to provide oversight of the nursing organization and nursing services of a healthcare delivery system.
   5.   Failure to practice within a modified scope of practice or with the required accommodations, as specified by the board in granting a modified license.
   6.   Conduct or any nursing practice that may create unnecessary danger to a client's life, health, or safety. Actual injury to a client need not be established.

f.   **Inability to Practice Safely** – demonstration of actual or potential inability to practice nursing with reasonable skill and safety to clients by reason of illness; use of alcohol, drugs, chemicals, or any other material; or as a result of any mental or physical conditions.

g.   **Unethical Conduct** – behavior likely to deceive, defraud, or harm the public or demonstration of a willful or careless disregard for the health, welfare, or safety of a client. Actual injury need not be established.

h.   **Misconduct** – actions or conduct that include, but are not limited to:
   1.   Failure to cooperate with a lawful investigation conducted by the board.
   2.   Use of excessive force upon or mistreatment or abuse of any client. "Excessive force" means force clearly greater than what would normally be applied in similar clinical situations.
   3.   Engagement in sexual conduct with a client, or conduct that may reasonably be interpreted by the client as sexual, or in any verbal behavior that is seductive or sexually demeaning to a client.

i.   **Drug Diversion** – diversion or attempts to divert drugs or controlled substances.

j.   **Failure to Comply with Alternative Program Requirements** – failure of a participant of an

Appendix 36.4 - National Council of State Boards of Nursing Model Nursing Practice Act cont.

alternative (to discipline) program to comply with terms of his /her alternative program agreement.

k.  **Other Drug Related** – actions or conduct that include, but are not limited to:
    1.  Intemperate use of alcohol or drugs that the board determines endangers or could endanger a client.
    2.  Use of any controlled substance or any dangerous drug or dangerous device or alcoholic beverages, to an extent or in a matter dangerous or injurious to himself or herself, any other person, or the public or to the extent that such use impairs his or her ability to conduct with safety to the public the practice authorized by his or her license.

l.  **Unlawful Practice** – actions or conduct that include, but are not limited to:
    1.  Knowingly aiding, assisting, advising, or allowing an unlicensed person to engage in the unlawful practice of registered or practical nursing.
    2.  Violating a rule adopted by the board, an order of the board, or a state or federal law relating to the practice of registered or practical nursing, or a state or federal narcotics or controlled substance law.
    3.  Practicing beyond the scope of practice as stated in this Act.

**Section 4.** *Procedure.* The board shall establish a disciplinary process based on the Administrative Procedure Act of the State of <NAME OF STATE >.

**Section 5.** *Immunity.* Any member of the board or staff and any person reporting to the board of nursing under oath and in good faith information relating to alleged incidents of negligence or malpractice or the qualifications, fitness, or character of a person licensed or applying for a license to practice nursing shall not be subject to a civil action for damages as a result of report such information. The immunity provided by this section shall extend to the members of any professional review committee and witnesses appearing before the committee authorized by the board to act pursuant to this section.

## Article X.  Emergency Relief

**Section 1.** *Summary Suspension.*
a.  Authority.  The board is authorized to temporarily suspend the license of a nurse without a hearing if:
    1.  The board finds that there is probable cause to believe that the nurse has violated a statute or rule that the board is empowered to enforce.
    2.  Continued practice by the nurse would create imminent and serious risk of harm to others.
b.  Duration.  The suspension shall remain in effect until the board issues a stay of suspension or a final order in the matter after a hearing or upon agreement between the board and licensee.
c.  Hearing.  The board shall schedule a disciplinary hearing to be held under the Administrative Procedures Act, to begin no later than < > days after the issuance of the summary suspension order. The licensee shall receive at least < > days notice of the hearing.

**Section 2.** *Automatic Suspension.*
Unless the board orders otherwise, a license to practice nursing is automatically suspended if:
a.  A guardian of a nurse is appointed by order of a court under sections <REFERENCE TO

Appendix 36.4 - National Council of State Boards of Nursing Model Nursing Practice Act cont.

GOVERNING STATE LAW>.

b. The nurse is committed by order of a court under <REFERENCE TO GOVERNING STATE LAW>.

c. The nurse is determined to be mentally incompetent, mentally ill, chemically dependent, or a person dangerous to the public by a court of competent jurisdiction within or without this state.

The license remains suspended until the nurse is restored to capacity by a court, and upon petition by the nurse, the suspension is terminated by the board after a hearing or upon agreement between the board and the nurse.

**Section 3.  *Injunctive Relief.***

a. Authority.  The board or any prosecuting officer upon a proper showing of the facts is authorized to petition a court of competent jurisdiction for an order to enjoin (injunctive relief):

1. Any person who is practicing nursing within the meaning of this Act from practicing without a valid license, unless exempted under Article XII.

2. Any person, firm, corporation, institution, or association from employing any person who is not licensed to practice nursing under this Act or exempted under Article XII.

3. Any person, firm, corporation, institution, or association from operating a school of nursing without approval.

4. Any person whose license has been suspended or revoked from practicing as an RN, LPN/VN, or APRN.

Such acts are declared to be a public nuisance and pose a risk of harm to the public health and safety.

b. The court may without notice or bond, enjoin such acts and practice.  A copy of the complaint shall be served on the defendant, and the proceedings thereafter shall be conducted as in other civil cases.  In case of violation of an injunction issued under this section, the court, or any judge thereof, may summarily try and punish the offender for contempt of court.

**Section 4.  *Preservation of Other Remedies.***  The emergency proceedings herein described shall be in addition to, not in lieu of, all penalties and other remedies provided by law.

# Article XI.  Reporting Required

**Section 1.  *Affected Parties.***

a. Hospitals, nursing homes and other employers of registered nurses, licensed practical/vocational nurses, or advanced practice registered nurses shall report to the board the names of those licensees whose employment has been terminated or who have resigned in order to avoid termination for any reasons stipulated in Article IX, Section 2.

b. Certifying nursing organizations shall report to the board the names of registered nurses, licensed practical/vocational nurses, or advanced practice registered nurses who have been denied certification or recertification for failure to meet certification standards.

**Section 2. *Court Order.***  The board may seek an order from a proper court of competent jurisdiction for a report from any of the parties stipulated in Section 1 of this Article if one is not forthcoming voluntarily.

Appendix 36.4 - National Council of State Boards of Nursing Model Nursing Practice Act cont.

---

**Section 3.** *Penalty.* The board may seek a citation for civil contempt if a court order for a report is not obeyed by any of the parties stipulated in Section 1 of this Article.

**Section 4.** *Immunity.*

a. Any organization or person reporting, in good faith, information to the board under this Article shall be immune from civil action as provided in Article IX, Section 5.

b. A physician or other licensed healthcare professional who, at the request of the board, examines a nurse, shall be immune from suit for damages by the nurse examined if the examining physician or examining healthcare professional conducted the examination and made findings or diagnoses in good faith.

# Article XII. Exemptions

No provisions of this Act shall be construed to prohibit:

a. The practice of nursing that is an integral part of a program by nursing students enrolled in board-approved nursing education programs.

b. An individual engaged in an internship, residency, or other supervised study/practice opportunity as defined by rules of the boards.

c. The rendering of assistance by anyone in the case of an emergency or disaster.

d. The practice of any registered nurses, licensed practical nurses, or advanced practice registered nurses currently licensed in another state, in the provision of nursing care in the case of emergency or disaster.

e. The incidental and gratuitous care of the sick by members of the family, friends, or companions; or household aides at the direction of a person needing such care who resides independently outside any hospital, nursing or healthcare facility, or other similar institutional setting.

f. Caring for the sick in accordance with tenets or practices of any church or religious denomination which teaches reliance upon spiritual means for healing.

g. The practice of any registered nurse, licensed practical nurse or advanced practice registered nurse, currently licensed in another state who is employed by any bureau, division, or agency of the United States government while in the discharge of official governmental duties.

h. The practice of any currently licensed registered nurse, licensed practical nurse, or advanced practice registered nurse who is employed by an individual, agency, or corporation located in another state and whose employment responsibilities include transporting clients into, out of, or through this state. Such exemptions shall be limited to a period not to exceed < > hours for each transport.

i. The practice of any registered nurse, licensed practical nurse, or advanced practice registered nurse currently licensed in another state who is in this state on a nonroutine basis for a period not to exceed < > days to:

    1. Provide care to a client being transported into, out of, or through this state.

    2. Provide professional nursing consulting services.

    3. Attend or present a continuing nursing education program.

    4. Provide other short-term nonclinical nursing services.

j. The practice of any other occupation or profession licensed under the laws of this state, provided that such care does not constitute the practice of nursing within the meaning of this Act.

Appendix 36.4 - National Council of State Boards of Nursing Model Nursing Practice Act cont.

# Article XIII.  Revenue, Fees

**Section 1.** *Revenue.*  The board is authorized to establish and appropriate fees for licensure by examination, reexamination, and endorsement and such other fees and fines as the board determines necessary.

**Section 2.** *Disposition of Fees.*  All fees collected by the board shall be administered according to the established fiscal policies of this state in such manner as to implement adequately the provisions of this Act.

**Section 3.** *Disposition of Fines.*  All fines collected shall be used by and at the discretion of the board for designated projects as established in the fiscal policy of this state.

# Article XIV.  Implementation

**Section 1.** *Effective Date.*  This Act shall take effect <DATE >.

**Section 2.** *Persons Licensed Under a Previous Law.*
a.  Any person holding a license to practice nursing as a registered nurse in this state that is valid on <effective date> shall be deemed to be licensed as a registered nurse under the provisions of this Act and shall be eligible for renewal of such license under the conditions and standards prescribed in this Act.
b.  Any person holding a license to practice nursing as a licensed practical/vocational nurse in this state that is valid on <effective date> shall be deemed to be licensed as a licensed practical/vocational nurse under the provisions of this Act and shall be eligible for renewal of such license under the conditions and standards prescribed in this Act.
c.  Any person eligible for reinstatement of a license as a registered nurse or licensed practical/vocational nurse, respectively, under provisions under the conditions and standards prescribed in the Act by applying for reinstatement according to rules established by the board of nursing.  Application for such reinstatement must be made within < > months of the effective date of this Act.
d.  Any person holding a lapsed license to practice nursing as a registered nurse or licensed practical/vocational nurse in this state on <effective date>, because of failure to renew, may become licensed as a registered nurse or as a licensed practical/vocational nurse, respectively, under the provisions of this Act by applying for reinstatement according to rules established by the board of nursing.  Application for such reinstatement must be made within < > months of the effective date of this Act.
e.  New applicants for advanced practice registered nurse as of <effective date of statute> shall meet requirements set forth in administrative rules.  Any individual authorized to practice in an advanced role prior to <effective date> may apply for licensure on the basis of the individual's prior education and practice as set forth in administrative rule.
f.  Those so licensed under the provisions of Article XIV, Section 2 (a) through (e) above, shall be eligible for renewal of such license under the conditions and standards prescribed by this Act.

**Section 3.** *Severability.*  The provisions of this Act are severable.  If any provision of this Act is declared unconstitutional, illegal, or invalid, the constitutionality, legality, and validity of the

Appendix 36.4 - National Council of State Boards of Nursing Model Nursing Practice Act cont.

remaining portions of this Act shall be unaffected and shall remain in full force and effect.

**Section 4.** *Repeal.*  The laws specified below are repealed except with respect to rights and duties that have matured, penalties that were incurred, and proceedings that were begun before the effective date of this Act.  <LIST STATUTES TO BE REPEALED, FOR EXAMPLE, THE CURRENT NURSING PRACTICE ACT OR APPROPRIATE SECTIONS>.

# Chapter 37: CERTIFICATION IN NURSING

Andrea Tacchi, BSN, MSN, RN

*"Be all you can be" is a familiar phrase, but what does it mean in nursing? Continuing education, self-development, and formal education are ways in which nurses strive to be all they can be. Formal and public acknowledgement of these efforts is provided by certification. Andrea Tacchi discusses the many issues related to certification, providing an insightful look at those many initials that follow so many nurses' names. – Linda Caputi and Lynn Engelmann*

## Introduction

There is a symbiotic relationship between the professions of teaching and nursing. At the heart of good teaching lie a distinct vision, a sense of purpose, a deep commitment to do right, and a deliberate goal to pass along knowledge and provide enthusiasm for learning. At the heart of nursing lies the same! Teaching, as well as lifelong learning, is vital to the profession of nursing. Nurse educators, despite a plethora of philosophies and styles of teaching, hold at least two ideals in common:

- A love for nursing.
- A desire to see nursing students transform from novices to experts as practicing clinicians.

### Educational Philosophy

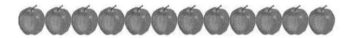

I believe that learning occurs in an atmosphere that is encouraging and non-threatening. As a clinical nursing instructor I see how fear and apprehension can hinder this. It is my goal then, as an instructor, to move students beyond this to foster learning and critical thinking. It is my personal priority to encourage them and to have my passion for nursing be evident to them as I teach at the bedside. – Andrea Tacchi

As the worldwide nursing shortage worsens, recruiting and retaining qualified, skillful nurses is a central issue in ensuring quality in the delivery of health care. Acquiring specialty certification is one way for nurses to validate their clinical competence and demonstrate this competence to the public, their employers, and the nursing profession as a whole. To this end, more research is needed to document this contribution of perceived value that certification brings to nursing practice (Frank-Stromborg, et al., 2002).

In all client-care environments, nurses must maintain clinical competence through lifelong learning. However, what motivates nurses to take that extra step past continuing education to certification? Does certification empower nurses, or do already empowered nurses seek validation for their clinical competency? Are client outcomes impacted when clients are cared for by nurses who are certified? These are the intriguing questions surrounding nursing certification. It is especially vital to explore these factors and assess the impact they have on our consumer-driven healthcare system.

By continually building on strengths and incorporating knowledge and mastery of skills into clinical practice, nursing care and, consequently, the profession of nursing are enhanced. To quote Aristotle, "We are what we repeatedly do. Excellence, then, is not an act but a habit" (*Aristotle Quotes*, 2003).

This chapter discusses certification among registered nurses (RNs) – the passage to expert clinical practice. RNs who choose to pursue and maintain certification in their area of specialty have a distinct vision, a sense of purpose, and a desire for excellence. It is important for faculty in all levels of nursing programs to be familiar with the process of certification and its implications for the profession and client care. Certification is an important consideration for graduating and practicing nurses as well as a requirement for nurses at the advanced practice level. Although many nursing faculty are certified in a nursing specialty, many faculty find it difficult – if not impossible – to meet the clinical hour requirement while maintaining a full-time academic appointment.

## Novice to Expert

Growth in clinical judgment, knowledge, and skill occurs gradually over time. The classic, timeless work of Patricia Benner (1984) provides a profound analysis of excellence in clinical nursing practice. Through dialogue with nurses, Benner identified five levels of competency in clinical nursing practice. These levels are:
- Novice.
- Advanced beginner.
- Competent.
- Proficient.
- Expert.

Nurses accrue clinical knowledge over time. It is a blending of theory, experience, and "know-how" that is central to good nursing judgment.

According to Benner (1984), clinical expertise turns out to be highly influenced by experience with similar client populations; hence, support for clinical specialization is realized. Higher client acuity, shorter hospital stays, unprecedented technological advances, and a competitive healthcare environment are among the many reasons clinical specialty recognition in nursing is especially necessary today as a safeguard for both the profession and the clients receiving care.

Like professionals in many other disciplines, the practice of nurses is regulated from the beginning. A state board of nursing awards an RN license upon satisfactory completion of a nursing program and successful completion of a mandatory national examination. The RN license assures the public that entry-level knowledge and skills to care for clients have been achieved.

Entry-level competence is measured by licensure; specialty knowledge, experience, and clinical judgment are measured by certification. It is an ethical and professional responsibility for nurses to obtain specialty knowledge and skill as their career progresses. In 1996, the National Council of State Boards of Nursing (NCSBN) issued a position paper titled *Assuring Competence: A Regulatory Responsibility*. In this paper, NCSBN identified that one of the greatest challenges to healthcare professionals is the attainment, maintenance, and advancement of professional competence in an evolving healthcare environment.

Advanced-level competence – competence beyond entry-level – can occur many ways. It can occur through formal education programs, continuing education, or clinical practice. Competence development is expected throughout a nurse's career – attaining certification is one way to document this achievement.

The American Nurses Association (ANA) in 1973 initially proposed certification as a way of recognizing superior performance in nursing practice. Over the years, experience and education have emerged as eligibility requirements for pursuing certification. In recognition that certification is an important method of enhancing the visibility and accountability of nurses to the public, the American Nurses Credentialing Center (ANCC), a subsidiary of the ANA since 1991, made certification in the 21st century accessible to all qualified RNs.

Experience, then, is requisite for expert clinical nursing practice. Clinical expertise is central to the advancement of nursing, nursing practice, and nursing science. Providing credentialing for nurses who have established and maintained standards of nursing excellence directly impacts the advancement of nursing.

# The Changing Healthcare Environment: Ensuring Care

The present-day healthcare environment has increased in complexity. Care in this new millennium is characterized by integrated systems, electronic and computer technology, specialization, and inter/transdisciplinary practice (Joel, 2002). The healthcare environment in the United States is currently multicultural, multigenerational, and consumer driven as the public's demand for accountability intensifies. This consumer-driven environment has prompted heightened vigilance from all providers amidst inescapable realities of reports of medication administration errors, unsafe care, escalating costs, and a nursing shortage that is predicted to become a national health crisis.

Clients are more informed and involved in their health care than ever before. Client satisfaction holds profound ramifications for healthcare providers and nurses. Because nursing care is the primary service or product of healthcare systems, it is logical and imperative to promote this resource and attain a positive relationship and balance between nursing, clients, and the various healthcare systems. When client satisfaction, job satisfaction, and professional development are valued, an institution can predict success and market leadership (Woods, 2002).

Nurses are of critical importance in determining the quality of health care, maintaining successful client outcomes, and helping a healthcare system differentiate itself from competitors. Therefore, a commitment to the promotion of nurse certification by a healthcare system helps ensure that nursing practices are consistent with national standards and insulate a facility from becoming myopic (Woods, 2002).

Certification is a venue for assuring quality care and for honoring nurses' stewardship to the public. Certification offers employers and clients an additional validation that a nurse possesses the specialty knowledge, skills, and experience to effectively and safely deliver care.

# A Potpourri of Certification in Nursing

The descriptions and definitions of certification examinations and eligibility criteria are as numerous as the number of certifications available. Criteria vary from each specialty and have changed over the years.

Smolenski (2002) differentiated and explained the six types of credentials that can be awarded to an individual. These include:

- Degree.
- License.
- State designation.
- National certification.

- Award or honor.
- Other certifications.

National certification credentials are awarded by nationally recognized, usually accredited, certifying bodies. Nurse certification credentials are usually linked to the profession, job role, or licensure. As of January 2001, RNs in the United States and Canada held more than 410,000 certifications in 134 specialties (Cary, 2001). Certification is a valued credential offered by the ANA and over 60 various specialty nursing organizations. Specialty organizations include medical-surgical, orthopedic, rehabilitation, occupational health, critical care, oncology, midwifery, neurology, and anesthesia, to name just a few. An RN who attains certification in a specialty-area displays the credentials of RN, C. Smolenski (2002) encouraged the displaying of credentials so clients know the qualifications of those providing care.

The process of certification requires:

- Obtaining considerable practical experience in a specialty area.
- Meeting eligibility criteria.
- Paying a fee, which can range from $150 to $300.
- Successfully completing a nationally administered examination.

A certification board, usually appointed by the parent nursing specialty organization, establishes the eligibility criteria and maintains the content validity of the certifying examination (Raudonis & Anderson, 2002). The content of the certification examination is based fundamentally on the nursing activities and knowledge of that nursing specialty.

Recertification requires rigorous continuing education requirements and hours of clinical practice. Validity periods for certification can vary from two to five years. Recertification represents an ongoing commitment of time, energy, and money. Regardless of the unique area of specialty or the credential sought, each nurse who seeks certification is committed to personal excellence as well as excellence for the nursing profession.

## Perceptions of Certified Nurses

Now more than ever, it is crucial to assess the certified nurse workforce's contributions to high-quality health care and to the profession of nursing. Cary's (2001) research reports on nurses' perspectives on the effect of certification attainment. The International Study of the Certified Workforce conducted by the Nursing Credentialing Research Coalition (NCRC) is the largest study to date on certification, based on a random sample of 19,452 nurses from the registries of 23 certifying organizations in the United States, Canada, and

United States territories.

Data revealed that certified RNs believed they were recognized as experts in their specialty area by their colleagues. Certified nurses were empowered in the domains of their personal and professional lives as well as in their careers and practice. Cary (2001) found that an impressive 77% of respondents experienced personal growth and 67% reported being more satisfied as professional nurses. Certified RNs reported serving as a resource to staff for client-care concerns and as a resource for organizational consultation. Certification brought about satisfaction with the RN's position as well as career aspirations.

What is most compelling are the responses Cary (2001) noted from certified RNs regarding their nursing practice. Certification enabled these RNs to experience:

- More competency with their skills as professional nurses.
- More regard as credible providers.
- More accountability as professional nurses.
- More confidence in their ability to make decisions and to detect early signs and symptoms of complications in their clients.

It is important to note that Cary's research is based on self-reports. There is a need for more research studies to support this data.

Foley, Kee, Minick, Harvey, and Jennings (2002) reported that autonomy, control over practice, and nurse-physician relationships were factors identified that foster clinical expertise and favorable work environments. These professional-practice attributes illuminate the profession of nursing and the best of nursing practice. Characteristics of certified nurses described parallel the essential characteristics of "magnet" hospital nurses (Aiken & Havens, 2000). The term magnet is used by the ANCC to denote a hospital that serves as a magnet – attracting a reputation for excellence in nursing that is among the finest in the nation. An in-depth discussion about the current "Magnet Movement" is beyond the scope of this chapter; however, the role that RN certification plays in the Magnet Movement certainly is not.

## RN Certification and the Magnet Movement

Magnet hospitals promote and sustain professional nursing practice by investing in the education and expertise of nurses. Supporting professional certification is one way this is accomplished. Magnet hospitals also excel at recruiting and retaining highly skilled, experienced, and professional nurses.

Employers need to support and sustain continued growth and learning for their nurses. This is the beginning of a successful strategy for developing a truly magnetic environment that fosters a culture of nursing professionalism and a culture that protects and safeguards the public it serves.

## Fostering Certification

Burdened with increasingly heavy client loads, nurses are tired of settling for less and simply making do (Mee & Robinson, 2003). In reality, burn-out among nurses has for too long permeated the profession.

This dissatisfaction is clearly evident from Aiken's study (cited in Mee & Robinson, 2003) – a multinational study of 43,000 nurses. More than 40% of respondents working in hospitals in the United States reported dissatisfaction with their jobs. A myriad of factors contributed to this dissatisfaction. The factors include a lack of a strong professional practice environment, inadequate collaboration, and lack of respect for the nursing role from employers and physicians. It is especially interesting that these are the same factors nurses who have achieved certification identified as benefits!

It is the collective attitudes and actions of individuals that can transform the feelings of burnout in the profession to feelings of hardiness. It is an important lesson for students to learn they must challenge themselves and strive to serve as a catalyst for change. This is evident in many Master's of Nursing programs where certification is part of the degree requirements.

Nurse educators must foster in students the commitment to lifelong learning. Nurse managers and administrators must view education of the nurse workforce in an institution as an organizational attribute. Staff nurses must support and mentor each other as they uphold elements of professional nursing practice as a priority. It becomes clear that every member of the healthcare equation can reap the rewards from professional nursing certification.

What are the reasons for nurses becoming certified or remaining uncertified? In Redd and Alexander's (1997) study of certified and noncertified nurses in several acute-care hospitals, personal achievement was the most frequently given reason, and professional growth was the second most frequently given reason for seeking certification. Lack of experience and lack of personal time were the most frequently given reasons for not becoming certified.

Similar results were documented by Coleman et al (1999). They also learned that the desire to be recognized as a specialist and a perception that certification is important to career development were additional reasons nurses sought certification. Reasons for not seeking certification included feelings that certification would not be relevant or financially rewarding.

Results from focus groups of certified critical-care nurses (American Association of Critical-Care Nurses [AACN], 2003) also revealed personal satisfaction as the most important reason for seeking critical care certification. The nurses, however, expressed strong dissatisfaction regarding the overall lack of recognition for their critical-carecertification by hospital administrators.

The literature reveals that a desire to keep current with the latest knowledge and best practices of nursing, along with an intrinsic desire to be the best one can be, serves as the motivation for nurses to become certified (Thew, 2003). The letter in Figure 37.1, submitted to *AACN News* (Kummer, 2001), illustrates one nurse's personal account of her process of pursuing and successfully achieving certification.

Figure 37.1 - One Nurse's Testimony

Dear AACN News,

Although I had been a nurse for about 12 years, the last 7 in critical care, I felt the need to learn more. I decided that studying for the CCRN exam was the best way to do this.

To prepare, I used critical care textbooks, review books, audiotapes, and practice tests, investing at least an hour or more daily for 4 months. I was shocked when, on the first practice test, I answered only about half the questions correctly. It seemed the more I learned, the more I needed to know, and the more I realized that I didn't know. It was quite an eye-opening process.

When the time came, I certainly did not feel ready to take the test. I had been sufficiently humbled by the people I had met and the material I had learned over my intense months of studying. To me, it seemed that everyone knew so much, and I knew so little. Although I was intimidated by the knowledge that I expected I should have learned, I was somehow happy and privileged to be sitting for such a prestigious exam.

When I received my test scores, I had not only passed; I had done quite well. I felt so proud that I had accomplished this goal in my life. Somehow, I knew that I would be able to deliver much better patient care with that added confidence.

I have renewed my CCRN twice and continue to read journals and attend conferences to maintain and add to the knowledge that I worked so hard to obtain. Now, as a CCRN liaison for my ICU, I am proud when one of my coworkers expresses an interest in taking the certification exam.

Making the decision to become certified is such an important step in a nurse's career. It means we have made the commitment to our specialty and to our patients. It is a part of me that I am extremely proud of.

Deborah Kummer, RN, BS, CCRN

### *Taking Action to Keep the Momentum Going*

Specialization and certification contribute to the professional growth of nursing as well as demonstrate competence to the public and employers. The number of RN candidates seeking certification increases annually (Woods, 2002). The call to action is for the entire healthcare industry to keep the certification momentum going. The members of the healthcare industry who can directly influence this goal include:

- RNs holding certification.
- Specialty organizations.
- Employers.
- Healthcare clients.

Certified nurses who enthusiastically promote the benefits of certification to uncertified colleagues can help keep the momentum going. The desire for certification can promote camaraderie, strengthen collegial relationships among staff, and promote staff unity.

Tenney, Golden-Baker, DeMoucell, and Wians (1993) described how the nursing department of a rehabilitation hospital developed a certification program to promote specialty certification among its nursing staff. A campaign was mounted promoting the professional organization and the certification program. Financial support and a review course were provided as incentives from the employer and proved to be important factors in the implementation process. A newly certified staff nurse shared her experience in preparing for the examination. She described the personal, renewed, commitment she experienced after attaining certification. She believed certification gives nurses the opportunity to interact with their peers, and be stimulated and energized.

### *Benefits at the Bedside*

Providing high-quality health care should be a major concern to all client-care professionals. Hospitals must look at nurses as a critical component to sustain successful client outcomes. Amid a vast array of system challenges, it is nursing's contribution that influences client care.

Research conducted by Needleman, Buerhaus, Mattke, Stewart, and Zelevinsky (2002) concludes that a higher proportion of hours of nursing care provided by RNs and a greater number of hours of care by RNs per day are associated with better care for hospitalized clients. Aside from staffing numbers and nurse-client ratios, Needleman, et al. point to other factors associated with quality care in hospitals that directly influence client outcomes. These factors include effective communication between nurses and physicians and a positive work environment. Promoting a professional culture in an institution can only prove to have a positive effect. Professional certification is one way to promote a professional culture, ensure quality care, and ultimately protect clients.

The NCRC study, referenced earlier in this chapter, found that certification has a dramatic impact on the personal, professional, and practice outcomes of certified nurses (ANCC, 2000). The study was based on the assumption that if certified nurses attribute favorable changes in their practice and professional development to certification, then the attainment of certification contributes to improved nurse, client, and system outcomes (Cary, 2001). Nurses in this study stated that certification enabled them to experience fewer adverse events and errors in client care. They reported experiencing more confidence in their ability to detect early signs and symptoms of complications. Redd and Alexander (1997) compared performance between certified and uncertified nurses and found that certified nurses performed better in the areas of teaching/collaboration and planning/evaluation than their uncertified colleagues.

The NCRC study (ANCC, 2000) revealed that certified nurses received high client satisfaction ratings and reported more effective communication and collaboration with other healthcare providers. Of particular interest, some of the nurses surveyed stated they experienced fewer disciplinary events and work-related injuries. These study participants reported that financial rewards for attaining certification included salary increases and bonuses. Many noted they were reimbursed for certification expenses.

The increased trust and professional visibility that certification can bring to the eyes of the public is vital for nursing as a whole. The ANCC (1999) reported that 87% of Americans would be more confident if they knew their nurses were certified. The above-mentioned data is significant and provides strong evidence linking nurse certification to positive client outcomes, increased public support, and nurse satisfaction.

## Conclusion

This chapter discussed nurse certification and the benefits that certification can bring to the nursing profession, clients, and employers. Advocating this distinctive credential must be in the forefront of healthcare discussions and is the responsibility of nurses, employers, and the public. Certification suggests superior performance, competence in a specialty area, and assurance of quality care.

## Websites

Following are two websites about ANCC. For easy launching, these website addresses are located on the CD accompanying this book. Simply launch your internet browser, put the CD-ROM in the drive, go to Chapter 37 on the CD, and then click on the website address.

To learn about ANCC go to:
http://www.nursecredentialing.org/index.htm
To learn about ANCC's Magnet Recognition Program go to:
http://www.nursecredentialing.org/magnet/magnet.htm

# Learning Activities

1. Explore the requirements for attaining nursing certification in your area of specialty.
2. Interview nurses in your student body and identify what motivating factors would influence their personal desire to seek or not to seek nursing certification, or perhaps renew their nursing certification.
3. Develop an implementation program for an institution-wide nursing certification promotion effort.

## References

Aiken, L. H., & Havens, D. S. (2000). The magnet nursing services recognition program. *American Journal of Nursing, 100*(3), 26-35.

American Association of Critical Care Nurses [AACN]. (2003). Safeguarding the patient and the profession: The value of critical care nurse certification. *American Journal of Critical Care, 12*(2), 154-164.

American Nurses Credentialing Center [ANCC]. (2000). Certified nurses report fewer adverse events. Retrieved April 21, 2003, from http://www.ana.org/pressrel/2000/ pr0211a.htm

American Nurses Credentialing Center [ANCC]. (1999). Americans support rigorous standards for nursing care. Retrieved April 21, 2003, from http://www.ana.org/ pressrel/1999/pr0507.htm

*Aristotle quotes*. (2003). Retrieved April 30, 2003, from http://www.ollympicpc.com/ quotes/aristotle.html

Benner, P. (1984). *From novice to expert*. Menlo Park, CA: Addison-Wesley.

Cary, A. H. (2001). Certified registered nurses: Results of the study of the certified workforce. *American Journal of Nursing, 101*(4), 44-52.

Coleman. E. A., Frank-Stromberg, M., Hughes, L. C., Gatson-Grindel, C., Ward, S., Berry, D., Oleske, D. M., & Miller-Murphy, C. (1999). A national survey of certified, recertified, and noncertified oncology nurses: Comparisons and contrasts. *Oncology Nursing Forum, 26*(5), 839-849.

Foley, B. J., Kee, C. C., Minick, P., Harvey, S. S., & Jennings, B. M. (2002). Characteristics of nurses and hospital work environments that foster satisfaction and clinical expertise. *Journal of Nursing Administration, 32*(5), 273-282.

Frank-Stromborg, M., Ward, S., Hughes, L., Brown, K., Coleman, A., Grindel, C., & Murphy, C. (2002). Does certification status of oncology nurses make a different in patient outcomes? *Oncology Nursing Forum, 29*(4), 665-672.

Joel, L. A. (2002). Reflections and projections on nursing. *Nursing Administrative Quarterly, 26*(5), 11-17.

Kummer, D. (2001). One nurse's testimony. *AACN News*, Aliso Viejo, CA: American Association of Critical Care Nurses.

Mee, C. L., & Robinson, E. (2003). What's different about this nursing shortage? *Nursing 2003, 33*(1), 51-55.

National Council of State Boards of Nursing [NCSBN]. (1996). Assuring competence: A regulatory responsibility. Retrieved April 29, 2003, from http://www.ncsbn.org/ public/resources/ncsbn_publicpro.htm

Needleman, J., Buerhaus, P., Mattke, S., Stewart, M., & Zelevinsky, K. (2002). Nurse staffing levels and the quality of care in hospitals. *New England Journal of Medicine, 346*(22), 1715-1722.

Raudonis, B. M., & Anderson, C. M. (2002). A theoretical framework for specialty certification in nursing certification in nursing practice. *Nursing Outlook, 50*(6), 247-252.

Redd, M. L., & Alexander, J. W. (1997, February). Does certification mean better performance? *Nursing Management, 28*(2), 45-49.

Smolenski, M. C. (2002, July). Playing the credentials game. *Nursing Spectrum.* Retrieved April 7, 2003, from http://community.nursingspectrum.com/Magazine Articles/article.cfm?AID=7126

Tenney, J., Golden-Baker, S. B., DeMoucell, P. J., & Wians, K. M. (1993). Empowerment through rehabilitation nursing certification. *Rehabilitation Nursing, 18*(4), 231-236.

Thew, J. (2003, March). Neuro nurses stretch their brains with certification exam. *Nursing Spectrum, 16*(61), 13.

Woods, D. K. (2002). Realizing your marketing influence, Part 3: Professional certification as a marketing tool. *Journal of Nursing Administration, 32*(7/8), 379-386.

## Bibliography

Hughes, L., Ward, S., Grindel, C., Coleman, E., Berry, D., Hinds, P., Oleske, D., Murphy, C., & Frank-Stromborg, M. (2001). Relationships between certification and job perceptions of oncology nurses. *Oncology Nursing Forum, 28*(1), 99-106.

# Legal Issues in Nursing Education

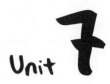

# Chapter 38: THE LAW AND THE NURSE EDUCATOR: A LOOK AT LEGAL CASES

Nancy J. Brent, MS, JD, RN

*Teaching nursing has so very many dimensions – one of which is legalities. As in all aspects of life, ignorance of the law is no excuse. Faculty must be cognizant of all the legal issues applicable to teaching nursing students and never unknowingly violate a student's legal rights. Knowledge of the laws applicable to education help guide faculty in developing curriculum, crafting program policies, and making decisions about individual student situations. This chapter is an excellent primer for all faculty, as well as a resource that can be revisited if the need arises. – Linda Caputi and Lynn Engelmann*

## Introduction

The rights of students in post-secondary institutions have developed over the years to include protections unheard of prior to the 1930s. Students in both private and public academic institutions simply "did the best one could" when it came to challenging the institution's decisions concerning – for example – admission, continuation in the school or program, or grading. Clearly, the development of student rights, albeit slow, has blossomed into a large body of legal theories and protections afforded students in all post-secondary schools. Although there are some clear distinctions of those rights based upon whether one is a student in a public or private school, the rights and protections of both student groups are real and firmly in place. Those rights and protections have been and continue to be shaped and refined by continued student challenges to almost every facet of post-secondary life.

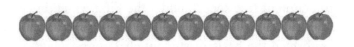

### Educational Philosophy

I believe that teaching in an interactive process. A student must be challenged if he or she is to learn. Learning can not take place unless both the teacher and the student actively participate in the process. – Nancy J. Brent

Faculty rights in post-secondary academic settings have also developed over the years but probably more slowly than those of students. Again, faculty in public institutions of higher learning enjoyed many more protections earlier than did their colleagues in private post-secondary schools. Even so, the protections and rights of faculty in both entities continue to exist and will continue to be shaped by recent developments in education, including distance learning, tenure, contract law, and intellectual property law.

This chapter provides an overview of the legal theories for students in nursing education programs in both public and private settings. Selected legal issues of concern to students in both types of education programs are also highlighted. Selected legal concerns for faculty in both types of educational programs are also explored, with an emphasis on the distinctions between faculty of public post-secondary schools and faculty teaching in private universities or colleges.

## Overview of Legal Theories for Students in Nursing Education Programs

### *Public Post-Secondary Institutions*

### *Constitutional Parameters*

The United States Constitution's Bill of Rights contains important and vital protections for all individuals vis-à-vis the federal and state government. Nursing students in public post-secondary academic institutions are no exception. For example, the First Amendment protects freedom of religion, press, speech, the right to assemble, and the right to petition the government for the redress of grievances. Students in public academic settings have attempted to use the Amendment's protections when adverse decisions were made against the student allegedly based on the First Amendment's areas of protection. As an example, a student who was a member of the Church of Jesus Christ of Latter-day Saints (Mormon) at the University of Utah unsuccessfully challenged the requirement of using profanity and disrobing during acting classes and acting performances.[1] Also, in *Orin V. Barclay*[2], Olympic Community College's arrest of a student at an anti-abortion protest organized by the student and based on his religious beliefs was held to be a violation of the student's protection of free speech under the First Amendment.

Likewise, the Fourth Amendment's protection against unreasonable searches and seizures has formed the basis of student challenges when dormitory or other living quarters were searched by public college or university officials.[3] The Fourth Amendment's protections have also been raised by students when drug or alcohol testing is initiated by the college or university. Perhaps the most important legal challenge to a public university or college's conduct with the student in its academic programs, however, rests in the Fifth and Fourteenth Amendments' protections of due process.

***Due process.*** The Fifth and Fourteenth Amendments protect individuals from a restriction or loss of certain rights by the federal and state government respectively. In addition to other protections in both Amendments, the concept of due process is an important one. The Amendments state that no federal or state government can take away "life, liberty, or property without due process of law." What life, liberty, or property are has been defined in both fixed and fluid ways. For example, there is no doubt that the term life means one's very existence. As a result, a government can not carry out the death penalty for a convicted criminal until and unless all due process protections are afforded the criminal. Property includes not only one's real property or personal items in one's possession but also the concept of entitlement. For example, a license to practice a profession has been interpreted as a property right. As a result, it can not be revoked, disciplined, or suspended without due process protections by the governmental agency empowered with enforcing and administering a state practice act.

The concept of due process is a complex and variable concept as well. It has different meanings and ramifications, depending upon the situation that is being evaluated by a court. For example, an individual facing incarceration due to the alleged violation of a crime (his or her liberty right thus at issue) faces far more due process rights than a student in a post-secondary program who faces dismissal from an academic program.

Even so, due process has generally been defined as what is fair in the circumstances.[4] Because it would be impossible to define each and every due process protection for every circumstance, courts have generally resolved the dilemma of what is fair by asking, "What process is due?" By evaluating the right that is being threatened and then identifying which protections should be afforded, the concept of due process continues to protect old as well as new rights.

In the educational setting, the due process rights of students in public schools were delineated in the 1961 case *Dixon v. State of Alabama.*[5] In this case, six students at the Alabama State College for Negroes in Montgomery, Alabama, were expelled from the school without notice and without a hearing for alleged misconduct, which many at the time believed was the students' participation in a civil rights demonstration.[6] The students filed a suit in federal court asking for a preliminary and permanent injunction against the school prohibiting it from expelling the students. The federal district court ruled in favor of the school, and the students appealed that decision. The Court of Appeals for the Fifth Circuit reversed the district court's decision and remanded (sent back) the case for further proceedings consistent with its opinion.

In its opinion, the Fifth Circuit Court of Appeals was specific in its requirements for public institutions and dismissals for alleged misconduct. It held that the due process protections of the Fourteenth Amendment applied to students in public institutions. As a result, the Amendment mandated that public academic institutions provide certain due process protections to its students **prior** to expulsion. Those protections are notice of the allegations against the students, notice of the hearing scheduled, and a hearing that allows both sides to present their respective positions (the exact nature being dependent upon the allegations the student is facing). Moreover, the appeals court held that a student should be provided with the names of any witnesses who would be called to testify against them in the hearing, what the witnesses would testify to, and an opportunity for the student to present his or her own witnesses and defenses to the charges. Last, if the hearing were held before an official body of the school (in this case, the board of education), the student was entitled to a written copy of the body's findings and decision.

The *Dixon* (1961) case was important, but it was not until the United States Supreme Court's decision in *Goss v. Lopez*[7] that its full significance was felt in the academic community. The Supreme Court held that the protections in *Dixon* (1961) applied to **all** students facing a suspension or explusion from a public institution, whether grade school, high school, or college or university. In addition to its support of the Fourteenth Amendment's due process protections, the Court also opined that students in public schools possess a liberty interest in their good name and reputation that is also protected by the Fourteenth Amendment. When a suspension or explusion occurs, the damage to the student's reputation may follow the student for the rest of his or her time in the school setting. As a result, the protections supported in both the *Dixon* and *Goss* cases provide some balance for the student when the school does take action against a student by requiring that the school not act in an arbitrary or unfair manner.

Due process protections are often paired with other constitutional shields as students make their way through academic programs. For example, the Fourteenth Amendment's Equal Protection Clause has been the basis of many suits alleging that a public entity made decisions differently for students similarly situated, as in *Cobb v. Rector and Visitors of the University of Virginia*[8].

In *Cobb*, Jonathan Cobb, who was African-American, was dismissed from the University in 1997 for cheating on an exam in his economics course. Cobb's position was that other students at the University were treated differently when charged with cheating on exams and that this was one of the reasons the Honor Committee found him guilty of cheating and recommended his removal from the program. He filed suit in federal district court, alleging many causes of action against the University. One of his claims was that the University violated his equal protection under the Fourteenth Amendment. The University asked the court to enter a summary judgment in its favor, as it argued there was no material issue of fact supporting Cobb's allegations.

The federal district court carefully analyzed Cobb's allegations. Cobb said that the Honor Committee had dismissed reported honor violations against several other students based on the length of time their cases had been pending before the Committee, yet did not do the same thing for his case, which had also been pending for some time. He alleged, therefore, that the Honor Committee practiced "racially biased prosecution" by litigating only certain students' cheating. The court held that because Cobb raised the concern that similarly situated students were treated differently based on their race, he should be permitted to go forward with this allegation at a trial. This allegation, therefore, was not summarily dismissed, and he was allowed to proceed to trial on this and other issues raised in his suit.

In addition to the constitutional parameters to which a public college or university must adhere, state and federal laws also exist that govern the student's academic journey from admission through attempted completion of the program. It is important to remember that none of the protections afforded students in public institutions are mutually exclusive; that is, one or more may be alleged in one suit challenging an institution's decisions or actions.

### *Admission to College or University*

In 1978, the United States Supreme Court decision in *Regents of the University of California v. Bakke*[9] (often called the "reverse discrimination case" because Bakke was White) held invalid procedures established by the University that considered race in its admission procedures. The Court characterized the procedures as establishing racial quotas. The University was ordered to admit Bakke into its medical school and enjoined the University from using race as a criterion in its admission procedures.

In two highly interesting cases dealing with admission policies at the University of Michigan, the issue of reverse discrimination or "affirmative action" has again raised its head. In the current cases, the focus is on whether White applicants are hindered in the admission process when a diverse student body is a goal of the academic institution. In *Gratz v. Bollinger*[10] and *Grutter v. Bollinger*[11], White students filed class-action suits against the University of Michigan alleging its affirmative action policies and admission customs discriminated against them because the University used different criteria to admit students of different races. The undergraduate and law schools both used race as one consideration in its admission procedure.

The U.S. District Court for the Eastern District of Michigan issued an opinion in the *Gratz* case that involves the undergraduate school. The judge held that diversity in higher education is a compelling interest sufficient to survive the constitutional mandate of strict scrutiny when evaluating whether discrimination is present and, therefore, upheld the University's current admission procedures. The case was appealed to the Sixth Circuit Court of Appeals, but the Court has not yet heard the case. In addition, attorneys for the plaintiffs have filed a request for review by the United States Supreme Court. The Court has not yet decided to review the case.[12]

The same U.S. District Court issued an opinion in the *Grutter* case in 2001, albeit by a different judge. The opinion stated that using race as one plus factor in addition to others that are evaluated in the admission process by the law school was not unconstitutional. In addition, the judge held that the law school's reason for utilizing race as a factor (diversity in the student body) is not a compelling state interest. The decision was appealed by the plaintiffs to the 6th Circuit Court of Appeals.

The Sixth Circuit Court of Appeals rendered its decision in May, 2002. The Appeals Court, in a 5-4 decision, held that diversity in higher education is a "compelling state interest" sufficient to survive the strict scrutiny test required by the U.S. Constitution. As a result, the race-plus admission process is constitutional. Further, the appeals court opined that the race-plus factor, with its intended purpose of enrolling a "critical mass" of underrepresented students, was not a quota system. Rather, the opinion continued, it was an appropriate, narrowly tailored method of achieving racial diversity required for students to have a broad-based education. Last, but also important, the opinion underscored the importance of deference to the law school's "educational judgment and expertise" when making admission decisions[13].

*Grutter* appealed to the United States Supreme Court. The decision will affect how institutions of post-secondary education manage their admission procedures.

### Continuation in University or College Programs

Often, a student's ability to successfully progress through a program and graduate meets with many roadblocks. Some of the obstacles are due to the student's inability to master the course or program requirements. When the student does not do so successfully, an academic dismissal of the student from the program and university can occur. Academic dismissals raise interesting legal issues for both the student and the academic entity and are discussed in the next section. When the student's inability to continue toward graduation is due to the academic institution's alleged discrimination and alleged violations of other federal laws, a federal lawsuit filed by the student can occur.

In *Gossett v. State of Oklahoma ex rel Board of Regents for Langston University*[14], a male nursing student believed he was the victim of gender discrimination that resulted in violations of his rights of equal protection, due process, and Title IX protections. Although Gossett had successfully completed the first semester in the school of nursing, during the second semester in the Process II course he did not fare as well. The instructors of the course were both female. When Gossett sought help from the instructors, he claimed that male students were not receiving the same academic help that female students were receiving. Gossett received a D in the class, and according to the nursing school policy, this grade resulted in his dismissal from the nursing program. He appealed the grade pursuant to school policy, but his appeal was denied. Moreover, his attempts to re-enter the nursing program were also met with denials.

Gossett filed suit in federal district court, alleging violations of 42 U.S.C. Section 1983[15] and Title IX[16]. Gossett's proof to support his allegations was interesting. He said that the instructors used the grade of incomplete to help students who were failing the course so they had more time to complete the required work, but female students were the main benefactors of this policy. He also stated that of the 24 students in the class, all the female students passed but only two of the five male students passed the course. Last, Gossett presented to the court two affidavits from a former student and a former instructor of the school. Both corroborated that special treatment was given to female students by the faculty and the dean of the nursing school.

The federal district trial court granted a summary judgment for the school, holding that there was no material issue of fact in Gossett's applications and the school was entitled to a judgment without going to a trial. The appeals court reversed the trial court, holding that Gossett had in fact presented sufficient evidence for a trial to determine whether his allegations were true. The case was sent back to the trial court for a trial.

## *Evaluation/Grading*

One of the largest areas of legal concern to students and faculty alike in the area of grading and evaluation are the consequences that flow from "not making the grade." When a student does not meet the academic requirements of a particular program, his or her continuation in the program, and indeed in the college or university itself, becomes highly questionable. Interestingly, faculty members believe that their ability to honestly grade a student's success in the classroom is greatly constrained by the student's threat of legal action if the grade earned is not what the student believes it should be. Moreover, when a program involves a clinical component to the overall passing requirement for the student, faculty members are often hesitant to give a grade for that portion of the student's overall grade that may result in the student's dismissal from the program and/or university.

Regardless of the origin of the misconceptions faculty members possess about grading, there is no question that the beliefs are incorrect. In 1978, the United States Supreme Court decided a landmark case that identified faculty rights when making **academic** decisions as opposed to **disciplinary** decisions, such as those in *Dixon* and *Goss*. The case, *Board of Curators of the University of Missouri v. Horowitz*[17], was particularly significant because it held that neither public or private academic institutions needed to provide a due process hearing prior to a dismissal for **academic** reasons.

Charlotte Horowitz was a student in the medical school at the University of Missouri, a public university. Ms. Horowitz had outstanding academic credentials. For example, she had graduated from Barnard College and Columbia University with a bachelor and master's degree respectively. Her testing scores during her medical school rotations at the

University of Missouri were also excellent. Even so, after the first year of medical school, the dean informed Horowitz in writing that she was being placed on academic probation. The reason for the probation was given as several specific deficiencies during her clinical rotation in pediatrics that included poor handwashing technique, inconsistent attendance during the rotation, and poor relationships with others. Ms. Horowitz was told that improvement was needed in the areas discussed with her, but that she would be allowed to continue to the next rotational unit in the curriculum.

Years two and three of medical school were completed by Ms. Horowitz, but the faculty was not satisfied with her improvement in the areas for which she had been placed on probation after her first year. The school's Council on Evaluation recommended that she not graduate. Ms. Horowitz was told that if she did not agree with the Council's decision, she could take a set of oral and practical exams by several of the medical school faculty who had no previous contact with her. She was also informed that their decision would be final as to her continuation or dismissal from the program. Unfortunately, the seven faculty could not agree as to Ms. Horowitz's student status. In fact, there was no majority decision by the faculty members as to what to recommend to the Council on Evaluation and the dean.

The Council on Evaluation decided not to allow Ms. Horowitz to graduate in May of 1973 and informed her of this decision in writing. In addition, the Council also decided to dismiss her from the program based on her lack of improvement in the areas identified after her first year in the medical school. The Council's decisions were processed through the University's required procedures and agreed to by the dean. Horowitz appealed the decision pursuant to the University's appeal procedures, but the decision was upheld.

Horowitz filed suit in federal district court alleging a violation of her Fourteenth Amendment rights of due process and a violation of her civil rights under 42 U.S.C. Section 1983. The federal district court, after a trial, dismissed the case, holding that all due process protections had been afforded Ms. Horowitz. She appealed, and the Eighth Circuit Court of Appeals held that because a dismissal from medical school can seriously jeopardize the student's ability to obtain work after graduation – framed as a liberty right by the Court – a due process hearing was required **before** dismissal[18].

The University appealed the Appeals Court decision to the United States Supreme Court. The United States Supreme Court unanimously reversed the Appellate Court decision. Characterizing the dismissal decision in Horowitz as an academic one, the Court held that there was no requirement of a hearing prior to dismissal. Academic decisions, the Court explained, are based on a subjective determination of a student's abilities and on a "continuing relationship between faculty and students"[19], whereas disciplinary decisions require a determination of the facts of the particular situation. The student-faculty relationship, according to the Court, is based on the expertise and evaluation of the faculty member who decides about a student's performance over a period of time. Because a court can not place itself in the shoes of a faculty member to evaluate academic performance, courts will not encroach upon those decisions unless the faculty makes a decision that is arbitrary, capricious, or in bad faith.

The Court also held that Ms. Horowitz's claims that her property and liberty rights were violated were unfounded because the dismissal was an academic one, not a disciplinary one. Moreover, the Court opined that even if one assumed these rights existed, Horowitz had been given as much due process as the Fourteenth Amendment would require.[20]

The *Horowitz* decision is still good law today and stands for the ability of faculty to make reasoned and careful academic decisions about a public or private student's progress in a program of academic study. Clearly, no hearing prior to an academic dismissal is required, although if a school decides to provide one, that can occur.

*Horowitz* also safeguards students as well. Adequate notice must be given to the student concerning his or her progression or lack thereof in the program, along with clear parameters concerning where improvement must occur and by when that improvement must be demonstrated. The ramifications of not meeting the necessary improvements must also be told to the student.

The Court did not resolutely define the difference between disciplinary dismissals and academic ones that might not be as clear as the *Horowitz* case, however. Students and faculty in public academic institutions can be assured, though, that when there is a doubt as to the nature of a dismissal, the prudent course of action would be to grant a hearing prior to the dismissal.

### Graduation/Granting of Degree

Successfully completing a program of study and obtaining one's degree is the goal of most, if not all, students in post-secondary institutions. Students in public schools can use the Fourteenth Amendment and other constitutional provisions when that goal is thwarted, as has already been discussed. Students whose degrees are not granted or who do not graduate can also use the theories of a breach of an express or an implied contract. Contract law is the most common allegation available to students in private academic institutions, but those in public post-secondary schools benefit from such a cause of action as well.

For example, in *Grine v. Board of Trustees*[21], Michael Grine was a doctoral student at the University of Arkansas's marketing program. Grine had a deadline of October 1995 to finish his doctorate in order to take a teaching position in Oklahoma. Although a faculty member had assured Grine that he could finish by that date, as the start of the academic year in September 1995 drew near, Grine was told it was doubtful he could finish by October of that year.

Grine's problems in meeting his deadline were due to one faculty member, a Dr. Dub Ashton. According to Grine, Ashton did not read the drafts of his dissertation in a timely manner. When Grines complained to the department head, he returned the drafts with comments that were negative rather than positive, as his comments had been on earlier drafts. After Ashton told him that he was angry that he had gone to the department head and informed him that it was clear that Grine had no idea what a dissertation was supposed to look like, Grine took his dissertation to several other faculty members. Their response was similar to Ashton's.

Grine was not able to finish his dissertation by October due to the faculty members' responses to his dissertation. Moreover, the University's seven-year requirement for the completion of a dissertation had expired. Grine sued the university and several faculty members, including Ashton. Grine alleged fraud and breach of contract against the defendants. He also asked that the university be enjoined from enforcing the seven-year requirement. Last, Grine also asked for damages.

The state trial court dismissed the case against the University and the faculty members, holding that the University and its officials were entitled to sovereign immunity under the Arkansas Constitution. Grine appealed the decision to the Supreme Court of Arkansas.

The Arkansas Supreme Court held that Grine was not entitled to injunctive relief. Only the University and its board could exercise such a power. Moreover, Grine's allegations that the University and the faculty members' decisions were capricious, in bad faith, and arbitrary were without a basis in fact. The Court found no merit in those allegations and upheld the lower court's decision based on the defendants' constitutional and statutory sovereign immunity. The Court also dismissed the count in the complaint against Dr. Ashton, but did so without prejudice in the event Grine wanted to proceed against him individually.

*Grine* illustrates the difficulty students have in obtaining relief from public academic institutions. It also illustrates the ability of the faculty to make reasoned and careful decisions involving a student's progress toward the completion of the program and a degree, so long as the decisions are well documented, within the expertise of the faculty, and not arbitrary, capricious, or in bad faith.

Other case decisions have also upheld a school or program's change in requirements prior to graduation or the granting of a degree. Although such cases are decided on a case-by-case basis, in *Mendez v. Reynolds*[22], for example, the court upheld a change by Hostos Community College's curriculum committee from the requirement of one exam that tested a student's ability to understand how to write to another exam, then reversed itself, and said that the first test, the CUNY Writing Assessment Test, must be passed prior to graduation. The passage of the test before graduation was an emergency resolution and was made without prior notice to the students. Several students who had taken the first exam but not the CUNY Writing Assessment Test, filed suit, alleging that the decision of the College was arbitrary and capricious. In addition, the students alleged that because they had relied on the College's faculty's advisement as to which test to take, they requested that the College be stopped from not awarding them a degree (equitable estoppel).

The trial court granted the students their request for equitable estoppel and ordered the students graduated who had completed all of the College's requirements except the passing of the CUNY Writing Aptitude Test. The decision was appealed by the College.

The appeals court reversed the trial court, holding that regardless of the change from one writing test to another, the college curriculum committee that recommended the change could simply **recommend** changes. Because the College retains the right to enforce such changes, the committee's recommendation was of no legal effect. The court also held that it would be against public policy to order students be graduated when they had not fulfilled all of the academic requirements set by the College. Last, no arbitrary and capricious decision making by the College trustees was found.

### *Private Post-Secondary Institutions*

#### *Contract Law*

Contract law has been a protector of students in private institutions for some time. Although not the only legal source of support for students in private institutions, it has been extremely helpful for students who clearly do not have the protections of a state or the federal constitution. The use of the contract theory for students in post-secondary private entities was greatly aided by the states' reduction of the age from 21 to 18 as the legal age of capacity to enter into contracts[23].

Traditional contract theory applied to students in post-secondary academic institutions is rooted in the student-college relationship and the many obligations, either express or implied, that surround that relationship. One of the first items a student receives when contemplating applying to a particular school or program is its school catalogue. The school catalogue becomes an implied contract with the student, setting parameters, requirements, expectations, and so forth during the time the student is enrolled at the school or college, should the student be admitted. Obviously, the language in the catalogue is extremely important in terms of what the student relies on and what the university will or will not do during that relationship. Interestingly, in recent years, school catalogues have contained disclaimers noting that the catalogue is **not** a contract, express or implied, and that the school or program reserves the right to make changes in its terms as it sees fit. Even so, the value and effect of such a disclaimer is often a legal issue that is decided by a court when a student alleges that a breach of the implied contract occurred by the academic institution or specific program into which the student is admitted.

Implied contract theory has also been applied to program syllabi and school or program policies and procedures. When a student is not evaluated as specified in the syllabus or assignments are not graded as listed in the syllabus, for example, and the student is adversely affected by a deviation from this written material, the student can use the implied contract theory to challenge adverse decisions by faculty. Likewise, if a policy allows a student to grieve a grade received, not following the policy can create a potential breach of implied contract allegation by the student if he or she files a suit challenging the school or program's decision.

Students also enjoy the benefit of express contracts with institutions of higher learning. The housing contract between the student and the school, for example, stands "at the core" of that relationship.[24] Other express contracts that define the student-school relationship include, as examples, work-study agreements, confidentiality and code of conduct agreements, and teaching assistantship contracts.

Remedies available under contract law are numerous. When an alleged breach of a contract occurs – defined as one party to the contract failing to perform, with no legal justification, a major obligation in the contract[25] – the breaching party is able to file a suit asking for compensatory damages (money covering the losses suffered by the non-breaching party); specific performance (non-breaching party asks that the court require the breaching party to perform its obligations under the contract); an injunction (prohibiting or requiring something); and reformation (court amends or refashions contract based on intent of the contract)[26].

The school or program has several defenses to attempt to thwart a student's allegation of its breach of contract. Defenses include fraud (party makes representations that are knowingly false and intends to have the other party rely on the misrepresentation); inability to enter into a contract (e.g., mental illness); and public policy violation (contract is illegal or against public's best interest)[27].

Contract law has not been the exclusive remedy for students in private academic institutions, however. Additional causes of action include many of those that their public-school sector colleagues use: discrimination, arbitrary decision making, and requests for injunctive or equitable estoppel relief. And, as with students in public post-secondary institutions, students can allege several theories of potential liability in one suit.

### *Admission to College or University*

In *Keles v. Yale University*[28], the question of whether or not an implied contract existed between a student applicant and the University was at issue. Resat Keles wanted to attend the Mechanical Engineering graduate school at Yale. Dr. Sreenivasan, a faculty member at Yale, suggested that Keles submit a formal application, which he did for the 1988-1989 and 1989-1990 school years. The graduate school denied Keles admission on both applications.

Keles told Dr. Sreenivasan of the results of his application process. Sreenivasan informed Keles that there were no openings in the graduate school, but he offered Keles a laboratory assistant position for the 1990-1991 academic year. He also told Keles that if "things worked out," he would recommend Keles for admission to the graduate school for the 1991-1992 academic year. Sreenivasan also told Keles that because he had been admitted to the University of Illinois' program, he should accept that offer.

Keles did not do well in the lab assistant position. Several research assistants and another faculty member complained that Keles did not have the academic preparation nor laboratory skills to work effectively.

In the fall of 1990, Keles composed a letter of recommendation for himself and sent it to Sreenivasan to sign. The letter described Keles's work as satisfactory and also included a recommendation for a scholarship. Dr. Sreenivasan neither signed nor sent the letter; neither did he submit his own letter. Sreenivasan did not believe Keles was a viable candidate for graduate school.

Keles applied to the Yale program a third time, and he was rejected again. Even so, Sreenivasan allowed Keles to continue working at the lab and to take on a class a semester as a special student during the 1991-1992 academic year. However, Sreenivasan continually encouraged Keles to apply to other graduate programs.

During the Fall 1991-1992 session, Keles did not show up for several class meetings. As a result, Sreenivasan did not make arrangements for him to continue as a special student. Moreover, Keles could no longer receive his salary for the laboratory position.

Keles applied a fourth time to the graduate school, and that application was not processed because the University had a policy that only three applications were possible. Keles then filed suit against Yale University, alleging a breach of an "implied educational agreement" because he was not accepted in the graduate school and for fraudulent inducement because he believed that Sreenivasan had him work in the laboratory for an eventual exchange of admission to the graduate school program.

The federal trial court ruled against Keles on both of his allegations. The court evaluated the implied educational agreement by using traditional contract law. Before an agreement can be breached, an agreement or contract must first exist. In this case, the court held, there was neither such an agreement nor a suggestion of such an agreement. Further, the court held that there was no fraudulent inducement by the University. Time and time again, Sreenivasan had encouraged Keles to accept the University of Illinois offer and to apply to other programs. He also conditioned any action that might admit Keles into the University with if things worked out.

Interestingly, the court also awarded Yale attorney fees in this case. Keles had sued every other college or university he had attended, and the attorney who handled this matter for Keles knew of his history of suing other academic institutions. Because Rule 11 of the Federal Rules of Civil Procedure mandates that an attorney who files frivolous suits be sanctioned, Keles's attorney was sanctioned and ordered to pay Yale University's costs and attorney fees.

## *Continuation in University or College Program*

Nursing students and other students in professional programs must not only successfully pass the classroom portion of a particular course, they must also successfully pass the clinical portion of the same course. It is not unusual for a student to perform well in the clinical segment of the course but not perform as well in the classroom. The reverse is also true. This learning model, although necessary, often brings with it legal challenges by students who are not able to complete both aspects of the course work.

In *Southwell v. University of the Incarnate Word*[29], Southwell, a nursing student, had done well in the academic portion of a required nursing leadership management course but failed its clinical portion due to compromising the safety of a client during the clinical rotation. The college of nursing offered the student to complete the clinical portion by undergoing an independent assessment of her clinical skills. The vice president of Academic Affairs sent Southwell a letter informing her that if she passed the clinical by meeting the course objectives, she would pass the course. If she did not meet the course objectives, however, she would have to apply for retention in the nursing program.

Southwell failed the independent assessment as well. She did not apply for retention, however. Instead, she filed a suit against the University alleging breach of contract, violation of the state Deceptive Trade Practices Act, and unfair grading in the independent assessment.

The Appeals court opined that an implied contract existed via the University and the College of Nursing's catalogue and its policies and procedures. It held, however, that Southwell did not meet her obligations under the implied contract. The requirement of a minimum of C or better in the required nursing courses was clearly included in the catalogue. Additionally, the catalogue clearly stated that in addition to a minimum grade of C, a student must receive a recommendation from the nursing faculty in order to graduate. Because Ms. Southwell had met neither of these requirements, she had not fulfilled her obligations under the implied contract.

The Appeals court also ruled in favor of the University on the former student's Deceptive Trade Practices allegations. According to the Act, Southwell was required to prove that she was a consumer, that the University or college engaged in false, misleading, or deceptive acts, and that she was damaged as a result of those acts. The court held that Ms. Southwell met none of these requirements. The College of Nursing and the University were clear about what was required of her and what the ramifications of her failure would mean for her continuation in the program. Moreover, the court continued, the only damage Ms. Southwell suffered was the result of her receiving a failing grade in the required course. Also, as the court stated, the student never applied for retention.

The college's actions in this case paralleled the *Horowitz* case discussed earlier. Despite the fact that the cases alleged different causes of action, in both situations, the faculty attempted to provide an objective evaluation of the students' clinical abilities through the use of an independent evaluation. Moreover, the students were informed of what would happen to them throughout the process as well as what the ultimate outcome would be if a passing grade were not achieved. Neither *Horowitz* nor *Southwell* were victories for the students. Even so, they stand for the right of students to obtain as much information as they can as to their progress in a program and what the ramifications will be if objectives are not met. Perhaps most importantly, both require that faculty treat students fairly and with careful and deliberate decision making when students' continuation in an educational program is at stake.

### Evaluation/Grading

Students in private academic institutions can allege that failure to obtain a passing grade in a particular course or a required exam is a breach of their particular contract with the school. Depending on the facts in the case, such a claim may be successful, although in other instances, it is not a winning allegation. Such was the case in *Harris v. Adler School of Professional Psychology*.[30]

Eleanor Harris and Bronwyn Raines were students in Adler School's doctoral program. One of the requirements of the program was the passing of a first-year written qualifying examination. Adler's student catalog characterized the examination as assessing the student's knowledge of the first-year courses and the basic foundations of psychology[31]. Harris took the exam two times, and Raines took it three times. Each student failed the exam every time it was taken, according to the faculty member who graded the examinations. Due to their failure of the required qualifying exam, both students were dismissed from the program.

Both students sued the School and alleged several breach-of-contract claims. The trial court dismissed the case and an appeal was taken by the students.

The appellate court held that the student's claims of breach of contract by the School were without merit. One of the former students' claim was based on the allegation that the qualifying exam did not test subject matter from the first year. The court recognized that the student catalog did create a contract upon which this claim could be based. However, the court continued, the alleged breach was an academic issue, and as such, it was not able to determine if the exam did or did not accurately reflect and test the first-year curriculum material.

Moreover, the court, in dismissing the other two claims of the students, opined that it was not capable of determining whether the standards used to evaluate the students' work during the first year were the same as those used to evaluate the results on the qualifying examination.

The appeals court also dismissed additional claims alleging breach of contract causes of action not germane to the grading of the exams. The trial court's decision dismissing the case was upheld in its entirety.

The *Harris* case is interesting in that it again shows that courts are reluctant to judge academic decision making by faculty. Had the students been able to allege and prove, for example, that the school never allowed them to sit for the required exam for a reason unrelated to the faculty's expertise in terms of the subject matter being tested, they would have been more successful alleging a breach of the school's contract with the students. Such an allegation would not have been based on the expertise of the faculty in determining what is and is not a successful passage of an exam but, rather, would be a decision that probably fell outside the protected realm of academic decision making.

## Graduation

In the case *Harwood v. John Hopkins University*[32], a denial of graduation and an earned degree due to unusual circumstances that occurred after degree and graduation requirements were met by the student resulted in a decision in favor of the University. Robert Harwood completed his degree requirements at the end of his last fall term. However, graduation ceremonies were held at the University once a year at the end of the spring term. As a result, Harwood returned to his native Rhode Island and, while there, received several letters from the dean informing Harwood that he had received several disturbing complaints about him and his harassment of a fellow student. The dean also informed Harwood that, based on these complaints, he would have to notify the dean whenever he returned to campus. Harwood informed the dean that he would be on campus on a specific day to attend a political rally that was going to be held there.

Harwood came to campus and attended the rally. He passed out opposition literature aimed at the student he had harassed earlier, who was running for a campus office. Harwood shot and killed the student after the rally was over. He was charged with and pled guilty to murder and several weapons violations.

The dean informed Harwood that because he had pled guilty to the murder and weapons violations, disciplinary action against him was being initiated because the conduct violated the University's code of conduct. Despite Harwood's defense of the allegations, the decision was to expel him, a decision that was upheld within the University's appeal process. Harwood filed suit against the University, asking for a declaratory judgment against the University to require it to grant him his degree. He also alleged that he was not subject to the University's student code of conduct and discipline because he had completed all degree requirements. Furthermore, he alleged that the University arbitrarily refused to grant him his degree.

The court held that the University did have the right to withhold the student's degree and thus not graduate Harwood, notwithstanding the completion of the degree and graduation requirements. Moreover, the court held that the University did not act arbitrarily in expelling him.

The court based its opinion on principles of contract law. Initially, the court opined, the student handbook clearly provided that approval for graduation required a student to resolve "any outstanding charges of misconduct" and "comply with any penalties imposed as a result of misconduct." The handbook also stated that the awarding of degrees was conditioned upon adherence to university and divisional regulations and performance that meets the "bona fide expectations of the faculty"[33]. The court further stated that murder was clearly against the student code of conduct and that Harwood had never been given notice by the University that he was going to graduate. In addition, when Harwood informed the dean that he would be on campus on the day of the rally, he was still subject to the University code.

Last, the court held that the University did not act arbitrarily in dismissing the student. Harwood was given adequate notice concerning the suspension pending the outcome of his criminal trial and was given an extension for the opportunity to prepare a defense of which he did not take advantage. In short, the procedures complied with the student handbook and "adequately protected" his rights.[34]

This case illustrates the importance of the contract law in private secondary education and the mandate that an academic institution abide by its adopted rules and regulations. Had the University not followed its own requirements, whether in terms of the dismissal or the code of conduct, a different result would have occurred. The case also underscores the importance of students in private institutions reading carefully and completely any and all written documents that impinge upon the student's relationship with the school or college.

## Selected Legal Issues Applicable to All Nursing Students

Many laws protect students, regardless of what type of post-secondary academic institution they attend. In other words, those laws protect students without a concern for whether it is a public or private institution. The application of those laws does, at times, depend upon the status of the student, however. For example, drug testing of students in public institutions of higher learning must still conform to the United States Constitutional mandates of the Fourth Amendment's protection against unreasonable searches and seizures. Likewise, student privacy, a right of all students, takes on special meaning within the expanded protections of the Fourteenth Amendment's due process requirements. Table 38.1 compares and contrasts selected legal issues applicable to all nursing students.

Table 38.1 - Selected Legal Issues Applicable to All Students in Post-Secondary Institutions

| Protections Afforded | Law | Illustrating Comment/Case |
|---|---|---|
| Freedom from sexual harrassment | Title IX of Education Amendments: Title VII of Civil Rights Act of 1964[35] | Institution liability occurs when school officials have "actual notice of . . . and deliberate indifference to teacher's conduct" under Title IX, based on USSCT decision in *Gebser v. Lago Vista Independent School District*;[36] Title VII liability for hostile environment of *quid pro quo* treatment of student by faculty (e.g., offensive jokes or requiring sexual favors for good grades or graduation). |
| Freedom from discrimination based upon disability | Section 504 of the Rehabilitation Act of 1973; Americans with Disabilities Act (ADA)[37] | *Southeastern Community College v. Davis*:[38] a nursing student with bilateral hearing loss not admitted to nursing program because not "qualified" for program and could not "reasonably accommodate" her in program without altering program drastically (Section 504); *Larson v. Snow College*:[39] a "wellness contract" requiring certain behaviors of a student treated for a mental illness upon her return to the College after treatment held to be intentional discrimination in violation of ADA because College treated student as an "embarrassment" rather than helping her make the most of her education once she returned from treatment. |
| Limitations on drug searches and seizures for students in pubic institutions; case law for students in private institutions | Fourth Amendment of U.S. Constitution | Basic premise: "reasonable" testing prohibition against unreasonable and "unobtrusive" testing of students when a high likelihood of drug use exists (e.g., school sports) probably okay by recent USSCT decisions[40]; for college students, test would be acceptable if academic institution had "probable cause" to believe drug use occurring; voluntary program of drug testing more acceptable than mandatory one. |
| Protection of student unconsented education records | The Family Educational Rights and Privacy Act's (FERPA) Buckley Amendment;[41] various state laws and case decisions | FERPA prohibits unconsented disclosures except in limited circumstances (e.g., when health care needed by student); newly passed USA Patriot Act[42] now allows academic institution to release educational records if court order for same is obtained pursuant to investigation or prosecution of terrorism. |

**Sources:**   Brent, N. J. (2001). *Nurses and the law: A guide to principles and applications* (2nd ed.). Philadelphia, PA: W. B. Saunders Co
Kaplin, W., & Lee, B. (1995). *The law of higher education: A comprehensive guide to legal implications of administrative decision making* (3rd ed.). San Francisco, CA: Jossey-Bass.
Springer, J. D. (2002). Do students have a right to privacy? *Academe.* Retrieved on September 7, 2002, from www.aaup.org

# Overview of Selected Legal Issues of Concern to
# Faculty in Nursing Education Programs

## *Faculty in Public Post-Secondary Academic Institutions*

### *United States Constitution Applications*

Like the students they teach in public academic post-secondary institutions, faculty members enjoy the protections of the United States Constitution's Bill of Rights and its Fifth and Fourteenth Amendment's protections of due process. As a result, freedom of speech (First Amendment), freedom from unreasonable searches and seizures (Fourth Amendment), and due process protections (e.g., dismissal from a tenured position), for example, all work to provide the faculty member with additional protections that private faculty members do not enjoy in the same way.

***Employment/tenure.*** Faculty employed in a public academic setting have their relationships with the institution regulated in one of two ways: through an employment contract (non-tenured) or through tenure. In addition to the application of traditional contract law when an employment contract exists, state statutes and administrative regulations also govern faculty positions in public post-secondary institutions insofar as personnel decisions are concerned.[43]

When a contract of employment exists, the law requires that the institution and the faculty abide by long-standing principles of contract law when a dispute arises within the employment relationship. For example, in *University of Alaska v. Fairbanks*[44], the federal court held that the notice requirement in the University's personnel regulations requiring a notice of the non-renewal of a faculty member's contract was part of the contract with the faculty member. Because the University had not provided notice to the faculty member as was required in the regulations, the court held that the University had breached it contract with the instructor.

When a contractual faculty member attempts to obtain tenure, in addition to contract law being applicable, institutional procedures (again, using contract law principles) and/ or state laws may also apply. In *Dugan v. Stockton State College*[45], the issue of *de facto* tenure was highlighted when a faculty member employed by the College for 13 years (some of which she held a non-faculty position) asked for tenure based on her years of service. Interestingly, Ms. Dugan was hired when the state law clearly stated that if one was constructively employed for five years in a state college, the person was tenured. The College opposed her position by stating that the state board of higher education had passed regulations granting the board exclusive power to confer tenure. The New Jersey appellate court decided in favor of Ms. Dugan, opining that the regulations were contrary to the statutory language. Therefore, the court continued, the board had no power to issue such regulations.

The United States Supreme Court has carefully analyzed a faculty member's interest in continued employment in a public post-secondary institution. This interest is manifested in a contract of employment because the contract provides the faculty member with an expectation of continued employment unless the faculty member is terminated "for cause." Likewise, tenure, at least in theory, provides the faculty member with procedural protections when allegedly adequate cause exists to terminate the faculty member's employment (e.g., incompetency). In addition, tenure affords the faculty more academic freedom because it limits the ability of the academic institution to dismissal for "no-cause" situations.[46]

Because of the faculty's continued employment expectation in these situations, faculty can not be terminated from a position that is seen as a property interest by the courts without the benefit of the Fourteenth Amendment's due process protections. Moreover, if a termination results in a deprivation of the faculty member's "liberty interest" in continued employment or employment at another academic institution with his or her reputation in tact, the termination, if it occurs, must meet constitutional requirements. In short, terminations involving those faculty under continuing employment contracts that state they can be terminated prior to the term of the contract only for cause and terminations of faculty with tenure must be handled with strict adherence to constitutional mandates of due process.

It is important to note that the Fourteenth Amendment's protections are not limitless. For example, it is possible for a contract not to be renewed at the end of its term (e.g., three years) unless the institution is discriminating against the faculty member (e.g., on the basis of gender or race) or the faculty member can prove that the institution is violating his or her constitutional rights in some way.[47]

Likewise, a tenured faculty member can be dismissed or terminated due to reasons unrelated to cause. For example, if a program or school is discontinued or there is no ability to continue a program due to financial exigency, no 14th Amendment protection exists.

Faculty members in public academic institutions must be ever vigilant in reviewing and understanding their rights of employment. Reviewing the contract of employment and any institution regulations and state law that apply to continued employment is absolutely essential for the contractual employee. If a faculty receives a notice indicating that the contract of employment is to be terminated prior to the end of the contract term, the faculty should obtain legal counsel to help in determining his or her next step in fighting the termination. Likewise, tenured faculty must exercise whatever legal avenues are available in order to defend themselves against such an action and, at the same time, ensure that any termination action by the academic institution is handled in a fair manner and consistent with due process mandates.

***Academic freedom.*** Individual faculty academic freedom within higher education was defined by the American Association of University Professors (AAUP) and the Association of American Colleges and Universities in 1940 in the organizations' *1940 Statement of Principles on Academic Freedom And Tenure*. According to the *Statement*, teachers are entitled to several privileges. The first is full freedom in research and the publication of the results of the research (subject to the faculty member's other academic duties). Second, faculty should have the freedom to discuss their subject(s) in the classroom (as long as the introduction of controversial matters that have no relation to their subjects are not introduced). Third, the freedom to speak and write without institutional censorship or discipline is vital, remembering that due to their status as citizens, scholars, and educational officers, they must be accurate, respect others' opinions, exercise restraint, and indicate that they are not speaking for the institution.[48]

Although the *Statement's* protections for faculty members seem broad, it is not as absolute a safeguard as it first appears. For example, there is some controversy over the scope of the First Amendment to the United States Constitution's "coexistence" with academic freedom[49]. Although it has been interpreted by the United States Supreme Court as providing the faculty member freedom from state regulation (e.g., state requirement to sign a loyalty oath or governmental inquiry into faculty member's lectures), the Court has yet to define the scope of its protections[50]. Moreover, whatever its protections, its protection neither is absolute nor does it protect a faculty member in a private institution in the same way it may shield a teacher in a public institution of higher learning. In addition to the constitutional safeguards of academic freedom, contract law (e.g., faculty handbook) and academic usage and custom, sometimes referred to as "academic common law," also protect academic freedom for the individual faculty.[51]

The concept of individual faculty academic freedom is further impacted upon by the institution's own academic freedom. Indeed, legally these two types of academic liberty are incongruous. The United States Supreme Court, in *University of Michigan v. Ewing*[52], characterized this conflict: "Academic freedom thrives not only on the independent and uninhibited exchange of ideas among teachers and students, . . . but also, and somewhat inconsistently, on autonomous decision making by the academy itself"[53].

There have been many interesting cases testing the parameters of academic freedom in the public post-secondary academic institution. For example, how teachers teach their subject matter raises the issue of academic freedom. In *Bonnell v. Lorenzo (Macomb Community College*[54]), the Appeals Court upheld the College's suspension of Professor Bonnell, who taught English, because he created a hostile learning environment in his classroom. One of Bonnell's female students' sued the professor because he consistently used "lewd and graphic language" in his class. The Appeals Court opined that although academic freedom and freedom of expression are vitally important in the classroom, neither is absolute, especially when the language used is not "germane to the subject matter."

Likewise, course content and syllabi have also been the focus of academic freedom for faculty members in public colleges and universities. *Edwards v. California University of Pennsylvania*[55] involved a media studies tenured professor's suit against the University for allegedly limiting his choice of classroom materials for his media course. The new syllabus for the course, which emphasized "bias, censorship, religion, and humanism," was not approved by the department. An earlier syllabus had been accepted, however. The suit was dismissed, and the United States Supreme Court refused to grant *certiorari* to review the case. In so holding, the Court based its decision on not using the standard of whether the course content and the syllabus was "reasonably related to a legitimate educational interest" because "a public university professor does not have a First Amendment right to decide what will be taught in the classroom."[56] In all likelihood, the reason for both of the courts' decisions rested on the fact that an earlier syllabus had been approved and the professor refused to use it rather than his new syllabus.[57] Other selected cases focusing on academic freedom and faculty in public colleges and universities are presented in Table 38. 2.

### *Intellectual Property Issues*

The law of copyright, one of the categories of intellectual property law, is found in the United States Constitution, Article I, Section 8, Clause 8. Its language clearly reflects its purpose "to promote the Progress of Science and useful Arts, by securing for limited Times to Authors and Inventors the exclusive Right to their respective Writings and Discoveries." Basically, the law guarantees the owner of the copyright exclusive rights to his or her works and, at the same time, encourages others to build upon the ideas and information contained in the copyrighted work.[62] The mechanics of the copyright law's protection are located in the federal Copyright Act.[63]

Copyright law does not protect any and all original works, however. For the law to apply, several conditions must be met. First, the work must fit into one of the designated groups of works protected: literary, musical, dramatic, pantomimes and choreographic, pictorial, graphic and sculptural, motion picture and other audiovisual, sound, and architectural.[64] Next, the work must be "original" and "fixed in any tangible medium of expression."[65]

Copyright law is easily applicable to higher education. Writings, research, course syllabi, plays, distance-learning programs, and other examples of faculty original works are generated consistently and regularly by faculty in public post-secondary institutions. It is understandable, then, that many cases have tested the limits and the protections of faculty works within the framework of the Copyright Act and within the internal framework of the academic institution's control over such works, including the academic institution's policies and the faculty member's employment contract or tenure status with the institution.[66] To discuss all of the applications and protections of the Act to faculty is beyond the scope of this chapter. Two applicable areas of copyright law that are important and impact upon

Table 38.2 - Selected Bases on Academic Freedom in Public Academic Institutions

| Issue | Case | Outcome/Comment |
|---|---|---|
| Faculty research and publications | *Levin v. Harleston*[58] | Faculty member's writings and publications espouse that Blacks are less intelligent on average than Whites and opposed affirmative action; among other actions, college threatens faculty member with dismissal; court rules in favor of faculty member, supporting faculty research by using the U.S. Constitution as a "basic source of protection."[59] |
| Expression of ideas outside of classroom | *Jeffries v. Harleston*[60] | Tenured professor and chair of Black Studies department expresses controversial off-campus statements reforming educational system in order to promote diversity and unfavorable remarks made about certain individuals and ethnic groups; college removes faculty member from chair position; court holds removal a violation of faculty member's constitutional right of free speech. |
| Grading of students | *Wozniak v. Contry (University of Illinois at Urbana-Champaign)*[61] | Tenured professor's refusal to use established grading policies (submitting student materials for review) could be basis of discipline against professor; no violation of faculty member's constitutional rights. |

*Source*:   Euben, D. (2002). *Academic freedom of individual professors and higher education institutions: The current legal landscape.* Retrieved October 15, 2002, from http://www.aaup.org

Kaplan, W. A., & Lee, B. A. (1995). *The law of higher education: A comprehensive guide to legal implications of administrative decision making* (3rd ed.). San Francisco, CA: Jossey-Bass.

faculty in public post-secondary institutions are the work-for-hire doctrine and whether a work was done "in the scope of one's employment."

***Work-for-hire doctrine.*** In a landmark case, the United States Supreme Court established one of the boundaries of the Law's protections, that of the work-for-hire doctrine, which has applicability to higher education. In *Community For Creative (CCNV) Non-Violence v. Reid*[67], the Court was asked to determine if a sculptor commissioned by an organization for the homeless to sculpt a statue was the owner of the copyright he filed for his work. CCNV also filed for copyright protection of the statue. The Court held that the work-for-hire doctrine – a doctrine stating that the employer and not the author is the holder of the copyright of the work – did not apply to Reid because he was an independent contractor and not an employee. As a result, as an independent contractor, the assumption did not apply to him.

In contrast, the Court continued, a work-for-hire is done by an employee within the scope of his or her employment or is part of a larger work (e.g., a textbook) in which all agree in writing that it is a work-for-hire. Practically, this means that only when one is considered an employee can the doctrine provide protection for an employer.

This analysis was a departure from previous appellate court decisions interpreting the work-for-hire doctrine because those courts had applied the doctrine based upon whether or not the employer had control over its production, not on whether the author of a work was an employee. However, the United States Supreme Court did not define what scope of employment meant in terms of its applicability to the doctrine.[68]

Although the case is considered a seminal one, it has not resolved all the questions of who owns the copyright when one is an employee. For example, whether a faculty member does create a work within the scope of employment, thus allowing an application of the work-for-hire doctrine is a difficult determination in many instances, one that can probably only be decided when the issue is litigated.[69] Indeed, the work-for-hire doctrine must, of necessity, include an analysis of whether the work prepared was done as part of a faculty member's duties.

***Work done within the scope of employment.*** The initial premise under this analysis is that an employer, including an academic institution, does not automatically own every piece of work done by its faculty.[70] In another landmark case, *Miller v. CP Chemicals, Inc.,*[71] the court identified the factors necessary for a project prepared within the scope of employment. Those factors are:
- It is the kind of work the employee is employed to do.
- It occurs substantially within authorized work hours and space.
- It is actuated, at least in part, for a purpose to serve the employer.[72]

The three-pronged test in *Miller* is often difficult to satisfy when looking at scholarly work done by faculty. To begin with, there is some argument as to what kind of work a faculty member is hired to do. For example, one expert author argued that the only kind of work faculty are hired to do is scholarly activities, a course exam, or a course syllabus.[73] When a faculty member prepares an educational program for a community organization on the weekends but is asked to do the program because of her faculty status at the local college, is the program owned by the college because it in some way served the employer?

Adding to the debate is the issue of tenure. What criteria are used to grant tenure to faculty? Is it scholarly activity alone? Or service to the employer? Are both important but not where and when the work is done? And what about computer courses developed by a faculty member? Are they required as part of the faculty member's duties and for which he or she was hired under the *Miller* test?

Because it is difficult to meet all three of *Miller's* requirements, it would appear that most faculty projects would not belong to the academic institution. Because the issue will continue to haunt the faculty-academic institution relationship, it has been recommended that a better approach might be for the faculty and institution to define as clearly as possible their respective intentions concerning original works by faculty.[74] This intention can be formalized in the facility's policy on copyright ownership, its contract of employment with faculty, and its tenure granting procedures.

## *Discrimination*

There are a plethora of laws prohibiting discrimination against faculty that are applicable in post-secondary institutions, not the least of which is the United States Constitution. In addition, other federal laws governing discrimination in employment are numerous and generally take precedence over any state law protections that might be afforded. The controlling federal laws are listed in Table 38.3.

One interesting case that illustrates Title VII's application to public post-secondary schools is *Scott v. University of Delaware*.[75] In this case, a Black professor filed a suit alleging that he and other Black faculty were discriminated against due to a policy that required applicants for faculty positions at the University to possess a Ph.D. Specifically, Scott alleged that such a policy had a disparate impact on Blacks because they were underrepresented among those with Ph.D.s. Under Title VII, this theory means that though not intentional, the policy adversely affects a protected group, and as a result, its effect results in discrimination. The court rejected this argument, holding that the requirement of a Ph.D. for University faculty is a necessary requirement because universities have as one of their missions the goal of conducting research and the Ph.D. is an indication of such training in scholarly inquiry.

Table 38.3 - Federal Antidiscrimination Laws Applicable to Faculty

| Law | Protections Afforded | Comment |
|---|---|---|
| Title VII of the Civil Rights Act of 1964[76] | Adverse employment decisions (e.g., refusal to hire or a discharge based on race, sex, color, creed, national origin) | Additional protections added by amendments include pregnancy, sexual harassment, abortion; applies to employers with 15 or more employees. |
| Title IX of the Education Amendments of 1972[77] | Discrimination on the basis of sex | Applies to public and private institutions receiving federal funds; administered by Office of Civil Rights (OCR); plaintiffs must prove discrimination on part of employer intentional. |
| Equal Pay Act[78] | Discrimination in payment of wages based on sex | Protection is for equal work of equal skill, effort, and responsibility done under similar working conditions. |
| Age Discrimination in Employment Act[79] | Discrimination against employees 40 and older in all employment decisions | Applies to employers with 20 or more employees; prohibits mandatory retirement except in limited circumstances (e.g., bona fide seniority system). |
| Rehabilitation Act of 1973[80] | Discrimination against **qualified** person who can do essential job qualifications with reasonable accommodation | Section 504 applies to any entity receiving federal funds; exceptions to mandate include disabled applicant or employee not qualified and accommodation not reasonable and too costly to employer. |
| Americans with Disabilities Act[81] | Discrimination against *qualified* person on basis of disability if able to do "essential job" functions with or without reasonable accommodation | Title I governs employment when 15 or more employees; prohibits questions about disability in pre-employment interview. |

***Source:*** Brent, N. J. (2001). *Nurses and the law: A guide to principles and applications* (2nd ed.). Philadelphia, PA: W. B. Saunders Company.

Kaplin, W. A., & Lee, B. A. (1995). *The law of higher education: A comprehensive guide to legal implications of administrative decision making* (3rd ed.). San Francisco, CA: Jossey-Bass.

Rothstein, M., Craver, C., Schroeder, E., & Shoben, E. (1999). *Employment law* (2nd ed.). St. Paul, MN: West Group.

Sovereign, K. (1999). *Personnel law* (4th ed.). Upper Saddle River, NJ: Prentice-Hall.

The Equal Pay Act's protection applies equally to male and female faculty. In *Board of Regents of the University of Nebraska v. Dawes,* [82] the University had established a formula that served as a means of determining the average salary for male faculty members. The University also used the formula as the basis for the **minimum** salary for female faculty members. The male faculty believed this formula was discriminatory in that they were paid less than what the minimum salary was for female faculty. The University filed a declaratory judgment action against the court to interpret the Act and its adopted formula. The court held that the formula and resulting pay scales violated the Equal Pay Act because the male faculty were paid less, despite their substantially equal qualifications.

The Rehabilitation Act of 1973 provided support to all faculty with a contagious disease, regardless of the level of academic institution within which they worked in *School Board of Nassau County v. Arline.* [83] In the case, the Court set forth four factors that employers must use to determine whether employees (in this case, a school teacher) with a potentially contagious disease (in this case, the disease was tuberculosis) pose a danger to others and therefore are unable to continue in their position. The four factors were:

1. The nature of the risk (how the disease is transmitted).
2. The duration of the risk (how long is the person a carrier).
3. The severity of the risk (the potential harm to third parties).
4. The probabilities that the disease will be transmitted and will cause varying degrees of harm.

The Court did not specifically address additional contagious diseases in its opinion. Moreover, the decision was reached before the Americans with Disabilities Act was passed. Even so, it set the parameters for the protections of other employees, including faculty in post-secondary institutions, with contagious diseases and the prohibition of discriminating against them unfairly, not only under the Rehabilitation Act of 1973 but also under the future Americans with Disabilities Act and those faculty who are HIV-positive or who suffer from AIDS.

### Faculty in Private Post-Secondary Institutions

### Contract Law Protections

Because private post-secondary faculty who teach in private institutions do not enjoy the same constitutional protections that their colleagues in public post-secondary institutions enjoy, faculty in private academic settings must rely on established legal principles applied to the many issues they face in their relationship with the academic entity. One established area of the law that is often used by the faculty in such settings is, of course, contract law. Similar to the student in a private post-academic institution, faculty use actual contracts of employment (express contract), faculty handbooks, adopted academic institutional policies, the law of implied contracts, and the parameters of tenured status. Academic custom and usage can also help faculty in a private academic setting receive fair treatment in all employment decisions.

***Employment/tenure.*** In *Upadhya v. Langenburg,*[84] a faculty member had been employed under a contract of employment for several years. The duration of each contract was one year. Pursuant to the contact provisions during the third year, the faculty member was notified that his contract would not be renewed for a fifth year. The faculty member believed the terms of the prior contracts stated that he would be employed for five years, so he sued the college alleging a breach of his contract. The Seventh Circuit Court of Appeals disagreed with the faculty member, holding that the language in the contract regarding a fifth-year review at the end of five years of employment was not contractually binding and that each prior contract was for a year's duration only. Furthermore, the court continued, the college faculty handbook clearly disclaimed a guarantee of the renewal of a contract for probationary faculty members.

It is a well-established principle of contract law that the "black-letter" language of the contract takes precedence over oral or other representations, either before or after the contract is entered. In a case wherein a faculty member's two-year contract was not renewed, the faculty member asserted the position that the head of his department had orally promised him a full four-year contract with the college. Suing for a breach of contract, the Pennsylvania court evaluated the contract's language and the faculty handbook parameters. It held that the contract did not guarantee the faculty member continued employment. The court also reviewed the faculty handbook for any guarantees inconsistent with the contract terms. The court held that the contract and the handbook simply gave the faculty member a right to be considered for reappointment. As a result, the faculty member's claim for breach of contract was denied.[85]

In *Howard University v. Best,*[86] the issue of tenure confronted Ms. Best, a faculty member who initially had a three-month non-faculty appointment at the University. Subsequent to the non-faculty appointment, she was given a three-year faculty appointment. When that appointment was near its completion, the University notified Best that the appointment would not be renewed but did not do so within the contract's one-year requirement. Ms. Best sued the University, alleging a breach of contract, and argued that because of its untimely notice, she was entitled to tenure. She also argued that the three-year faculty appointment was in reality a reappointment. Best based this argument on the faculty handbook that stated when a faculty member was reappointed, the faculty member received tenure status. The court analyzed the custom and practice of the University's granting of tenure to renewed appointment faculty from a non-faculty appointment. It found no pattern of such decisions and therefore denied Best's claim of an entitlement to tenure. It did, however, affirm the trial court verdict in favor of Ms. Best for a second three-year appointment without tenure, noting that the University had a custom and practice of granting reappointments in other instances when its notice was untimely. In addition, it affirmed the trial court's grant of $155,000.00 in damages.

*Academic freedom.* Academic freedom in private academic settings has seen fewer case decisions than in the public academic setting because it is difficult to defend in the same way it can be defended by faculty in public academic settings due to the application of the United States Constitution. Even so, faculty in private post-secondary institutions can challenge threats to their academic freedom when established institutional policies are violated, when a faculty member's contract's provisions governing academic freedom are not honored, or when guidelines from such organizations as the AAUP are not followed. Additionally, despite the direct non-applicability of the United States Constitution to private academic settings, the decisions involving academic freedom in public post-secondary institutions are valuable guideposts for private academic entities to use when dealing with academic freedom in its setting.

Interestingly, academic freedom in private academic settings has been receiving attention in relation to the use of computers by faculty in those settings. In a situation involving Duke University, Professor Gary Hull had developed a web page on which he posted an article called *Terrorism and Its Appeasement*. The article supported military action in response to the September 11, 2001, terrorist attacks in the United States. The University apparently disabled the website on numerous occasions. Eventually, the web page was reinstated after Professor Hull agreed to place a disclaimer on the website that the views expressed in the article were not those of the University.[87] The disclaimer addition was consistent with the AAUP *1940 Statement of Principles on Academic Freedom and Tenure* discussed earlier in this chapter. The *Statement* clearly declares that when faculty speak as citizens, they remain scholars and educational officers and should therefore make "every effort to indicate that they are not speaking for the institution."[88]

### Intellectual Property Issues

In addition to the issues discussed in this section for faculty in public academic institutions, another interesting issue in copyright law and faculty is the issue of grant writing. Grant writing is one of the many expectations of faculty in institutions of higher education, especially in tight economic times. The process is long and arduous at best, and the time spent on the finished grant is in addition to the other tasks and expectations of faculty by the post-secondary institution. Additionally, the issue of who owns the completed work is often a concern to the faculty member, who may want to leave the current employer for a faculty appointment elsewhere.

The general rule of thumb for grant writing and copyright ownership is that the funding source's document controls the ownership issues when the funding comes from outside sources and is a work-for-hire.[89] If, however, the work on the grant and its results are seen as "specially commissioned" under the Copyright Act of 1976, and the grant document so indicates, the copyright ownership rests with the funding entity, whether that be an outside agency or the college or university.

## *Discrimination*

The antidiscrimination laws protecting faculty in public post-secondary institutions also protect faculty in private academic settings. For example, in *Roebuck v. Drexel University*[90], a Black professor filed a suit alleging he had been discriminated against under Title VII and another federal law (Section 1981). He alleged that the department chair and the president of the university did not give him full credit for his service in the local community (one of the responsibilities he was hired for). Professor Roebuck also alleged that the university made selective use of his teaching evaluations, resulting in an overall level of teaching as satisfactory rather than outstanding. The trial court returned a verdict in favor of the university and found no violation of Title VII. The appeals court, however, remanded the case back to the trial court for a new trial.

## Summary and Conclusions

Post-secondary institutions are places in which various sources of the law have applicability to almost every phase of student and faculty life. Whether the setting is a public or private one, the law constantly impacts upon academic life. It is certain that this application will continue in the future in increasing instances. With the rapid development of distance learning, the use of computers in post-secondary education, and the need to preserve academic freedom for both students and faculty as world affairs continue to create conflict and divergence of opinion, the legal issues inherent in these and other developments in the academic area will be spotlighted. The law must and will continue to shape the lives and responsibilities of students and faculty as they go about their respective roles in the academic setting.

## Learning Activities

1. Compare and contrast a reported case involving a student in a public institution with that of a student in a private academic institution involving the same issue (e.g.,

admission to the school, dismissal from the school). Identify the legal issues identified in each case regarding as the student's respective rights, theories upon which the suit was filed, and success with the case. Develop various legal arguments that might have been used in one or both cases. Indicate how the legal issue(s) in both cases could be solved without resort to the court.

2. Interview a faculty member who is tenured. Determine the process of applying for tenure in his or her academic institution, criteria required, length of time until a decision was made, and any other factors considered crucial to the process. Write an evaluation of the process, indicating its strengths and weaknesses. Where improvements could be instituted, identify what those might be. Then develop a proposed policy and procedure for tenure from the information gathered.

3. Research the topic of academic freedom for faculty. Identify cases other than those cited in this chapter and compare and contrast how the legal concept has expanded from its inception until the current time, using modern teaching/learning techniques, such as distance learning and computers. Write a position paper supporting or rejecting academic freedom for faculty.

4. Evaluate the effectiveness of one federal law's prohibition of discrimination against a faculty member or student, and write a paper on the topic. In the written paper, identify how the law has been helpful and where it has fallen short of protecting the victim of discrimination. Where the law has fallen short, identify suggestions for improving the law and propose language that would amend the statute to remedy the weaknesses in the law.

## Disclaimer

This chapter is intended to provide information on selected legal issues in nursing education programs. It is not intended, neither should it be taken, as specific legal advice. If such advice is needed, an attorney or other appropriate professional should be consulted.

# Endnotes

[1] *Axson-Flynn v. Johnson*, 151 F. Supp. 2d 1326 (2001).

[2] 272 F. 3d 1207 (9th Cir. 2001).

[3] See generally, Gehring, D. D. (Ed.). (1992). *Administering college and university housing: A legal perspective* (rev. ed.). Asheville, NC: College Administration Publications, Inc., pp. 13-38.

[4] Brent, N. J. (2001). The nurse in the academic setting. In (2nd ed.). *Nurses and the law: A guide to principles and applications* (2nd ed.). Philadelphia, PA: W. B. Saunders Company, p. 428.

[5] 294 F. 2d 150 (5th Cir. 1961), *cert. denied* 386 U.S. 930 (1961).

[6] Young, D. P., & Gehring, D. (1986). *The college student and the courts: Cases and commentary*. Asheville, NC: College Administration Publications, pp. 13-16.

[7] 95 S. Ct. 729 (1975).

[8] 69 F. Supp. 2d 815 (1999).

[9] 438 U.S. 265 (1978).

[10] The court did not issue a written opinion in *Gratz* but indicated it would issue a separate opinion. To date it has not. *AAUP Legal Docket*. The American Association of University Professors. Retrieved October 4, 2002, from http://www.aaup.org

[11] No. 01-1447/1516 (May 14, 2002).

[12] *AAUP Legal Docket* at 2.

[13] *AAUP Legal Docket* at 3.

[14] 245 F. 3d 1172 (10th Cir. 2001).

[15] This statute, passed after the Civil War, protects all the rights included in the United States Constitution, and federal statutory and administrative law. It allows damages or equitable relief (e.g., an injunction) to be awarded the plaintiff (person bringing the suit) if the violation was done "under color of state law" (governmental official).

[16] 20 U.S.C. Section 1681 (a) (1972). Title IX was passed to eliminate discrimination on the basis of sex in any education program or activity receiving federal funds.

[17] 435 U.S. 78, 98 S. Ct. 948 (1978).

[18] 538 F. 2d 1317 (8th Circ. 1978).

[19] 435 U.S. at 85-90.

[20] 435 U.S. at 92.

[21] 2 S.W. 3d 54 (Supreme Court of Arkansas, 1999).

[22] 681 N.Y.S. 2d 494 (1st Appellate Division 1998).

[23] Kaplin, W. A., & Lee, B. A. (1995) *The law of higher education: A comprehensive guide to legal implications of administrative decision making* (3rd ed.). San Francisco, CA: Jossey-Bass, p. 55.

[24] Miller, S. T. (1992). Contracts and their use in housing. In D. D. Gehring (Ed.), *Administering college and university housing: A legal perspective*. Asheville, NC: College Administration Publications, Inc., p. 61.

[25] Black, H. C. (1999). *Black's law dictionary* (7th ed.). St. Paul, MN: West Group, p. 318.

[26] Brent, N. J. (2001). Contract law. In (2nd ed.), *Nurses and the law: A guide to principles and applications* (2nd ed.). Philadelphia, PA: W. B. Saunders Co., Tables 10-12.

[27] Calamari, J., & Perillo, J. (1998). *The law of contracts* (4th ed.). St. Paul, MN: West Group.

[28] 889 F. Supp. 729 (S.D. New York 1995).

[29] 974 S.W. 2d 351 (Ct. App. 4th District 1998).

[30] 723 N.E. 2d 717 (1st District Appellate Court 1999).

[31] *Harris v. Adler School of Professional Psychology*. (2000). In D. Gehring & T. Letzring (Eds.), *The college student and the courts: Briefs of selected court cases involving student/institutional relationships in higher*

*education*. Asheville, NC: College Administration Publications, Inc., p. 1449.

[32] 747 A. 2d 205 (Md. Ct. Sp. Appeals 2000).

[33] *Harwood v. John Hopkins University*. (2000). In D. Gehring & T. Letzring (Eds.), *The college student and the courts: Briefs of selected court cases involving student/institutional relationships in higher education* (no page). Asheville, NC: College Administration Publications, Inc.

[34] *Harwood v. John Hopkins University*. (2000). In D. Gehring & T. Letzring (Eds.), *The college student and the courts: Briefs of selected court cases involving student/institutional relationships in higher education* (p. 1439). Asheville, NC: College Administration Publications, Inc.

[35] 20 U.S.C. Section 1681 *et seq.* (1972); 42 U.S.C. Section 2000e *et seq.* (1964).

[36] 118 S. Ct. 1989 (1998).

[37] 29 U.S.C. Section 794 (1973); 42 U.S.C. Sections 12101-12117 (1990).

[38] 442 U.S. 397 (1979).

[39] 115 F. Supp. 2d 1296 (2000).

[40] *Vernonia School District v. Action*, 515 U.S. 646 (1995); *Board of Education of Independent School District No. 92 of Pottawatomie County et al. v. Earles et al.*, 122 S. Ct. 2559 (2002). In both cases, the United States Supreme Court held that for students in middle and high schools, a drug policy requiring students in after-school sports programs, extracurricular activities, and competitive extracurricular activities could be tested without a prerequisite of suspicion so long as there was n identifiable drug abuse problem in the school, the drug testing was not overly intrusive, its purpose was to protect the health and safety of the students, and the drug testing policy was reasonable.

[41] 36 20 U.S.C. 1232g *et seq.* (1974).

[42] 37 P.L. 707-56, passed 10/26/01 (Bill No. HR 3162).

[43] Kaplin, W. A., & Lee, B. A. (1995). *The law of higher education: A comprehensive guide to legal implications of administration decision making* (3rd ed.). San Francisco, Ca: Jossey-Bass, p. 279.

[44] 794 P. 2d 932 (Alaska 1990).

[45] 586 A. 2d 322 (N.J. Sup. Ct. App. Div. 1991).

[46] Kaplin, W. A. & Lee, B. A. (1995). *The law of higher education: A comprehensive guide to legal implications of administration decision making* (3rd ed.). San Francisco, CA: Jossey-Bass, p. 23.

[47] Hollander, P., Young, D. P., & Gehring, D. (1995). *A practical guide to legal issues affecting college teachers*. Asheville, NC: College Administration Press, p. 8.

[48] American Association of University Professors [AAUP]. (2001). *Policy documents and reports* (9th ed.). Washington, DC: AAUP, pp. 3-4.

[49] Euben, D. (2002). *Academic freedom of individual professors and higher education institutions: The current legal landscape* (p. 2). Retrieved October 15, 2002, from http://www.aaup.org

[50] Euben, D. (2002). *Academic freedom of individual professors and higher education institutions: The current legal landscape* (p. 2). Retrieved October 15, 2002, from http://www.aaup.org

[51] Finkin, M. W. (1972,). Toward a law of academic status. 22 *Buffalo Law Review*, 575.

[52] 474 U.S. 214 (1985).

[53] 474 U.S. 214, 226 note 12 (1985).

[54] 241 F. 3d 800 (6th Cir. 2001).

[55] 156 F. 3d 488 (3rd Cir. 1998), *cert. denied*, 525 U.S. 1143 (1999).

[56] Euben, D. (2002). *Academic freedom of individual professors and higher education institutions: The current legal landscape* (p. 12, citing *Edwards v. California University of Pennsylvania*). Retrieved October 15, 2002, from http://www.aaup.org

[57] Euben, D. (2002). *Academic freedom of individual professors and higher education institutions: the legal landscape* (p. 12). Retrieved October 15, 2002, from http://www.aaup.org

58 770 F. Supp. 895, *affirmed* 966 F. 2d 85 (2d Cir. 1992).

59 Kaplin, W. A., & Lee, B. A. (1995). *The law of higher education: A comprehensive guide to legal implications of administrative decision making* (3rd ed.). San Francisco, CA: Jossey-Bass, pp. 314-315.

60 741 (S.D.N.Y. 1993), *motion to set aside jury verdict granted in part and denied in part, and permanent injunction granted*, 828 F. Supp. 1066 (S.D.N.Y. 1993).

61 236 F. 3d 888 (7th Cir.), *cert. denied*, 121 S. Ct. 2243 (2001).

62 McMillen, J. D. (2001). *Intellectual property: Copyright ownership in higher education: University, faculty, and student rights*. Asheville, NC: College Administration Publications, Inc., p. 3, citing *Feist Publication, Inc., v. Rural Telephone Co.*, 499 U.S. 340 (1991).

63 17 U.S.C. Section 102 *et seq.* (1976), *as amended*.

64 17 U.S.C. Section 102 (a) (1976).

65 17 U.S.C. Section 102 (a) (1976).

66 McMillen, J. D. (2001). *Intellectual property: Copyright ownership in higher education: University, faculty, and student rights*. Asheville, NC: College Administration Publications, Inc., pp. 11-20.

67 490 U.S. 104 (1989).

68 Kaplin, W. A., & Lee, B. A. (1995). *The law of higher education: A comprehensive guide to the legal implications of administrative decision making* (3rd ed.). San Francisco, CA: Jossey-Bass, p. 753.

69 McMillen, J. D. (2001). *Intellectual property: Copyright ownership in higher education: University, faculty, and student rights*. Asheville, NC: College Administration Publications, Inc., p. 30.

70 McMillen, J. D. (2001). *Intellectual property: Copyright ownership in higher education: University, faculty, and student rights*. Asheville, NC: College Administration Publications, Inc., p. 30.

71 808 F. Supp. 1238 (1992).

72 *Miller v. CP Chemicals, Inc.*, 808 F. Supp. 1239 (1992); *Restatement 2d of Agency* Section 228 (1958).

73 McMillen, J. D. (2001). *Intellectual property: Copyright ownership in higher education: University, faculty, and student rights*. Asheville, NC: College Administration Publications, Inc., p. 30.

74 McMillen, J. D. (2001). *Intellectual property: Copyright ownership in higher education: University, faculty, and student rights*. Asheville, NC: College Administration Publications, Inc., p. 31.

75 455 F. Supp. 1102 (Del. 1987), *affirmed on other grounds*, 601 F. 2d 76 (3rd Cir. 1979).

76 42 U.S.C. Sections 2000e-4 through e-9 (1964), *as amended*.

77 29 U.S.C. Section 1681 *et seq.* (1963).

78 29 U.S. C. Section 206 *et seq.* (1963).

79 29 U.S.C.A. Sections 701-794 (1973).

80 29 U.S.C.A. Sections 701-794 (1973).

81 42 U.S.C. Sections 12101-12233 (1991).

82 522 F. 2d 380 (8th Cir. 1975).

83 780 U.S. 273 (1987).

84 834 F. 2d 661 (7th Cir. 1987).

85 *Baker v. Lafayette College*, 504 A. 2d 247 (Pa. Super. Ct. 1986).

86 547 A. 2d 144 (D.C. 1988).

87 Euben, D. (2002). *Academic freedom of individual professors and higher education institutions: The current legal landscape*, p. 18. Retrieved October 15, 2002, from http://www.aaup.org

88 The Association also has a statement providing guidelines on the electronic communications in academic settings, *Academic Freedom and Electronic Communication*.

89 McMillen, J. D. (2001). *Intellectual property: Copyright ownership in higher education: University, faculty, and student rights*. Asheville, NC: College Administration Publications, Inc., p. 38.

90 852 F. 2d 715 (3rd Cir. 1988).

# Chapter 39: THE LAW AND THE NURSING STUDENT: ANSWERS YOU WILL WANT TO KNOW

Nancy J. Brent, MS, JD, RN

*Faculty everywhere are concerned about the legal implications of teaching and providing safe client care. Faculty and students alike want to know what they can do to be more proactive and avoid situations that are potentially fraught with legal pitfalls. Ultimately we strive for safe, competent client care. Perhaps the most important step faculty can take to avoid problems is to be well informed. We asked Nancy Brent to share her expertise and to respond to compelling issues that impact faculty and students so nurse educators may be well informed and prudent in their dealings with students and clients. – Lynn Engelmann and Linda Caputi*

## Introduction

Nurse educators face many challenges. Perhaps uppermost in their minds is the axiom, "Do no harm". The editors invited nurse educators to share questions about legal issues of interest to them in their teaching. Many nurse educators voiced similar concerns. This chapter, presented in a question and answer format, goes right to the heart of these concerns. It is the hope of these editors that faculty reading this chapter will glean valuable information that will help allay some of the anxiety associated with the legal aspects of nursing education.

### Educational Philosophy

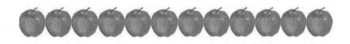

I believe that teaching in an interactive process. A student must be challenged if he or she is to learn. Learning can not take place unless both the "teacher" and the "student" actively participate in the process. – Nancy J. Brent

**Question: As a faculty, I am concerned about the potential for my liability when a student commits an error and a client is injured while providing care for the client that he or she is assigned as part of their clinical rotation. What is the liability of the student, if any? What is my liability?**

This question raises the issue of professional negligence of faculty and of students. Professional negligence is a type of tort and is actionable when the four essential elements of professional negligence are met: duty, breach of duty, proximate cause, and damages or injuries. When evaluating professional negligence, the overall standard of care becomes what the ordinary, reasonable, and prudent person would have done in the same or similar circumstances in the same or similar community. The concept of personal or individual liability is also essential to keep in mind when analyzing professional negligence. That concept states that everyone is responsible for his or her own behavior, including one's negligent behavior. As a result, if someone is professionally negligent, it is extremely difficult to shift the burden of liability or responsibility to someone else.

Students who injure a client during the provision of nursing care during a clinical rotation are responsible for their own conduct. As a result, if a client decides to sue for an alleged injury caused by a student, the student can be sued. The standard of care for the student is not what another nursing student would have done in the situation. Rather, it is a standard that compares the nursing student's conduct with that of a *graduate* nurse. As a result, it behooves students to be prepared for the client care assignment they are undertaking and to voice discomfort or concern about their abilities to handle the situation if such discomfort or concern exists.

Faculty who work with students in the clinical area are also subject to the principles of professional negligence and individual liability. As a result, they must be certain that the supervision, instruction, and other responsibilities they possess as a faculty are met in a non-negligent manner. A faculty may be sued for a situation involving a student if the allegations against the faculty are due to a breach of his or her responsibilities (e.g., not properly supervising the student, improper assignment of the student to that particular client). The standard of care for the nurse faculty becomes what the ordinary, reasonable, and prudent faculty would have done in the same or similar circumstance in the same or similar community.

It is important to note that the injured client (plaintiff) is not limited to suing only the student nurse and the faculty. He or she could also include the school of nursing and/or academic facility in the suit because under *respondeat superior*, the school employs the faculty. If the faculty is found negligent, the school may also bear vicarious liability because it controls the faculty through its policies and procedures, requirements of faculty, and work mandates (e.g., assignment of faculty to courses, hours of work). The school may also be included in the suit under the corporate theory of liability if the school or academic entity breached one of its own duties of care vis-a-vis the student (e.g., unqualified student).

The plaintiff could also include the healthcare facility in the suit as well. Again, this inclusion may be based on the unit manager's breach of a duty of care to the clients for whom the manager is responsible, that is, to prevent a foreseeable and unreasonable risk of harm to the clients. For example, if it were foreseeable that a student nurse's assignment was not appropriate for the particular client, due to either the client's healthcare needs and the student nurse's inexperience or the student not being prepared, the unit manager must intervene and prevent that client care assignment. The unit manager's duty in such circumstances, as is the case with every person's duty, is not necessarily actual knowledge. Rather, if the unit manager *knew or should have known* of this limitation, liability may result for the unit manager.

If a student enrolled in a graduate nursing program is involved in a client care situation that results in an alleged injury as a result of his or her care, the student, who is already licensed by the state, can also be included in the suit. The graduate student's standard of care in such a circumstance would not be what an ordinary, reasonable, and prudent *graduate* nurse would have done in the same or similar circumstances. Rather, the standard would be what another ordinary, reasonable, and prudent registered nurse in a graduate program would have done in the same or similar circumstances.

Because there is the potential for inclusion in a suit when a student nurse allegedly injures a client, the protection of professional liability insurance can not be underestimated. All those who work with student nurses in the clinical area and classroom should carry professional liability insurance, including the student nurse him- or herself. For the cost of the premium for the policy, the insurance company is obligated to defend the person insured and, if an event is covered under the policy, pay any judgment or settlement on behalf of the insured. Clearly, the yearly cost of the insurance policy is well worth this protection.

**Question: When a student nurse documents in a client's medical record concerning the care given, observations made, and so forth, is it required that I, as the clinical faculty, "co-sign" the student's notation in the record? If so, why?**

Whenever anyone "co-signs" another's documentation in a legal record (such as the client's chart), the co-signer is attesting to two things:

- The accuracy of the information contained in the documentation.
- The personal knowledge that the co-signer has of the information in the documentation.

An example in which the implications of co-signing can be seen is when one co-signs a narcotics count at the end of each shift. If there is a question about the accuracy of the information contained on the narcotics documentation form, both the initial signer and the co-signer will be called upon to speak to the accuracy or inaccuracy of the information in that record. The requirement of co-signing documents concerning the administration of controlled substances stems from federal and state laws governing the dispensing and administration of those substances.

Similarly, the answer to the question of co-signing a student nurse's documentation is to consult the state nurse practice act and its rules and regulations. Because no one, including a student nurse, can practice nursing without a valid, current license to do so, the provision of nursing services must be done by individuals who are licensed in the state to provide those services. Most, if not all, nurse practice acts contain an exception to this requirement when a student nurse is providing care as part of a bona fide nursing education program with faculty supervision. As a result, some nursing education programs and some clinical facilities in which students have their clinical rotations require clinical faculty to co-sign students' notations in the records to attest to the review of the students' care and the faculty approval of that care. The requirement of co-signing student nurse notations in the client records also helps the clinical facility meet its requirements under state licensing and certification laws. For example, a facility's documentation policies are developed to reflect, among other things, meeting its responsibilities under these laws.

Other nursing education programs and clinical facilities do not require co-signing of student nurse's notes by faculty because they believe the exception in the act does not mandate the co-signature. Rather, they rely on the fact that there is active supervision of the student nurse when in the clinical area. The supervision of the student nurse is established pursuant to the bona fide educational program's policies and procedures and is a part of the affiliation agreement between the nursing education program and the clinical facility.

Student nurses who are in a graduate program have already been licensed by the state. The concern about co-signing nursing notes for licensed graduate nurses, then, is to ensure supervision about their compliance with the graduate school program. If required, it also illuminates the faculty's knowledge of what the students are doing insofar as client care and its implications for their continued progress in the nursing education program.

It is important to keep in mind, then, that the requirement of co-signing a student nurse's entry is not necessarily a universal mandate. Clinical faculty should evaluate this issue with the legal counsel for the academic institution in order to comply with any nurse practice act requirements. Additionally, the issue must be raised with the clinical facility in order to determine its needs and requirements so that there is consensus between the facility and the educational program on this aspect of student clinical experience.

**Question: What is the "Good Samaritan" law, and how does it apply to student nurses and nursing faculty?**

A state's Good Samaritan statute provides protection for healthcare providers and others who provide care to an individual in an emergency without a fee and without prior knowledge of the person's injuries or diagnosis. The protection afforded is that of **immunity** from suit for professional negligence in the event the person who is provided care sustains an injury due to the care given in the emergency. Immunity from suit is limited, however, to instances of "ordinary negligence." If one acts in a "willfully and wantonly" negligent manner when providing care in the situation, no immunity exists, and the individual can be sued for injuries sustained as a direct result of breaching the standard of care in the situation. Willful and wanton negligence has been defined as an intentional disregard for the safety and well-being of a person.

Good Samaritan statues are usually broad based. Such a statute would apply to nursing faculty and a student nurse who, as examples, provide care at the scene of an accident or initiate CPR in the school or hospital cafeteria.

In some states, Good Samaritan statutes have also been interpreted by the courts as applying to certain healthcare providers who respond to emergent situations in a hospital setting, such as a code. For the most part, these cases have involved physicians responding to an emergency within the institution. The statutes have not been interpreted as applying, however, to situations in which there is an established physician-client relationship. Neither have they been interpreted to apply to situations in which there is an established student nurse-client or clinical faculty-client relationship.

Good Samaritan statutes may also contain immunity provisions for those healthcare providers who donate services at free clinics, health fares, or summer camps. Again, the requirements for the immunity to apply are the same as for providing services at the scene of an accident:

- No compensation.
- An emergent situation.
- No knowledge of the client's condition or diagnosis.

Good Samaritan statutes may also provide immunity from suit to those who administer CPR after successfully passing a certified CPR course. Additionally, those who teach CPR courses are also often granted immunity from suit against allegations that their teaching was negligent.

Student nurses and nursing faculty should review their state's Good Samaritan statute for the protections afforded them. Reliance on such a statute in the usual provision of care to clients as part of the nursing education program, either by the student nurse or the faculty, would be a misplaced assurance, however.

**Question: What is the potential liability of a nursing education program and/or its faculty and administration if a student nurse graduates from the school but is unable to pass the required NCLEX® for licensure?**

This question raises the vital concern surrounding what information is included and what language is used in a student handbook and other print information concerning the nursing education program and the college or university in which it is located. A student handbook and, as an example, a course syllabus become part of the implied contract among the students, the school, and the larger academic entity. Students can use any or all of those documents if they believe their lack of success in passing state boards are due to the program or academic entity's failure to do what it said it would do. When students are unsuccessful in passing the NCLEX®, they may attempt to evaluate that failure by placing blame on the institution, the faculty , and/or the overall nursing education program.

Students' blame of the school and faculty is easily fostered if the student handbook and other printed material contain assurances to the student that the program "prepares the student to successfully pass" the state licensure exam or prepares the student "to become a Registered Nurse." Likewise, if there is an emphasis on the pass rate of the nursing program's graduates to the extent that it is seen as an assurance that all students will experience the same result, students often believe that the fault for failing the exam rests outside of themselves.

Student handbooks, school catalogues, and other printed material that establish the implied contract between or among students, the academic program, and the entity must be carefully drafted by faculty and reviewed by its legal counsel prior to their dissemination to the student body or to applicants. Including a disclaimer in the student handbook and catalogue that neither implies nor establishes a contract between or among the student and academic organization and school is a good way to alert students "up front" that no express contract exists between or among the two or more parties. Moreover, if the disclaimer also reserves the academic entity's and school's right to change the handbook and catalogue specifics as they deem necessary, students are helped to see the relationship as a flexible one upon which they can not absolutely rely.

Despite the attempts of faculty and academic entities to protect against guarantees or assurances that can not be met, students may still seek legal recourse for their disappointment in the event that they are not successful in achieving licensure. In addition to suing the faculty and school for a breach of an implied or express contract, students may also add a count of educational malpractice to their suits. In such a count, students allege that they were not educated correctly as students and the lack of teaching by faculty – negligent teaching by faculty, to be accurate – is the reason they were not able to pass the NCLEX®.

Educational malpractice is a cause of action yet to be recognized by any court in the United States, despite attempts by students to make it successful. Courts to date have been reluctant to say what is and what is not "educational malpractice." There is a great deal of deference to faculty decisions, and the courts see reasoned decision making by faculty as to student learning or lack of learning as something not to be second guessed. Furthermore, the courts have continued, why and how a student learns or does not learn is not easily proven in a courtroom setting. Last, courts have consistently held that to identify a cause of action of "educational malpractice" would "open the floodgates" to litigation of every kind for every student who did not pass a course, did not graduate, or did not successfully pass a licensing or certification exam.

In the law, there are always exceptions to any principle. As the law pertains to the passing of NCLEX® or other such licensing or certification exam, there may be a situation wherein the school and faculty would be carefully scrutinized. If many students from a particular school failed NCLEX® and continued to do so, a review of the school's program by the state board of nursing would most certainly occur. If factors were present that indicated a need for the nursing education program to be placed on probation or take other corrective action in order to "cure" the poor pass rates on the licensing exam of graduates of that particular program and school, those would be enforced by the board. Depending on any deficiencies identified as contributing to the problem of low pass rates by graduates (e.g., unqualified faculty), several students could attempt to file a civil suit, perhaps a class action suit, to seek redress for their failure to successfully pass the NCLEX®. It is unclear what the outcome of such a suit would be, but nursing faculty and a nursing education program could well be at risk for inclusion in such a suit if a connection between the deficiency identified and the low pass rate could be linked.

**Question: What is the legal status of incident reports when an incident as defined by an employer policy occurs and must be filed? Should the fact that an incident report was filed be recorded in the client's record? Some students have told faculty they were instructed not to place any notation of the incident report in the client's record.**

Incident/occurrence reports are tools used by healthcare delivery facilities as part of their overall quality assessment program. Whether used by risk management, quality management, or utilization management, they help identify adverse client care and other adverse situations (e.g., visitor injury). They also help to "prevent" future client care problems and/or prepare for the possibility of a suit.

The process of filing and screening a report may vary from institution to institution. For example, a report may be filed initially with a risk manager or it may go to a risk management committee. In any case, the person or group receiving it carefully screens the information contained in the incident report.

Insofar as client care situations are concerned, an incident report is often generated by nursing staff, who, pursuant to the employer's adopted policies and procedures, use the formal document to notify risk management of an adverse client care situation. Information requested in an incident report usually includes the name of the client, a factual description of the incident or occurrence, injuries sustained by the client, and the occurrence's outcome. Others may include questions "evaluating" the incident. For example, the form may request an answer about how such a situation could be avoided in the future.

Common or statutory law considers incident reports to be "confidential and privileged communications" between the healthcare delivery institution and its legal representative. Because of this status, incident reports should not be placed in the client's record and notations that the report was filed should not be placed in the record. Although it is no secret that incident reports exist and are used when an adverse event occurs, nursing students and nursing faculty, along with nursing staff, must not weaken their protected status. Any contest concerning their existence, their discovery, and their use in a legal matter should be left for lawyers to resolve in court.

Such a privileged status does not mean, however, that the client record should not contain factual and complete information concerning the incident that did occur. The student nurse must ensure that information concerning what occurred, what interventions took place and by whom, the client's response, and any other information necessary to include in the client's record concerning the event be documented following the clinical facility's medical record documentation policy.

In addition to the healthcare facility's incident report, the policies of the nursing education program may also require that its own "incident report" be filed by the student nurse and the clinical faculty involved in the client care occurrence. This obligation should be taken seriously and done without delay in order to alert the nursing program, the academic entity, and its lawyers for the same purposes such a report is used in the healthcare facility.

**Question: Am I obligated to follow the student and course expectations in the syllabus or can I make exceptions?**

Because the course syllabus is considered part of the implied contract of the student with the nursing education program and academic entity, it is important that it be followed. When the syllabus is gone over with students at the beginning of a course or clinical rotation, it serves to let each student know what the parameters of his or her conduct, expectations, and requirements are within that course or clinical experience. The parameters also serve as a notice to each student that grading will occur for each student based on the criterion in the syllabus.

Because uncontrollable situations may arise that require faculty to alter identified criterion (e.g., no more than one clinical day can be missed), the syllabus should contain a statement that the faculty does reserve the right to alter course or clinical requirements if certain conditions are met by the student. For example, a death in a student's family may necessitate that student's absence from a clinical day or days or make the student unable to take an exam scheduled for a day the student is not in school due to the death. The syllabus can contain specific instructions for a student to follow when confronted with a situation that prevents the student from conforming to the syllabus's requirements (e.g., immediate notification of the faculty member). The instructions should also include a statement that it is the faculty who ultimately decides how and when the missed requirement will be met and what penalties, if any, will be assessed against the student for noncompliance with the stated requirements. When necessary, the student or other students would most likely not challenge such individualized, careful, and deliberate decision making. If, however, faculty rigidly enforce course requirements without regard for uncontrollable life situations or make capricious, discriminatory, or arbitrary exceptions to adopted course requirements as contained in the syllabus, students will more likely than not challenge such decisions.

If a student considers a decision by a faculty member concerning a change in the course requirements to be unfair, arbitrary, or in some other way not consistent with his or her rights in the situation, the student should be encouraged to grieve that decision. It should be pointed out to the student that his or her right to do so is included in the student handbook and the adopted policy should be followed. It will, of course, be important for the faculty member to be clear about his or her reasons for the decision made. Any necessary documentation by the faculty member concerning the situation will be helpful in resolving any challenge to his or her exception to the requirements stated in the syllabus.

Any major changes to the syllabus that are not affected by a student's particular uncontrollable situation (e.g., death in the family, illness of student) must be carefully evaluated by the faculty. Because the syllabus sets forth the guidelines and parameters of the course expectations, when a change is detrimental to a student's progression through the course, it must be analyzed before instituting such a change, despite the disclaimer concerning the faculty or school's reservation to change printed requirements and so forth that appear in the student catalogue and perhaps even the syllabus.

Most likely, a change over which the faculty had no control (e.g., a clinical rotation is suddenly not available) will be more "acceptable" to students and can be rectified by not penalizing the student for the change. Sometimes such a resolution requires a creative answer, but sharing the problem solving with the student may be a way in which to come to a consensus about how to handle the difficulty encountered. However, when a change occurs in "midstream" that "punishes" a student's progression through the course and program, he or she has every right to contest that change.

**Question: What is faculty required to do for a student who has a disability? What does "accommodation" mean within the context of the educational program?**

Titles II and III of the Americans with Disabilities Act (ADA) of 1990 prohibit discrimination by public entities relating to state and local governmental services, activities, or programs (Title II) and places of public accommodation (Title III) based on a disability. Title II's application to any governmental entity is clear; for example, a state school is included in its reach. Title III's application contains any privately owned enterprise and/or services – including a private college or university – that affects interstate commerce.

Not everyone who has a disability is covered under the ADA. In order to benefit from its protection, a student must meet the requisite, applicable definitions contained in the Act. Under Title II, for example, a student alleging a violation of the Act must prove:

1. That he or she is qualified individual,
2. With a disability,
3. Who, by reason of such disability,
4. Was excluded from participation in or denied the benefits of programs, services, or activities or subjected to discrimination,
5. Of or by a public entity.

Title III requires a student alleging a violation of the Act to prove that he or she has been discriminated against participating in the equal and full enjoyment of services, goods, programs, advantages, and other benefits of any place of pubic accommodation. A person or entity that owns, leases, or operates a place of public accommodation must base the discrimination on the student's disability.

As can be seen from the requisite elements of any case under the ADA, one of the pivotal hurdles a student alleging discrimination under the ADA must prove is whether his or her impairment meets the definition of disability under the Act. A disability is defined as a physical or mental impairment that substantially affects one or more major life activities of the individual (e.g., walking, breathing, talking) and that the individual has a record of such impairment or is regarded as having such impairment.

If a nursing student is able to meet the requirements of the Act and is therefore protected by it, the question of accommodation of the student during the educational experience may arise. Although the subject is well beyond the scope of this question, some general principles can be highlighted.

For example, a student's request for an accommodation must be supported by adequate and accepted medical proof (e.g., a thorough evaluation of the student and the need for the accommodation). Second, the requested accommodation must be reasonable. If, for example, a disabled student's request requires a total revamping of the entire course of study, such a request would not be accommodated. Exams for disabled students must be offered as frequently and as often as for non-disabled students. Additional time may be required for the disabled student to complete the examination as may a modification in the manner in which the test is given. Facilities in which exams are provided must be accessible to the disabled student (e.g., ramps, space for wheelchairs, if needed).

Auxiliary aids may also need to be provided to a disabled student to help with the taking of exams or with the successful completion of a course or educational program (e.g., taped cassettes of class lectures for a visually impaired student). If the provision of auxiliary aids would pose an undue burden on the educational program or fundamentally alter the course of study, they would not be required under the ADA.

Nursing education programs that have disabled students enrolled in their programs must ensure that the ADA's mandates are complied with, not only through adopted policies but also in carrying the policies out. Doing so involves an open line of communication with the program's attorneys in order to ensure compliance and, at the same time, respect the limitations of the ADA and its regulations. Because every student, including a disabled student, is an individual with unique strengths and weaknesses, there can be no blanket application or nonapplication of the Act and its rules. Indeed, there is a plethora of case law interpreting the ADA and its application to disabled students. Only by a careful analysis of those cases and compliance with their mandates and the limitations of the ADA (where they exist) can nursing faculty and nursing education programs ensure that discrimination against a disabled student in its program will not occur.

## Question: What should students be taught about documentation in the client record?

The fundamentals of good documentation is an essential and ongoing subject that nursing students must be exposed to and master. Because documentation serves so many purposes (e.g., third-party reimbursement, communication among and between staff, use in trials for professional negligence), students need to be exposed to basic principles of good documentation **and** their application to the clinical area.

In addition to specific issues in documentation (e.g., nursing notes must be done as soon after care is given as is possible, never leave empty spaces in the documentation), the student should practice simulated documentation in unique circumstances. For example, what would be included in a nursing note when a client wants to leave against medical advice (AMA)? What should be reflected in the record when a family member is abusive to the client? An interesting way to do simulated documentation is with the use of case studies. In addition, using actual court decisions that focus on poor documentation or helpful documentation blends the theoretical with real situations. The latter also reinforces the importance of nursing documentation in the courtroom.

Graduate nursing students must also learn to improve their basic documentation skills and to fashion nursing entries as a support of their increased level of expertise in the clinical area. Additionally, nurses in a graduate student role should be challenged to develop nursing documentation forms that can be used in the clinical areas. For example, a psychiatric/mental health nurse who is enrolled in a nurse practitioner program may develop a form for use with clients he or she is exposed to when doing an assessment in a mental health clinic or emergency department.

## Question: What is the "Buckley Amendment" and how does it apply to me as faculty working with students?

The federal Family Educational Rights Act and Privacy Act (FERPA) of 1974 was amended by the Buckley Amendment and is the controlling law concerning a student's confidentiality protections. Students covered by the Act are all students in primary, secondary, and post-secondary academic institutions. There are state laws that also govern a student's right of privacy (e.g., medical information release, notification of parents for treatment issues) that should be familiar to nursing faculty as well, although many of them govern students in grades 1 through 12.

The Buckley Amendment controls the access and release of information from a student's school files. Its enforcement is linked to the receipt by the academic institution of funds from the federal programs of the Department of Education. Moreover, the Act applies to both private and public academic entities.

For a student 18 years of age and older, the Act allows the student access to his or her academic dossier and the right to be informed of the school's policy concerning that access. In addition, the student has the right to challenge information in his or her file that is objectionable to the student. Also important is the student's right to provide consent or refusal of consent for information released from the files.

There are some exceptions to the need to obtain the consent of the student to release information from his or her student records. One exception is information that is shared by faculty within a school who has a "legitimate educational interest" in the information. For example, a faculty who is working with a student in a particular clinical area may seek information about the student's abilities in other clinical areas prior to the student taking the clinical rotation. Or a faculty may review a student's file for information concerning the need to take a course or clinical rotation a second time. It is important for faculty to keep in mind, however, that the information can not be further disseminated (e.g., to someone outside the nursing program) without the student's consent.

Nursing education faculty must develop and adhere to program policies concerning the confidentiality of student information. Student files should be stored where there is limited access to them, and a sign-out sheet should be kept to ensure compliance with the adopted policies. Sharing information about a student with other students is not permitted and may violate the Act and other state laws on student confidentiality and privacy.

## Summary

This chapter has explored common concerns that faculty face as they educate nursing students. Faculty liability in the case of student error, documentation issues – such as appropriate content and co-signing – incident reports , and application of the "Good Samaritan" Law have been addressed.  Nursing programs face challenges as well, not the least of which are use and application of the course syllabus, accommodations for students with disabilities, and ultimately, when students fail NCLEX® upon program completion. Armed with the knowledge of safe practice, nurse educators may be confident in their role.

## Learning Activities

1. Contact at least three professional liability insurance companies and determine their rates of coverage for nurse faculty. Compare and contrast the events covered under the policy, deductible amounts, types of coverage (occurrence or claims-made), and duties of the insured. Determine which company provides the best insurance for the premium and present a proposal for fellow faculty for their consideration to purchase the policy.

2. Research case decisions interpreting the obligation of higher education learning programs to accommodate a student with a disability. If possible, compare and contrast a student in a nursing or other medical field with that of a non-healthcare program student. Formulate an argument in favor or against the decisions researched. Identify how the law under which the decision was decided could be changed to support the argument developed.

3. Develop a documentation self-study module for nursing students to learn the basics of nursing documentation, using either an interactive computer program or a more traditional format. Base the examples in the module on actual court cases that were won or lost because of the nursing documentation.  In additional to more traditional modes of documentation, include cases and examples using computer documentation as well. Compare this method of learning documentation with the traditional method or methods of learning documentation by analyzing pass rates obtained by students using both methods of learning, assessing actual clinical documentation by students in clinical rotations, and evaluating students' comments concerning the learning method used. Write a paper for publication that summarizes the results obtained.

4. Research the Buckley Amendment's exceptions to the general consent requirement of the student for the release of information from a student's educational file. How have the exceptions changed, if at all, over the years? Are the exceptions overly broad or are they necessary exceptions with narrow applications? How could the exceptions be changed to still protect student confidentiality yet provide necessary information to be released when a situation required it? Propose written amendments that might allow faculty to better help students by sharing information with those who need the information.

# Disclaimer

This chapter is intended to provide information on the subject matter presented. It is not intended to be legal, or other, advice. If legal or other advice is needed, the services of a competent professional should be obtained.

## Bibliography

Brent, N. (2001). The nurse in the academic setting. (2nd ed), *Nurses and the law: A guide to principles and applications* (pp. 426-458). Philadelphia, PA: W. B. Saunders Company.

Hollander, P., Parker-Young, D., & Gehring, D. (1995). *A practical guide to legal issues affecting college teachers* (The Higher Education Administration Series). Asheville, NC: College Administration Publications, Inc.

Howard-Martin, J., & Hopper, D. (2002). *Public accommodations under the Americans with Disabilities Act: Compliance and litigation manual.* St. Paul, MN: West Group.

Kaplin, W., & Lee, B. (1995). *The law of higher education: A comprehensive guide to legal implications of administrative decision making* (3rd ed.). San Francisco, CA: Jossey-Bass.

Perritt, H. (1997). *Americans with disabilities handbook* (Vol. I, II, III) (3rd ed.). New York: John Wiley & Sons.

Roach, W., & Aspen Health Law And Compliance Center. (1998). *Medical records and the law* (3rd ed.). Gaithersburg, MD: Aspen Publishers, Inc.

# Organizations of Interest to Nursing Faculty

Unit 8

# Chapter 40: NATIONAL LEAGUE FOR NURSING (NLN)

Susan Abbe, MS, PhD, RN

*Throughout its long and flourishing history, the National League for Nursing (NLN) has witnessed many changes in nursing education. However, its fundamental mission never floundered. NLN always has been, and remains, committed to assisting schools of nursing to prepare nurses at all levels to meet current healthcare challenges. Its annual education summit, one of its many educational activities, is a stellar event that presents the latest in educational strategies and research. In this chapter, nurse educators can learn about NLN and the historic role it has played in the support of nursing education at all levels. – Linda Caputi and Lynn Engelmann*

## Introduction

In June 1952, the National League for Nursing Education ceased to function as an autonomous organization and became the nucleus for a new organization the National League for Nursing (NLN). NLN was formed by the consolidation of several professional nursing organizations to advance nursing education in the United States. Under the visionary leadership of Ruth Sleeper, NLN's first president, the organization addressed such issues as shortage of nursing faculty, limited availability of clinical facilities, and inadequate funding for nursing education. From the beginning, NLN's membership has been nurse educators, nurse practitioners, and non-nurses with the primary purpose of improving nursing education to prepare nurses to carry out client care. Fifty years later, NLN continues as a nursing organization that advances excellence in nursing education, representing nursing faculties from all types of nursing education programs.

## Educational Philosophy

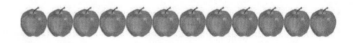

To facilitate student learning; to encourage inquiry and creativity; and to be a resource. – Susan Abbe

## History of NLN

The NLN bylaws in 1952 provided for two divisions: Division of Nursing Service and the Division of Nursing Education. The functions of the Division of Nursing Education were to be carried out through two departments: the Department of Baccalaureate and Higher Degree Programs and the Department of Diploma and Associate Degree Programs. In 1965, the Department of Diploma and Associate Degree Programs separated into their respective areas. In 1967, the Departments were renamed:

- Council of Baccalaureate and Higher Degree Programs.
- Council of Diploma Programs.
- Council of Associate Degree Programs.

In the 1960s, the Council of Practical Nursing was formed. The Councils remained in place until 2000 when they were incorporated under the Advisory Council of Nursing Education.

In June 1953, the first biennial NLN Convention was held in Cleveland, Ohio. The theme was *Concerted Action to Meet the Nation's Nursing Needs*. Sleeper, in a 1953 letter to *Davis' Nursing Survey*, stated the convention platform was "Working together through the National League for Nursing we can help – bring people everywhere in the United States well-organized nursing services, coordinated nursing programs, more nurses, well-prepared nurses" (Rodies,1998, p.262). NLN's biennial conventions continued until 1999 when the NLN Annual Education Summit replaced them.

As the 1960s emerged, many changes in education were occurring nationwide. The time was regarded as the years of crisis in nursing education. Nurse educators were divided over where nursing education should originate – in academic institutions or in service institutions. It was during this period that the entry-into-practice issue exploded. With the rapid growth of junior and community colleges, there was growing declaration by nursing leaders that professional nursing needed to be in colleges and universities. NLN spoke to the need for community planning for nursing education and in Resolution #5 stated,

> NLN . . . strongly supports the trend toward college-based programs of nursing . . and implement[s] the orderly movement of nursing education into institutions of higher education . . . to the end that through an orderly development, a desirable balance of nursing personnel with various kinds of preparation become available to meet the nursing needs of the nation (Fondiller, 1983, p. 55).

The entry-into-practice issue continues currently.

As an outgrowth of the Fourth Nursing Education Conference held in Philadelphia in 1987, a mandate was put forth for the "transformation of nursing curricula from a training model to a schema that would educate caring, critically thinking, healthcare professionals" (Donley, 1989, p. 1). The curriculum revolution began in 1989. The debate began – to teach students to think or to teach students technical skills. The climate was right for change. The movement for curriculum revolution focused on aspects such as:

- Faculty-student and faculty-faculty relationships.
- Multicultural, multiracial, and diversity of individual and family lifestyles.
- Current healthcare systems and future needs.
- Broadening view of what is quality nursing education.
- Innovative teaching strategies.

As the 1990s emerged, the NLN became a leader in the outcomes movement. Accreditation criteria were developed for all nursing program types addressing student academic outcomes within the curriculum. Each NLN Educational Council was absorbed in efforts to determine outcome measures for their nursing education programs.

During all these events and others over the years, the NLN never lost sight of the advancement of nursing education for the excellence of client care. The present-day NLN continues to focus on nursing education, faculty development, and nursing education research. In addition, the organization continues to provide a national comprehensive nursing workforce database and comprehensive strategies to evaluate educational outcomes, student achievement, and nursing workforce competencies.

## Present-Day NLN

### *Mission and Goals*

NLN's (2001) mission is "to advance quality nursing education that prepares the nursing workforce to meet the needs of diverse populations in an ever-changing healthcare environment". Supporting the mission are five goals:

- NLN will lead in setting standards, advancing quality and innovation, and will advocate for all types of academic and lifelong learning programs in nursing.
- NLN will lead in promoting the professional growth and continuous quality improvement of educators for the nursing workforce.
- NLN will lead in promoting evidenced-based teaching in nursing and the ongoing development of research that informs and improves nursing education.
- NLN will be the authority in providing and interpreting comprehensive nursing workforce supply data.
- NLN will lead in developing and providing comprehensive strategies to evaluate educational outcomes, student achievement, and nursing workforce competencies.

## Structure

The NLN is governed by a voluntary 17-member Board of Governors. Each governor is elected at large to serve a three-year term. The four officers and 13 governors-at-large are responsible for the policy setting and general management procedures of NLN. The organization also has a chief executive officer. Together the chief executive officer and Board of Governors work to accomplish the goals of the organization. In addition, there are 38 constituent leagues providing an avenue for members to share best practices and advance legislation and policy. The constituent leagues have formal representation to the NLN through the Constituent Organizations Advisory Council.

The NLN has established four advisory councils:
- Nursing Education.
- Nursing Workforce Development.
- Nursing Education Research, Technology, and Information Management.
- Constituent Organizations.

These councils promote opportunities for addressing and influencing significant issues in nursing education, workforce development, and technology in education. All NLN members are eligible to participate in one or more of the councils.

Membership in NLN is through one of the following three categories:
- Agency membership.
- Faculty membership.
- Individual membership.

Agency membership represents either educational, healthcare, or allied/public agencies. Faculty membership is for all full-time faculty at NLN-member educational agencies. Individual membership is open to nursing educators, policymakers, and interested members of the public, along with nursing students and retired nursing faculty.

## Activities

NLN offers the following activities through the NLN Professional Development Unit:
- Annual Education Summit.
- Faculty development institutes.
- On-line learning modules.
- NLN journal – *Nursing Education Perspectives*.
- Continuing Education Provider Program.

Additional activities are provided through the NLN Research Unit:

- The annual survey dealing with student admissions, enrollments, and graduations and the dissemination of data obtained from the survey.
- Management of grants to support nursing education research.
- Development and distribution of tests.
- The encouragement and support of research in the areas of nursing education.

## *Headquarters*

The NLN headquarters is located at 61 Broadway, New York, NY 10006. Telephone: 800-669-1656 or 212-363-5555. Website: www.nln.org.

For easy launching of the NLN website, the URL is located on the CD accompanying this book. Simply launch your internet browser, put the CD-ROM in the drive, go to Chapter 40 on the CD, and then click on the website address.

## Learning Activities

1. Research the academic outcomes developed by NLN and discuss how they might impact curriculum development.
2. Examine the Curriculum Revolution in light of what was happening within society during the same time period. Consider such influences as the arts, religion, politics, health care, and education.
3. Interview NLN members in service and in education. Ask them to discuss how NLN is beneficial in their professional roles.

### References

Donley, R. (1989). Curriculum revolution: Heeding the voices of change. In National League for Nursing (Ed.), *Curriculum revolution: Reconceptualizing nursing education*, (p. 1-8). New York: Author.

Fondiller, S. H. (1983). *The entry dilemma: The National League for Nursing and the higher education movement, 1952-1972*. New York: NLN.

National League for Nursing [NLN]. (2001). *Shaping the future of nursing education*. New York: Author.

Rodies, K. E. (1998). Concerted action to meet the nation's nursing needs: The first convention. *Nursing and Health Care Perspectives, 19*, 262-263.

Rodies, K. E. (1999). Together we stand: Ruth Sleeper and the early years. *Nursing and Health Care Perspectives, 20*, 6-7.

Tanner, C. A. (1990). Introduction. In National League for Nursing (Ed.), *Curriculum revolution: Redefining the student-teacher relationship*, (p. 1-4). New York: Author.

# Chapter 41: THE AMERICAN ASSOCIATION OF COLLEGES OF NURSING (AACN)

### Geraldine "Polly" Bednash, MSN, PhD, RN, FAAN, and Robert Rosseter, BA

*We are pleased to present this overview of the American Association of Colleges of Nursing (AACN), a national organization whose main purpose is to advance nursing education at the baccalaureate and graduate levels. Central to the mission of AACN is faculty development and curricular enhancement. Dr. Geraldine "Polly" Bednash and Mr. Robert Rosseter address the Essential series, a rich resource for curriculum standards and faculty practice and research. Recently, AACN has set curriculum standards relative to student needs, alternatives to face-to-face learning, inclusion of women's health issues, and nurse practitioner competencies in specialty areas. AACN is indeed a rich resource for faculty. – Lynn Engelmann and Linda Caputi*

## Introduction

The American Association of Colleges of Nursing (AACN) was established in 1969 to advance nursing education at the baccalaureate and graduate levels, and it remains the only national organization dedicated exclusively to achieving this goal. With more than 570 institutional members, AACN represents the interests of the entire academic unit, including 10,000 nursing school deans and faculty and more than 150,000 students enrolled in

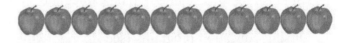

### Educational Philosophy

I strongly believe that there is a connection between education and quality patient care. As the practice of nursing grows more complex, nurses are expected to know more and operate on a highly sophisticated level. I am committed to raising awareness of the need for lifelong learning in the interest of preparing a more highly educated nursing workforce. – Geraldine "Polly" Bednash

Learning is a dynamic process fueled by communication, challenge, and commitment. Teachers and students are true partners on the journey to higher education. Their shared experience is enriched by a free-flowing exchange of information, ideas, and perspectives. – Robert J. Rosseter baccalaureate, master's, and doctoral programs in nursing. The Association's mission extends to assisting nurse educators in preparing a workforce well equipped to meet the demand for innovative and expanded nursing care. (See: *Accreditation: Commission on Collegiate Nursing Education (CCNE),* a chapter in this book by Mary Collins.)

Though representing a variety of constituent groups, AACN's programming is focused on four key areas:

1. Establishing quality standards for nursing education at the baccalaureate and graduate levels.
2. Assisting deans, directors, and faculty to implement those standards.
3. Influencing the nursing profession to improve health care.
4. Promoting public support of baccalaureate and graduate education, research, and practice in nursing.

Because all nursing faculty teaching in entry-level and advanced practice programs are the products of the institutions that AACN represents, the association is committed to providing programs and resources that support nurse educators and enhance faculty practice.

## A Brief History

Over the past three decades, AACN has evolved from a small organization of dedicated volunteers to an internationally recognized professional force representing a broad array of comprehensive and liberal arts institutions, research universities, and academic health centers. The association has achieved a host of key firsts throughout its brief history. AACN produced the first national guidelines to define the essential knowledge, skills, and values expected of new baccalaureate-prepared nurses, the first comprehensive standards for master's degree education of advanced practice nurses (APNs), and the first indicators of quality for doctoral nursing programs. Other milestones include:

- Establishing the Commission on Collegiate Nursing Education (CCNE), the nation's only agency focused exclusively on accrediting baccalaureate and graduate-degree nursing education programs (see *Accreditation: Commission on Collegiate Nursing Education*, a chapter in this book by Mary Collins).
- Creating the first comprehensive database on master's, doctoral, and postdoctoral preparation of nurses, including data on faculty salaries and demographics.
- Leading the drive in the House of Representatives that gave the National Institute of Nursing Research full institute status within the National Institutes of Health.
- Launching a series of executive development workshops to train junior and senior faculty for careers in academic administration, and instituting a parallel executive development series for new and aspiring deans.

- Partnering with the People's Medical Society to publish *Ask A Nurse: From Home Remedies to Hospital Care* (Bednash, 2001), a comprehensive reference book that celebrates the unique expertise of nurses.

AACN is governed by an 11-member Board of Directors. Board members serve three-year terms and are charged with representing the interests of the association's more than 570 institutional members. The association has standing committees on government affairs, membership, programs, and other areas of AACN operations; maintains task forces on such professional concerns as faculty development; and sponsors interest groups in six areas of nursing education, practice, and scholarship. The work of recent AACN task forces has resulted in the creation of several white papers that provide an in-depth analysis and recommendations for action related to key issues impacting professional nursing education. These white papers include *The Role of the Clinical Nurse Leader* (AACN, 2003b), *Faculty Shortages in Baccalaureate and Graduate Nursing Programs* (AACN, 2003a), *Hallmarks of the Professional Nursing Practice Environment* (AACN, 2002), *Distance Technology in Nursing Education* (AACN, 1999b), and a revised position statement on the *Indicators of Quality in Research-Focused Doctoral Programs in Nursing* (AACN, 2001).

In addition to its own initiatives, AACN works closely with other nursing, healthcare, and higher education organizations in a range of coalitions on federal appropriations and other issues of mutual concern. Many of the Association's advocacy efforts are conducted in partnership with the Tri-Council for Nursing, which, in addition to AACN, includes the American Nurses Association, American Organization of Nurse Executives, and National League for Nursing. AACN is an active member of the Federation of Associations of Schools of the Health Professions and the Call to the Profession Steering Committee. The Call to the Profession is a group of 60 top leaders from national nursing organizations who are working together to ensure safe, quality nursing care and to define the nursing profession's agenda for the future. The Association also plays a major role in the Health Professions and Nursing Education Coalition, a group of professional, education, and practice organizations and other constituency groups that advocate for education funding. In addition, AACN's executive director serves as vice president for nursing of the Health Professions Education Council of the Association of Academic Health Centers.

## Enhancing Faculty Practice

AACN's mission extends to developing resources to strengthen faculty practice and facilitate success in faculty roles. By providing faculty with networking and training opportunities, AACN is working to create a community of scholars to steer the nursing profession, build nursing's science base, and improve client care. The organization achieves these goals through its educational programming, leadership development initiatives, and advocacy efforts.

The association provides several platforms to showcase the work of nursing faculty and highlight innovative teaching strategies. AACN hosts faculty conferences each year for nurse educators in baccalaureate, master's, and doctoral programs. These events focus on the latest trends in faculty practice and emerging issues in nursing education. AACN conferences give nurse educators personal contact with key decision makers in health care, higher education, and government. Association meetings offer a stimulating source of continuing education and professional development that builds leadership and administrative skill.

The organization's scholarly publication, the *Journal of Professional Nursing* (JPN), provides a forum for faculty to share research findings, publish policy papers, and stimulate discussion on any number of hot topics. Now in its 20th year, JPN strives to keep pace with continuing changes and professional standards that affect nursing education, research, and practice. This bimonthly publication presents observations by nursing leaders on the diverse roles of baccalaureate-and-graduate-prepared nurses, as well as insightful columns on clinical, legislative, regulatory, and ethical issues of vital interest to stakeholders within the nursing profession. AACN also works to shine the spotlight on the key contributions nursing faculty make in preparing the nursing workforce through e-mail newsletters, monthly publications, and biannual issue bulletins.

Nursing faculty interested in pursuing the role of dean or director of a nursing program look to AACN for leadership development programs designed to facilitate this transition. The annual Executive Development Series welcomes faculty looking to increase the knowledge and skills needed to manage a school of nursing at a time of complex and accelerating change in health care. New deans, faculty, and administrative staff who aspire to the deanship become oriented to the dean's role in academic, financial, and student affairs.

In a related initiative, the Leadership for Academic Nursing Program, AACN is working to enhance the leadership capabilities of individuals aspiring to lead academic nursing organizations. Supported by the Helene Fuld Health Trust, this year-long program provides participants with a focused assessment experience, a range of content and case studies related to successful leadership, and the opportunity to establish networks of mentors or peers for the development of long-term partnerships that facilitate shared growth and development. This program currently accommodates up to 60 Fellows selected by an advisory panel each year.

In the advocacy arena, AACN is a leading voice for federal support for nursing faculty practice and research. The organization works closely with Congress and federal agencies to ensure funding and regulatory policies that provide stable and sufficient support for nursing education. AACN has been effective in securing sustained federal funding for nursing education and research, in shaping legislative and regulatory policy affecting nursing school programming, and in ensuring continuing financial assistance for nursing students. The association played a pivotal role in the creation of a new nurse Faculty Loan Program contained in the Nurse Reinvestment Act that was enacted in August, 2002. Through this program, nurses prepared at the graduate level are entitled to educational loan repayment in exchange for a commitment to serve as nursing faculty. Beyond this important initiative, AACN's governmental affairs staff works to maintain funding for Title VIII nursing education programs, support funding for the National Institute of Nursing Research, and encourage legislation to alleviate the growing shortage of registered nurses.

Through its outreach efforts, AACN strives to generate interest in academia as a career option for nurses. The association identifies and shares best practices related to promoting the faculty role to diverse nursing populations and enhancing cultural sensitivity of nursing faculty. AACN's role in sparking interest in faculty careers is gaining in importance in light of the intensifying nursing faculty shortage, which is severely limiting efforts to expand all types of entry-level nursing programs.

In fact, faculty shortages at nursing schools across the country are contributing to the overall decline in new enrollments at a time when the need for nurses is continuing to grow. Budget constraints, an aging faculty, and increasing job competition from clinical sites have contributed to this emerging crisis. To minimize the impact of faculty shortages on the nation's nursing shortage, AACN is leveraging its resources to help secure federal funding for faculty development programs, collect data on faculty vacancy rates, and identify strategies to alleviate the shortage and bridge the faculty gap.

In an effort to focus federal attention on the nursing faculty shortage and raise public awareness, AACN's Research and Data Center has become a clearinghouse for key statistics and research findings related to the nursing faculty population. Every year, the data center surveys baccalaureate and graduate nursing schools to collect information related to the total faculty population, including demographic and salary information. Supplemental surveys are also used to collect data on retirement patterns, future faculty supply, career plans, practice issues, and related concerns. The results of these surveys are disseminated to key policymakers, the media, and all stakeholders within the healthcare community to raise awareness and generate support for programs designed to increase the faculty pool.

## Setting Curriculum Standards

AACN's curriculum standards provide a framework for positioning baccalaureate-and -graduate-degree nursing programs to meet the healthcare challenges of a new century. Nursing deans and faculty nationwide have implemented AACN's guidelines in designing curricula used to prepare professional nurses to thrive in a healthcare system marked by continual change. Together with nursing faculty and an interdisciplinary panel of stakeholders, AACN, through its *Essentials* series, developed curriculum standards for baccalaureate and master's programs in nursing and outlined the critical elements of clinical support needed for the entire nursing academic mission to flourish.

## The Baccalaureate Essentials

First released by AACN in 1986, *The Essentials of Baccalaureate Education for Professional Nursing Practice* is a comprehensive set of core standards for baccalaureate-degree nursing education programs. This publication, which provides a central framework for designing baccalaureate nursing programs, was the first national effort to define the fundamental knowledge, values, and professional behaviors expected of baccalaureate-degree nursing graduates.

The *Essentials of Baccalaureate Education* (AACN, 1998) provides direction for the preparation of professional nurses for practice in the 21st century. The publication is the outcome of a series of roundtable conferences and regional hearings held throughout 1997 and coordinated by an AACN task force. Created by the AACN Board of Directors, the task force reviewed the 1986 document for its relevance to current and future nursing practice and found that major revisions were necessary.

In a two-phase review process, AACN sponsored two invitational roundtable meetings assembling nurses and other experts in areas of primary concern to nursing presently and in the foreseeable future, including:

- Genetics.
- Gerontology.
- Rural health.
- Interdisciplinary practice.
- Healthcare financing.
- Integrated healthcare delivery.

Participants identified the core knowledge and skills that baccalaureate-prepared nurses must attain to practice in the present-day changing health system.

Following the roundtables, five regional meetings invited comment on a draft *Essentials of Baccalaureate Education* document – developed from the roundtables – from nurse educators, clinicians, administrators, and researchers representing a broad range of educational programs, specialties, and organizations. More than 770 individuals – representatives of 49 states, the District of Columbia, and Puerto Rico, as well as representatives from 349 schools of nursing, 23 professional organizations, and 19 healthcare delivery systems – participated in the consensus-building regional hearings.

The new realities of health care require nurses to master complex information, coordinate a variety of care experiences, use technology for healthcare delivery and evaluation of client outcomes, and assist clients with managing an increasingly complex system of care. The *Essentials of Baccalaureate Education* (AACN, 1998) focuses on preparing entry-level registered nurses (RNs) to deal effectively with, among other new trends, technological advances that have a profound effect on disease prevention and detection, information management, and clinical decision making. Nurses also must address the needs of an increasing aging population that brings new challenges related to lifelong health promotion, management of the chronically ill, and end-of-life issues.

In addition, the increasing diversity of the U.S. population requires a fuller understanding of how health is influenced by such factors as age, gender, culture, ethnicity, religion, lifestyle, and functional ability level. At the same time, AACN believes nurses must understand how a more interconnected global environment affects the health of individuals and the delivery of care.

The *Essentials of Baccalaureate Education* (AACN, 1998) details standards for preparing bachelor-degree nurses to assume roles as care providers; as designers, managers, and coordinators of care; and as members of a profession. Within these roles, the document provides specific standards for educational components that are essential for all baccalaureate nursing programs, including liberal education, professional values, core competencies, core knowledge, and role development.

To build core competencies, the *Essentials of Baccalaureate Education* (AACN, 1998) recommends a range of coursework and clinical experiences in such areas as critical thinking, communication, assessment of clients' health status, and technical skills. Under core knowledge, AACN suggests specific course content in key areas, including:

- Health promotion, risk reduction, and disease prevention.
- Management of illness and disease.
- Ethics.
- Human diversity.
- Information management and client care technology.
- Global healthcare issues.
- Healthcare systems and policy.

For example, the *Essentials of Baccalaureate Education* urges that baccalaureate nursing students:

- Acquire the skills to initiate community partnerships in health promotion programs.
- Understand how healthcare systems are organized and financed.
- Use communication technology to improve the accessibility of care.
- Provide care that addresses the needs of diverse populations across the life span.
- Identify the political and economic factors that influence healthcare services.

The *Essentials of Baccalaureate Education* (AACN, 1998) not only recommends the content of what is taught but also suggests strategies for how to teach it. For example, to motivate students to be active, creative learners, AACN encourages educators to use actual communications, such as written or verbal testimony to legislative bodies, that are more engaging or relevant than those based on data on unknown individuals, which are impersonal and non-engaging.

### The Master's Essentials

Released by AACN in 1996, *The Essentials of Master's Education for Advanced Practice Nursing* outlines a standardized core curriculum for APNs and all other registered nurses who are prepared at the master's-degree level. This publication was developed following 18 months of regional, consensus-building conferences with participation by nurse educators, clinicians, administrators, and researchers from a broad array of specialties, states, and organizations. The curricular model was created in response to the AACN (1993) position statement, *Nursing Education's Agenda for the 21st Century,* which called for a common educational core to ensure that America's master's-educated RNs are sufficiently prepared to practice in a health system marked by rapidly changing technologies and dramatically expanding knowledge.

In developing the curriculum, AACN's Task Force on the Essentials of Master's Education convened the regional conferences to provide a national forum for developing a document that would be backed by wide professional support. The original intent of the project was to focus mainly on the education of APNs. However, soon after deliberations began, a consensus emerged that two separate but related components of the master's essentials were needed – a statement of the essential core content for all master's-educated nurses and a statement of the core curriculum for all APNs who work in direct care roles. The model AACN curriculum has three main components:

1. A graduate nursing core, the essential foundation for all students who pursue a master's degree in nursing, regardless of specialty. The curricular elements in the graduate core are consistent with standards established by the Council of Graduate Schools.
2. An advanced practice nursing core, content deemed essential for all nurses who provide direct care at an advanced level.
3. A specialty curriculum comprised of clinical and classroom learning experiences defined by nursing organizations that represent nurse practitioners, clinical nurse specialists, certified nurse-midwives, and certified registered nurse anesthetists.

The *Essentials of Master's Education* (AACN, 1996) not only calls on master's programs to give all graduates – regardless of specialty – a firm understanding of the roles and requirements of advanced practice nursing, but also to be solidly grounded in such areas as healthcare policy, organization, and financing. Moreover, the *Essentials of Master's Education* points out that programs in nursing administration and community health also should include AACN's core master's curriculum in their teaching. The reasoning here that advanced practice RNs should be able to provide quality care that is also cost-effective and have the skills for leadership roles to manage the human, financial, and physical resources of health care.

Specifically, coursework at the master's level should provide graduates with the knowledge and skill to:
- Analyze the results of policy research that impact upon healthcare delivery.
- Be familiar with health services across a variety of systems, including acute and out-patient care as well as managed care and integrated care settings.
- Understand the interaction between quality controls and regulatory controls.

Graduates also should understand the economic implications of health planning, the organization of personnel and resources, and the design of payment systems. In addition, the *Essentials of Master's Education* stresses the need for graduates to work both in collaborative and interdependent relationships with other health professionals, design and deliver healthcare that is culturally relevant, and develop holistic plans of care that address the health promotion and disease prevention needs of clients.

Finally, as healthcare technology expands and the demands for cost-containment increase, ethical decision making must be a core component of all master's-degree nursing education, the *Essentials of Master's Education* urges. This not only includes the ability to counsel clients as ethical issues arise, but for nurses to participate in discussions of healthcare ethics as they affect one's community, society, and the health professions overall. Although AACN views the *Essentials of Master's Education* as the foundation of all master's-degree preparation for nursing, it is expected that educators will individualize the model to their schools' own missions and to the needs of their regions and student populations.

### *The Clinical Essentials*

Changes in healthcare financing are exerting new pressures on the ability of students and faculty to be assured sufficient access to training sites. The *Essential Clinical Resources for Nursing's Academic Mission* (AACN, 1999a), the latest in AACN's Essentials Series, defines the clinical elements crucial to supporting the full spectrum of academic nursing – undergraduate and graduate education, faculty practice, and research. Released in April 1999, the volume identifies factors that facilitate and hinder educators' access to clinical sites, describes essential on-site learning experiences for undergraduate and graduate nursing students, and details the clinical resources needed for faculty practice and nursing research to develop and thrive.

In this landmark publication, AACN (1999a) identifies the facilitators and barriers to clinical access in nursing education, describes essential clinical-site learning experiences for preparing skilled nurses for basic and advanced practice. The *Essential Clinical Resources* recommends strategies for reshaping the relationship between education and practice to ensure that essential clinical resources are accessible and achievable. To remain relevant and appropriate, present-day clinical nurse training requires even more than providing students with such current skills as case management, interdisciplinary experience, and access to the latest information technologies. Indeed, the changing dynamics of health care, especially its financing, are threatening the conventional means of access to clinical practice sites and require a re-thinking of how nursing schools can provide students with clinical learning experiences.

Produced by an AACN task force of distinguished educators and nurse executives, the *Essentials of Clinical Resources* (AACN, 1999a) provides direction for the preparation of professional nurses into the 21st century. The task force was established in 1997 out of growing concern over changes in healthcare delivery and health profession education that significantly altered the number and types of clinical resources available for nurse education, faculty practice, and nursing research.

Nursing schools now must vie for clinical training slots not only with other area nursing schools but also with medical and physician assistant programs that are placing students for primary-care experiences in the same health centers used traditionally for nursing education. For example, an AACN (1997) issue bulletin reported that although applications remained strong, some schools had cut admissions to nurse practitioner programs because of a tightening supply of training locations. Many schools nationwide continue to report problems placing undergraduate nursing students for clinical experiences due to a shrinking availability of training sites.

In the *Essentials of Clinical Resources,* AACN (1999a) notes that the healthcare system is moving from an array of disconnected agencies to integrated systems run increasingly by the private sector, with an increasing emphasis on cost and the bottom line. Moreover, as care has shifted from hospitals to more outpatient treatment, the tremendous cost-cutting and re-engineering of acute-care delivery sites have diminished educational support from these agencies.

Throughout the *Essentials of Clinical Resources* (AACN, 1999a), educators, administrators, and other policy leaders explore:

- How the shifting focus of healthcare delivery has changed the level of educational support by clinical agencies.
- Essential clinical-site learning experiences for both undergraduate and graduate nursing students.
- Regulatory, financial, competitive, and other barriers impeding nursing schools'

access to clinical training sites.

- How nursing's academic culture, including reward systems, must change to incorporate clinical practice into the faculty role.
- Funding, intra- and interdisciplinary, and other resources of clinical environments that successfully support and foster nursing research.

In addition, AACN's (1999a) *Essentials of Clinical Resources* features an extensive resource listing of creative collaborations among nursing schools, healthcare institutions, and community agencies to provide on-site clinical nurse education as well as research and faculty practice opportunities. Among the nearly 50 innovative programs highlighted are academic-corporate partnerships, contracts with government agencies and managed care companies, alliances with academic health centers, partnerships between communities and local governments to establish nurse-managed primary care clinics, and collaborations with healthcare institutions to create joint nursing research centers.

## Specialized Curriculum Standards

Throughout its history, AACN has worked with the generous support of healthcare foundations to produce specialized sets of curriculum standards and guidelines that influence how nurses are educated across the country.

### *Curricular Guidelines for End-of-Life Nursing Care*

In recognition of the universal need for humane end-of-life care, AACN, supported by the Robert Wood Johnson Foundation, convened a roundtable of expert nurses and other healthcare professionals in 1998 to stimulate scholarly discourse and initiate change on this important reality. This action was taken in accord with the International Council of Nurses' (1997) mandate that nurses have a unique and primary responsibility for ensuring that individuals at the end of life experience a peaceful death.

The United States is facing the realities of an aging population, a recognition of the limits and inappropriate use of technological resources, and concerns about the capabilities of healthcare providers. Additionally, the increase in demand for assisted suicide, as well as apprehensions of the public about suffering and expenses associated with dying that may be prolonged unnecessarily by technology, contribute to a renewed interest in humane end-of-life care. Increased awareness of the success of hospice as an alternative model of care has served as a catalyst for integrating palliative care into traditional models of care delivery.

Precepts underlying hospice care are essential principles for all end-of-life care. Such precepts include the assumptions that individuals live until the moment of death; that care until death may be offered by a variety of professionals; and that such care is coordinated, sensitive to diversity, offered around the clock, and gives attention to the physical, psychological, social, and spiritual concerns of the client and the client's family. These precepts provide guidance to the development of the educational preparation of nurses. However, educational preparation for end-of-life care has been inconsistent at best, and sometimes neglected within nursing curricula. Given the likelihood that care will be given by a variety of healthcare professionals, it is essential that such preparation be interdisciplinary in its approach to preparing students for the end-of-life practice in which they will engage.

Armed with this understanding, the roundtable's group of healthcare ethicists and palliative care experts developed end-of-life competency statements, which every undergraduate nursing student should attain. The group made recommendations concerning the content areas where these competencies could be addressed in the publication *Peaceful Death: Recommended Competencies and Curricular Guidelines for End-of-Life Nursing Care* that was released by AACN and the John A. Hartford Foundation Institute for Geriatric Nursing in 1998. These guidelines have served as a catalyst for strengthening end-of-life nursing care content in undergraduate programs and provided the foundation for AACN to further develop nursing's expertise in this key area through the End-of-Life Nursing Education Consortium.

### End-of-Life Nursing Education Consortium

The End-of-Life Nursing Education Consortium (ELNEC) is a comprehensive, national education program to improve end-of-life care by nurses. The primary goal of this project is to develop a core of expert nursing educators and to coordinate national nursing education efforts in end-of-life care. This project is supported by a major grant from the Robert Wood Johnson Foundation.

This three-year project began in February 2000 and is administered through a partnership between AACN and the Los Angeles-based City of Hope National Medical Center (COH). ELNEC is a consortium of many organizations that are represented on an advisory board, including the Oncology Nursing Association, the Hospice and Palliative Care Association, American Nurses Association, and the Veterans Administration Health System. This diverse group insures that the ELNEC project brings together leading nursing groups and perspectives to form a collaborative approach to improve end-of-life education and care. AACN is coordinating the project, and nurse researchers at COH developed and continue to revise the curriculum, as well as evaluate the educational program.

The ELNEC project also has representation from the national program Educating Physicians on End-of-Life Care (EPEC) to foster strong collaboration with medical colleagues. The ELNEC core curriculum has been developed through the work of highly qualified subject-matter experts serving as consultants, with extensive input from the advisory board and reviewers. Courses are designed to prepare educators to disseminate this important subject matter into nursing schools and healthcare agencies.

Originally five courses were planned, but the call for applicants for the first course elicited an overwhelming response from the nursing education community. Supplemental funding by the Robert Wood Johnson Foundation resulted in a total of eight ELNEC courses sponsored by AACN and COH during the three-year project. Five additional courses were also provided in conjunction with Last Acts Regional Conferences.

The 13 total courses sponsored by the ELNEC project were designed to meet the unique needs of specific groups of nursing educators:

- Baccalaureate and associate degree nursing faculty who will facilitate integration of end-of-life care in basic nursing curricula.
- Nursing continuing-education providers and clinical staff development educators who will offer educational activities to improve the end-of-life care by practicing nurses. This group includes nurses providing continuing education in colleges and universities, state and specialty nursing organizations, and independent businesses, as well as continuing education/staff development in clinical settings such as hospitals, hospices, home care, and long-term care.

With new courses planned over the next few years, the project is reaching out in new directions. Subject-matter experts are adapting the ELNEC curriculum for faculty teaching in graduate nursing programs and introducing new content on pediatric end-of-life nursing care.

AACN and COH hope to continue this effort to offer training opportunities for undergraduate faculty and continuing education providers and expand overall end-of-life nursing education. To date, the ELNEC training program has reached over 16,000 nursing students and clinicians, with representatives from all 50 states. Over the next few years, project leaders estimate that ELNEC-trained educators will touch the lives of six million clients and their families facing the end of life.

### *Curricular Guidelines for Geriatric Nursing Care*

Currently, there are 25 million Americans over the age of 65, with America's older adults comprising the fastest growing segment of the U.S. population. Nurses play an essential role in providing acute and chronic care, health education, and health promotion to these older Americans. The need for geriatric nurses is growing as the nation's baby boom generation nears retirement, yet the country is challenged to prepare geriatric nurses at a time when the number of individuals entering the healthcare disciplines is diminishing.

In light of these realities, AACN believes that nurses who graduate from bachelor-degree programs should have the skills to recognize the complex interactions of acute and chronic conditions common in the elderly; use technology to enhance older adults' independence and safety; and assess older adults' physical, cognitive, psychological, social, and spiritual status. To support this recommendation, AACN and the John A. Hartford Foundation Institute for Geriatric Nursing released a set of curricular guidelines for geriatric nursing care in 2000, titled *Older Adults: Recommended Baccalaureate Competencies and Curricular Guidelines for Geriatric Nursing Care*. This joint publication calls for a curriculum infusion in geriatric care and recommends that related content be integrated throughout baccalaureate nursing curricula.

Despite a 30-year effort on the part of academic and professional nursing organizations, the number of master's prepared geriatric nurses remains quite small. Approximately 1,800 nurses nationally are certified by the American Nurses Credentialing Center (ANCC) as geriatric nurse practitioners, and only 500+ are certified as gerontological clinical nurse specialists. Their small numbers prevent geriatric nurse specialists from providing care to those older persons who are at high risk or whose needs are extremely complex. In addition, because nurses tend to cluster in urban areas, few advanced practice geriatric nurses are available to care for older persons living in rural areas.

*Older Adults* (AACN & the John A. Hartford Foundation Institute for Geriatric Nursing, 2000) was developed in collaboration with the project's National Expert Panel for Baccalaureate Competencies in Geriatric Nursing, a 25-member task force of leading nurse educators, clinicians, and nursing and other healthcare organization representatives to address this gap in nursing education. The publication's competencies, curricular guidelines, and teaching strategies are designed to work hand-in-hand with AACN's (1986) *Essentials of Baccalaureate Education for Professional Nursing Practice*, the association's comprehensive standards that define the fundamental knowledge, values, and core competencies expected of bachelor-degree nursing graduates. The *Essentials of Baccalaureate Education* stresses the need for course work and clinical experiences to prepare graduates to deliver care across the lifespan, with particular attention to changes due to aging.

*Older Adults* (AACN & the John A. Hartford Foundation Institute for Geriatric Nursing, 2000) defines 30 clinical competencies necessary for nurses to provide high-quality care to older adults and their families. In addition, the publication suggests content and teaching strategies in critical thinking; communication; assessment; health promotion, risk reduction, and disease prevention; healthcare system and policy; and nine other core competency areas identified in the *Essentials of Baccalaureate Education*, and recommends steps for incorporating these concepts throughout the nursing curriculum. This baccalaureate geriatric nursing competency document is organized as follows:

- Competencies necessary for nurses to provide high-quality care to older adults and their families.
- Geriatric competencies in relationship to the AACN's (1986) *Essentials of Bacca-*

*laureate Education,* with suggestions for content and teaching strategies.

- Suggestions for including competencies, content, and teaching strategies in the curriculum.
- Resources to facilitate implementation of content and teaching strategies.

Nursing faculty are encouraged to use these guidelines to strengthen specialized nursing content in an effort to better equip the nursing workforce to meet the growing demands for geriatric nursing care.

### *Geriatric Nursing Education Initiatives*

The work of the AACN and Hartford Foundation continues in the area of geriatric nursing care through three grant-funded projects that are of special interest to nursing faculty. The first effort, the annual Awards for Exceptional Baccalaureate Curriculum in Gerontologic Nursing is a national awards program created to recognize model baccalaureate programs in nursing with a strong focus on geriatric nursing. Awards are presented to nursing programs that exhibit exceptional, substantive, and innovative baccalaureate curriculum in this subject area. Beyond innovation, programs must also demonstrate relevance in the clinical environment and have the ability to be replicated at schools of nursing across the country. New categories have recently been added to recognize nursing faculty who demonstrate a special commitment to infusing geriatric content into their coursework.

The second initiative, Enhancing Geriatric Nursing Education for Undergraduate Baccalaureate and Advanced Practice Nursing Programs, is designed to increase geriatric nursing content in baccalaureate and APN programs by providing grants to baccalaureate and higher degree schools of nursing. This program enables nursing students to develop the specialized skills needed to provide high-quality care to older adults.

In the area of undergraduate education, grants assist nursing schools in adapting their gerontology curriculum based upon national education and practice standards, such as those developed by the John A. Hartford Foundation Institute for Geriatric Nursing in collaboration with AACN. Funds were disseminated to institutions to provide an innovative plan of action that reflects these nationally recognized benchmarks for effective gerontological nursing education. In a parallel initiative for graduate programs, the grant allows for the development of a set of core gerontological competencies for all APNs who provide care to older adults but are not specialists in gerontology. In addition, funds were awarded to schools to integrate these newly identified competencies into APN programs and to develop models of excellence that may be adopted by the broader graduate nursing education community. Innovative curriculum developed through this project will be disseminated to the full body of nursing schools, who will be encouraged to adapt their curriculum accordingly.

The final initiative, Creating Careers in Geriatric Advanced Practice Nursing, provides scholarship monies to schools of nursing to expand opportunities for nursing students to choose a career in geriatric advanced practice nursing. The need for geriatric APNs is growing as the nation's older adult population continues to expand, with baby boomers nearing retirement age. Geriatric APNs are expert nurses prepared at the master's-degree level who provide, direct, and influence the care of older adults and their families in a variety of settings. These nurses are uniquely prepared to improve outcomes of care, promote quality of life, and provide comprehensive care for older adults.

Although the need for geriatric nurses has been identified, the number of students pursuing this field of expertise has neither expanded sufficiently nor been distributed appropriately to various geographic regions and healthcare settings. The reasons behind the lack of student interest include a limited number of master's programs in this area, few scholarship opportunities, and the lack of visible leadership to attract new students to this career path.

Through this grant-funded initiative, AACN provides scholarship monies to schools of nursing with geriatric APN programs to expand their student base. In addition to eliminating financial barriers to education, the project provides for networking, mentorship, role modeling, and leadership activities between scholarship awardees and experts in geriatric nursing. Stronger links between students and clinical leaders will help to solidify the role of the geriatric APN and attract new students to the field. Faculty are encouraged to steer promising students into careers in geriatric care to help meet the national need for expertly prepared nurses in this important specialty area.

### *Emerging Areas in Nursing Education*

AACN's work in setting curriculum standards extends to emerging areas of nursing education and practice. Since the year 2000, AACN has released several sets of competencies and statements that impact how nurses are educated at the baccalaureate and graduate levels, including:

- Revising the *Indicators of Quality in Research-Focused Doctoral Programs in Nursing* (AACN, 2001), first released in 1986, to ensure that graduates of professional-degree programs are prepared to function in advanced practice roles, as well as administrative, executive, public policy, and teaching roles.
- Working with the Alliance on Nursing Accreditation to release a statement on the need for nursing education programs delivered solely or in part through distance-learning technologies to maintain the same academic program and learning support standards and accreditation criteria as programs provided in face-to-face formats.
- Collaborating with five federal agencies on a project to describe women's health content in bachelor-degree nursing curricula, cite best practices, and recommend

strategies for strengthening women's health perspectives in preparing new baccalaureate nurses.

- Creating a guidebook and CD-ROM to assist nursing faculty in transitioning to community-based pedagogy through a project supported by the Helene Fuld Health Trust.
- Partnering with the National Organization of Nurse Practitioner Faculties to publish *Nurse Practitioner Primary Care Competencies in Specialty Areas: Adult, Family, Gerontological, Pediatric, and Women's Health* (National Organization of Nurse Practitioner Faculties & AACN, 2002), a project supported by the federal Division of Nursing.

AACN staff are currently working on a set of recommendations for preparing nurses to respond to mass casualty incidents, including acts of bioterrorism. These new competencies are to be released in 2003.

## Summary

Since its inception, AACN has helped schools of nursing to remain as adaptable and attuned to change as the healthcare environment itself. AACN's curriculum standards, position statements, issue bulletins, and other educational resources serve as rich resources for nurse educators wishing to stay abreast of emerging issues and curricular innovations. The association's website (www.aacn.nche.edu) serves as the portal to this information, which may be accessed and circulated to augment both student and faculty learning. AACN encourages nursing school faculty to continue their professional development and encourage students to embrace education as a means of developing strong competencies in nursing-care delivery and exploring new horizons within the nursing profession.

For easy launching of the AACN website, the URL is located on the CD accompanying this book. Simply launch your internet browser, put the CD-ROM in the drive, go to Chapter 41 on the CD, and then click on the website address.

## Learning Activities

1. Read an AACN white paper of your choice (see www.aacn.nche.edu), summarize the issue, and outline the action steps needed to influence the national agenda related to this concern.
2. Describe how your nursing education program supports or counters the recommendations made in either the *Essentials for Baccalaureate Education (AACN, 1998)* or

*Essentials for Master's Education (AACN, 1996).*

3. What are some of the key issues presently facing professional nursing education? What steps can be taken to rally support to advance the profession and embrace change?

4. Interview the coordinator of the gerontology program at your school and identify the action steps that are being taken to address the needs of the aging population. Are they sufficient? What would you recommend?

5. Identify the ways in which nursing curriculum has changed over the past 30 years to meet client needs. Describe how you envision it changing in the future. What role will national nursing organizations play to make this change happen?

## References

American Association of Colleges of Nursing [AACN]. (1993). *Position statement: Nursing education's agenda for the 21ˢᵗ century.* Washington, DC: Author.

American Association of Colleges of Nursing [AACN]. (1996). *Essentials of master's education for advanced practice nursing.* Washington, DC: Author.

American Association of Colleges of Nursing [AACN]. (1997). *Issue bulletin: As schools produce for primary care, training sites grow slim.* Washington, DC: Author.

American Association of Colleges of Nursing [AACN]. (1998). *Essentials of baccalaureate education for professional nursing practice.* Washington, DC: Author.

American Association of Colleges of Nursing [AACN]. (1999a). *Essential clinical resources for nursing's academic mission.* Washington, DC: Author.

American Association of Colleges of Nursing [AACN]. (1999b). *White paper: Distance technology in nursing education.* Washington, DC: Author.

American Association of Colleges of Nursing [AACN]. (2001). *Position statement: Indicators of quality in research-focused doctoral programs in nursing.* Washington, DC: Author.

American Association of Colleges of Nursing [AACN]. (2002). *White paper: Hallmarks of the professional nursing practice environment.* Washington, DC: Author.

American Association of Colleges of Nursing [AACN]. (2003a). *White paper: Faculty shortages in baccalaureate and graduate nursing programs: Scope of the problem and strategies for expanding the supply.* Washington, DC: Author.

American Association of Colleges of Nursing [AACN]. (2003b). *White paper: The role of the clinical nurse leader.* Washington, DC: Author.

American Association of Colleges of Nursing [AACN] & The John A. Hartford Foundation Institute for Geriatric Nursing. (1998). *Peaceful death: Recommended competencies and curricular guidelines for end-of-life nursing care.* Washington, DC: Author.

American Association of Colleges of Nursing [AACN] & John A. Hartford Foundation Institute for Geriatric Nursing (2000). *Older adults: Recommended baccalaureate competencies and curricular guidelines for geriatric nursing care.* Washington, DC: Author.

Bednash, G. D. (Ed.). (2001). *Ask a nurse: From home remedies to hospital care.* New York: Simon & Schuster.

International Council of Nurses. (1997). *Basic principles of nursing care.* Washington, DC: American Nurses Publishing.

National Organization of Nurse Practitioner Faculties & American Association of Colleges of Nursing

[AACN]. (2002). *Nurse practitioner primary care competencies in specialty areas: Adult, family, gerontological, pediatric, and women's health*. Washington, DC: U.S. Department of Health and Human Services, Health Resources and Services Administration.

**Bibliography**

Alliance for Nursing Accreditation. (2002). *Statement on distance education policies*. Washington, DC: Author.

American Association of Colleges of Nursing [AACN]. (2000). *White paper: Guidelines for accommodating students with disabilities in schools of nursing*. Washington, DC: Author.

American Association of Colleges of Nursing [AACN]. (2002). *Moving forward with community-based nursing education*. Washington, DC: Author.

Berlin, L. E., Stennett, J., & Bednash, G. D. (2003). *2002-2003 enrollment and graduations in baccalaureate and graduate programs in nursing*. Washington, DC: AACN

Berlin, L. E., Stennett, J., & Bednash, G. D. (2003). *2002-2003 salaries of instructional and administrative nursing faculty in baccalaureate and graduate programs in nursing*. Washington, DC: AACN.

# Chapter 42: NATIONAL ORGANIZATION FOR ASSOCIATE DEGREE NURSING (N-OADN)

Elizabeth Hilbun Mahaffey, MS, PhD, RN

*In 1986, as a new nursing faculty, I became fascinated with the chance to be involved with the birth of a state chapter of a new nursing organization. This was an incredible experience – took about 9 months – at times it was difficult but the results were very rewarding. In this chapter Dr. Mahaffey provides a succinct overview of the birth of the national organization for which I was working at the state level. After reading her chapter, I now see that, although I thought we had accomplished much within the state, working at the national level must have been an incredible adventure! – Linda Caputi*

## Introduction

The National Organization for Associate Degree Nursing is one of the youngest professional nursing organizations in the United States. Established in 1986, the National Organization for Associate Degree Nursing (N-OADN) has had substantial growth in membership and in representation opportunities. "N-OADN is the only national professional nursing organization whose goals and strategic plan are focused on associate degree nursing education and maintaining registered nurse licensure of graduates from associate degree nursing programs" (Mahaffey, 2002, p. 6).

As the leader in associate degree nursing education, N-OADN provides many benefits for nursing educators and nursing education administrators. N-OADN members benefit from the national exposure enjoyed by leaders in the organization, and from the ongoing efforts of the board of directors. Communication between the board of directors and members is dynamic through state and national meetings, a quarterly newsletter, and an active listserv.

### History of the National Organization for Associate Degree Nursing (N-OADN)

N-OADN was founded during a time of controversy in the nursing profession. The American Nurses Association (ANA) and the National League for Nursing (NLN) had both published position statements that promoted the baccalaureate degree as the minimum entry-level for professional nursing practice. Graduates from associate degree and diploma programs were identified as technical nurses. Distinct licensing exams, either totally different or the addition of an exam for baccalaureate graduates, were promoted.

Although similar entry-level issues had been discussed since the mid-1960s, delegate actions from both ANA and NLN in the mid-1980s created further controversy. With a stand by NLN representatives and funding by ANA to implement the ANA position statement, many associate degree educators became disenfranchised with the two leading nursing organizations (Mahaffey, 2002).

In 1984, after discussing the need for someone to speak out in support of associate degree nursing education, three Texas associate degree nursing leaders and educators identified the necessity for a new nursing organization. With the leadership of these three women, Naomi Brach, Mary Hardy, and Mary Moses, the Texas Organization for the Advancement of Associate Degree Nursing was organized in June, 1984. The following year, the Texas organization was asked to host a national meeting. Thirty states were represented at this meeting; representatives included a mix of nursing educators, nursing education administrators, and community college presidents (Singer, 1992).

A national steering committee was formed during this meeting with the composition of the steering committee reflecting the national interest in forming a new organization (B. Anderson, personal communication, May 28, 2003). See Table 42.1.

Table 42.1 – National Steering Committee of 1984

| National Steering Committee<br>To Form a National Organization for Associate Degree Nursing |
|:---:|
| Mrs. Bobbie Anderson, Mississippi, Chairperson<br>Mrs. Naomi Brach, Texas, Vice-Chairperson<br>Mrs. Faith Rierson, Washington, Secretary<br>Mrs. Peggy Saxton-Isaac, Arizona, Treasurer<br>Mrs. Patricia Bayles, Kansas, Director-at-Large<br>Dr. Linda Spink, Massachusetts, Public Relations<br>Mrs. Catherine Natzke, Michigan, Bylaws |

The National Organization for the Advancement of Associate Degree Nursing was organized in 1986. The name of the organization was later changed to the National Organization for Associate Degree Nursing (N-OADN). As noted by Mary Moses (N-OADN 2000, p. 2) very quickly, "N-OADN became the voice for Associate Degree Nursing Education nationwide. We joined forces with other professional organizations to be sure that associate degree concerns were being heard" (p. 1). The first chair, and later president, Naomi Brach (1986) described the National Organization for the Advancement of Associate Degree Nursing as "a new organization with a clear mission – retain R.N. title, R.N. licensure, and the same level scope of practice for A.D.N. graduates" (p. 1).

Throughout the years, distinguished leaders have served as President of N-OADN. See Table 42.2 for a listing of those presidents.

Table 42.2 – Past and Current Presidents of N-OADN

| N-OADN Presidents |
| --- |
| Mrs. Naomi Brach, Texas, 1986-1988 (Chair) |
| Mrs. Bobbie Anderson, Mississippi, 1988-1990 |
| Dr. Jodie Parks, Florida, 1990-1992 |
| Dr. Carol Singer, Florida, 1992-1994 |
| Dr. Carol Caresio-Haas, Illinois, 1994-1996 |
| Dr. Deanna Naddy, Tennessee, 1996-1998 |
| Dr. Sue Ochsner, Texas, 1998-2000 |
| Dr. Libby Mahaffey, Mississippi, 2000-2002 |
| Dr. Sharon Bernier, Maryland, 2002-2004 |

The early mission and goals of the organization have remained a consistent influence on the mission, goals, and strategic plans in subsequent years. President Bobbie Anderson emphasized the goals of the new national organization:

- Act as a national organization in speaking for associate degree nursing education and practice.
- Reinforce to the public the value of associate degree nursing education and practice.
- Retain the title, RN, and no less than the current scope of practice for the registered nurse.
- Maintain endorsement of registered nurse licensure from state to state for the associate degree nurse.

- Retain registered nurse licensure exam for graduates of associate degree nursing programs.
- Promote the development of associate degree nursing through recruitment, education, and practice (Anderson, 1988, p.1).

Early organization activities focused on incorporation of state chapters, attending meetings of interest, and communicating with members. Newsletters and the journal, *AD Nurse*, were used to inform members of early organization activities and local, regional, and national issues. Review of early N-OADN newsletters illustrates efforts on national issues. Numerous networking activities and collaborative efforts were also ongoing.

Over the past seventeen years, N-OADN has worked closely with numerous professional nursing organizations. President Naomi Brach (1989) emphasized the importance of ongoing professional relationships, "We each have responsibilities in other nursing organizations and I hope as we move from one professional group to another, we can assume the role necessary to be accountable to the group and to ourselves" (p. 2).

There have been national nursing organizations and other health-related organizations that have not welcomed N-OADN. Some groups have viewed N-OADN as divisive, but no other organization has consistently represented associate degree nursing education and the practice of registered nurses who are graduates of associate degree nursing programs. N-OADN has been a part of several national nursing consortiums; however, it has been excluded from others. As noted by the N-OADN president in 2002:

> "The future of nursing has been the subject of many groups over the past fifty years. In recent years, these groups have attempted to be inclusive of the various education program types, and multiple practice groups. Unfortunately, through timing, degree of involvement, or number of participants, associate degree nursing has not enjoyed equal inclusion in many of these endeavors. Participation involves risks, but is essential if a group or organization is to have a voice in what the future of nursing will be. For associate degree nursing, it is our responsibility to articulate the educational outcomes of our programs, and the competencies of our graduates. Models of nursing practice that compliment the efficacy of associate degree nursing education must be identified or designed." (Mahaffey, 2002, p.10)

From the earliest stages of the organization, N-OADN has worked closely with the American Association of Community Colleges (AACC). AACC leaders have joined N-OADN in representing associate degree education and practice to multiple groups, and were instrumental in the establishment of both the national organization and state chapters. For many years, the N-OADN president has served as a member of the Licensure Committee of AACC, and an AACC Director has been an appointed board member of N-OADN.

## N-OADN Mission and Strategic Plan

Although there have been minor changes in the N-OADN mission statement throughout the years, the mission focus has been a constant since its inception. The current mission statement is: "N-OADN is the leading advocate for associate degree nursing education and practice, and promotes collaboration in charting the future of health care education and delivery" (N-OADN, 2003, p. 1).

N-OADN operates through a strategic plan that is reflected in the following statements: "N-OADN strives to:

- Maintain eligibility for registered nurse licensure for graduates of associate degree nursing programs.
- Educate students and promote AD nursing programs at community colleges nation-wide.
- Provide a forum for discussion of issues impacting AD education and practice.
- Develop partnerships and increase communication with other professional organizations.
- Increase public understanding of the role of the associate degree nurse.
- Participate at national and state levels in the formation of healthcare policy.
- Facilitate legislative action supportive of the goals of N-OADN." (N-OADN, 2003, p. 1)

Table 42.3 highlights a few of the activities included in each strategic plan component.

## Organization Activities

A Board of Directors that includes a president, president-elect, secretary, treasurer, immediate past-president, and five directors governs the activities of N-OADN. Directors have designated responsibilities in the areas of AACC liaison, bylaws, education, membership/marketing, and public relations. All board members are elected by the membership through a formal nominations and elections process.

Board members and individual members represent the organization in multiple venues, including information sharing, policy shaping, and leadership development. A position statement approved by the membership in 1998 provides a brief and effective overview of the organization's views. N-OADN's *Position Statement in Support of Associate Degree Nursing as Preparation for the Entry-Level Registered Nurse*

Table 42.3 – Components of the N-OADN Strategic Plan

| N-OADN Strategic Plan | |
| --- | --- |
| Strategic Plan Component | Activities |
| Advocacy | • Provide a voice for associate degree nursing programs and their graduates.<br>• Promote efficacy of associate degree nursing.<br>• Promote strategies to provide an adequate supply of registered professional nurses.<br>• Collaborate with the N-OADN Foundation. |
| Administration | • Demonstrate organizational and fiscal accountability.<br>• Promote membership growth. |
| Communications/Networking | • Maintain information regarding N-OADN and associate degree registered nursing on the N-OADN web site.<br>• Enhance communication with members through the web site, listserv, and a potential new journal.<br>• Promote the active involvement of members. |
| Education | • Provide N-OADN members with educational opportunities, including the annual meeting program.<br>• Recognize excellence among associate degree education faculty and students. |
| Research | • Serve as a resource for accurate data regarding associate degree professional nursing education and practice.<br>• Participate in research activities collaboratively with other organizations. |
| Policy | • Shape policy regarding associate degree nursing education and practice within the healthcare delivery system. |

asserts:

> Associate Degree Nursing (ADN) education provides a dynamic pathway for entry into registered nursing (RN) practice. It offers accessible, affordable, quality instruction to a diverse population. Initiated as a research project in response to societal needs, ADN education is continually evolving to reflect local community needs and current health care trends. ADN graduates are prepared to function in multiple health care settings, including community practice sites.
>
> Graduates of ADN programs possess a core of nursing knowledge common to all nursing education routes. They have continuously demonstrated their competency for safe practice through National Council Licensure Examination for Registered Nurses (NCLEX-RN®) pass rates. These nurses provide a stable workforce within the community. The majority of ADN graduates are adult learners who are already established as an integral part of the community in which they live. They exhibit a commitment to lifelong learning through continuing education offerings, certification, credentialing, and continued formal education.
>
> Nurses prepared at the ADN level are caring, competent, and committed health care providers who fill a vital need in local communities. Accordingly, the National Organization for Associate Degree Nursing supports ADN preparation as the entry level into registered nursing. (N-OADN, 1998, p.1)

A more recent policy statement, adopted by the N-OADN Board of Directors in 2001, identifies the influence of associate degree nursing education on the current nursing shortage. N-OADN's *Policy Statement on the Nursing Shortage* (2001), emphasizes the commitment of associate degree educators:

> The current nursing shortage is most acute in hospitals; the initial setting for practice for the majority of registered nursing graduates. Therefore, associate degree nursing educators continue to be committed to provide educational programs that produce the nurses necessary to meet the demands of the nursing shortage.
>
> Associate degree programs provide a sound foundation for the delivery of safe client care in the current complex health care delivery system. The programs are a reasonable investment of time and money for the student, allowing for licensure and employment in two years from the time of admission to the nursing program. Evidence of this can be seen by: the number of students who seek associate degrees in nursing; the strong passage rate on the NCLEX-RN® exam by associate degree nursing graduates, which exceeds or equals that of other

graduates; and the success of the associate degree graduates in nursing practice. (N-OADN, 2001, p. 2)

In 2002, N-OADN membership accepted a N-OADN Model for Nursing Education/ Practice, which is being finalized for publication on the N-OADN website.

## Membership Benefits

The National Organization for Associate Degree Nursing is a chartered, not-for-profit national organization with state chapters. The membership of N-OADN is comprised of individuals and institutions. Membership categories include:
- Individual Membership:  composed of individual members.
- Associate Membership:  composed of retired individuals.
- Agency Membership:  composed of colleges and institutions.

The majority of individual and associate members are involved in nursing education as teachers or administrators. Membership is open to practicing nurses and other interested individuals. Agency membership is again primarily education institutions, but does also include healthcare organizations.

Membership benefits include:
- Quarterly issues of the N-OADN newsletter.
- Networking through a members-only listserv.
- Networking and educational opportunities sponsored by national and state chapters.
- Reduced member rates at the annual convention, which offers an opportunity to earn valuable continuing education credits.
- Annual scholarship opportunities.
- Annual opportunity for Educator of the Year Award.
- Opportunities for leadership development, authorship, public speaking, legislative activity, and more!  (N-OADN, 2002, p. 1)

One of the most popular benefits is the listserv, where members regularly pose questions to gather feedback, or share important news. This is available for members only, and, since its inception, has been used frequently by the national board of directors and N-OADN members.

# N-OADN Contact Information

Current information about N-OADN activities and communication with the board of directors can be accomplished through the following means:

National Organization for Associate Degree Nursing

| | |
|---|---|
| Mailing Address: | P.O. Box 3188 |
| | Dublin, OH 43106-0088 |
| Phone: | 614.451.1515 |
| Fax: | 614.538.1914 |
| E-mail address: | noadn@noadn.org |
| Web Address: | www.noadn.org |

For easy launching of the N-OADN website, the URL is located on the CD accompanying this book. Simply launch your internet browser, put the CD-ROM in the drive, go to Chapter 42 on the CD, and then click on the website address.

## Learning Activities

1. Visit the N-OADN website. Read one of the items listed under *Nursing Issues*. Analyze the item and respond with pros and cons to its contents.
2. Compare and contrast the mission of N-OADN with the American Association of Colleges of Nursing (AACN), representing baccalaureate and higher education. See the chapter in this book by Polly Bednash and Robert Rosseter.

### References

Anderson, B. B. (1988). President's message. *National Organization for the Advancement of Associate Degree Nursing Newsletter*, 3:2, 1.

Brach, N. (1986). Message from the chairman – fight the good fight. *National Organization for the Advancement of Associate Degree Nursing Newsletter*, 1:3, 1.

Brach, N. (1989). National OADN history. *National Organization for the Advancement of Associate Degree Nursing Newsletter*, 4:1, 2.

Mahaffey, E. (2002). The relevance of associate degree nursing education: past, present, future. *Online Journal of Issues in Nursing, 7*. Retrieved February 17, 2003, from http://www.nursingworld.org/ojin/topic18/tpc18_2.htm

National Organization for Associate Degree Nursing [N-OADN]. (1998). Position Statement in Support of Associate Degree as Preparation for the Entry-Level Registered Nurse. Retrieved February 25, 2002, from http://www.noadn.org/positionstatement.htm

National Organization for Associate Degree Nursing [N-OADN]. (2000). Closing Luncheon Speech by Mary Moses. Retrieved February 25, 2002, from http://www.noadn.org/positionstatements.htm.

National Organization for Associate Degree Nursing [N-OADN]. (2001). Policy Statement: Associate Degree

Nursing Response to the Nursing Shortage. Retrieved April 29, 2002 from the World Wide Web: http://www.noadn.org/NursingShortage.pdf

National Organization for Associate Degree Nursing [N-OADN]. (2002). Membership. Retrieved April 24, 2003 from the World Wide Web: http://www.noadn.org/membership.htm

National Organization for Associate Degree Nursing [N-OADN]. (2003). About N-OADN. Retrieved February 17, 2003 from the World Wide Web: http://www.noadn.org/about.htm

Singer, C. (1993). Associate Degree Nursing: Past, Present, & Future, as presented at the Second Annual Convention of the Louisiana Organization for Associate Degree Nursing, Baton Rouge, Louisiana.

# Chapter 43: NATIONAL ASSOCIATION FOR PRACTICAL NURSE EDUCATION AND SERVICE, INC. (NAPNES)

Helen M. Larsen, BS, JD, LPN

*Dr. Larsen walks us through the prolific history of the National Association for Practical Nurse Education and Service, Inc. (NAPNES). Her thorough and sensitive coverage provides us with a clear and detailed view of the inception and growth of both NAPNES and the Practical/Vocational Nurse. As Dr. Larsen so adeptly states, "I encourage readers to develop and implement projects and programs that reach and raise the knowledge level of those who practice the art and science of nursing at any level." We believe this chapter will appeal to all those who teach the art and science of nursing! – Lynn Engelmann and Linda Caputi*

## Introduction

The National Association for Practical Nurse Education and Service, Inc. (NAPNES) is the oldest organization focused on the education and practice of licensed practical or vocational nurses (LP/VNs) in the United States. NAPNES was founded in 1941 by a group of registered nurse (RN) educators for the purpose of improving and extending the education of the practical nurse to meet the critical need for more nursing personnel.

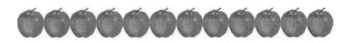

## Educational Philosophy

Teaching is the process of providing return on investment. Each person given the opportunity to acquire knowledge and experience is privileged to share that investment with students and colleagues. The ability to enrich the life of others, thereby enriching the lives of those they impact, multiplies the return on investment in education. The more knowledge and experience shared, the more acquired producing the impact of better understanding, more fulfillment, and especially in nursing, better care at all levels of delivery. – Helen Larsen

Within a few years, after professionally planned curricula had been established and duties of the practical nurse defined, NAPNES expanded its activities to include a broad program of service to schools of practical nursing and practitioners. Important among these was the establishment in 1945 of the first accrediting service for programs of practical nursing education officially recognized by the U.S. Commissioner of Education. The accreditation program was discontinued in 1986.

NAPNES activities include:

- Conducting workshops and seminars to keep LP/VNs abreast of new nursing and medical techniques.
- Sponsoring of continuing education programs.
- Evaluating such programs sponsored by other agencies for continuing education credit.
- Disseminating recruitment materials.
- Interpreting LP/VN education and practice to the public.

NAPNES speaks for LP/VNs at federal and state levels on such matters as licensing, laws governing LP/VN practice, educational opportunities for the LP/VN, and matters of general welfare. Additionally, NAPNES publishes the *Journal of Practical Nursing* quarterly.

Individual membership in NAPNES is open to all, including:

- LP/VNs.
- RNs.
- Nurse educators.
- Physicians.
- Hospital and nursing home administrators.
- Lay citizens interested in LP/VN's role in the health field.
- Students in schools of practical/vocational nursing are welcomed as student members.
- Agency membership is open to hospitals, nursing homes, schools of practical/vocational nursing, alumni groups, civic organizations, and others interested in the objectives of NAPNES.

The early history of NAPNES is in itself a history of the occupation of LP/VNs. NAPNES leaders were catalysts for the creation of this new vocational occupation, which emerged in the 1940s. As new one-year courses for practical nurses were opened, the concept of the practical nurses as glorified "domestics" skilled in simple nursing duties disappeared, and in its place came the reality of a well-prepared practitioner with sound clinical experience. NAPNES leaders secured funds to establish the first model schools of practical/vocational nursing outside of New York and so gave national prominence to this new standard of education for nurses.

In 1944, NAPNES spearheaded an historic conference in Washington, D.C., bringing together representatives of NAPNES, vocational educators throughout the country, and public health nurses at the call of the U.S. Department of Vocational Education. After a week of debate, it was voted unanimously to add practical nursing to the list of vocational programs, and practical nursing students became eligible for federal funds. The fight for mandatory state licensing laws, as well as formulation of curricula and analysis of functions that came with the admission of practical/vocational nursing to the list of vocational studies, was all part of the early history of NAPNES – the history of the birth of the occupation of the LP/VN.

## The Work of NAPNES

The objectives of this Association are directed toward the development of sound practical/vocational nurse education and the promotion of LP/VNs as important members of the health team, concerned with the health and welfare of all people. In furtherance of its objectives, the work of the Association is to:

- **Establish** sound standards for practical/vocational nurse education and service.
- **Initiate and foster** research in practical/vocational nurse education and service.
- **Promote** the philosophy and the opportunity for continuing education among LP/VNs.
- **Further** recognition by health agencies of practical/vocational nursing services, especially their substantial contribution to communities at a local level.
- **Endeavor** to increase the number of dedicated and well-prepared LP/VNs.
- **Represent** the interests of practical/vocational nurse education, and service on committees concerned with health, education, and service.
- **Advise** LP/VN associations on matters pertaining to organization activities.

## History

The history of NAPNES is an extraordinary example of teacher mentoring and impartation of knowledge for a higher cause – the service of nursing. Present-day, well-educated, competent practitioners of licensed practical/vocational nursing owe a deep debt of gratitude to the dedicated RNs from the 1940s who made it all possible. The 63-year tradition of open membership and teamwork between the two distinct levels of licensed nursing, RN and LP/VN, is a sacred trust that the current NAPNES protects and promotes at every possible turn. From the 1940s to the present day, the NAPNES story is replete with acts of unselfish sharing of knowledge and expertise from RNs to LP/VNs, and it is cherished. The NAPNES founders set the stage for the long-term success of NAPNES by incorporating the expertise of faculty in the practical nursing schools, hospital administrators, and lay citizens to create the organization that is the living record of their faith, support, and perseverance. This NAPNES tradition continues to benefit LP/VNs and the people for which they provide the service of nursing.

The vastly condensed information presented here comes from over 60 years of NAPNES corporate records. To help readers understand the progress from "new occupation" to the present-day professional licensed practitioner, highlights of the challenges and how NAPNES continues to meet them gives an idea of the steel determination that is alive and well in the hearts and souls of NAPNES members. Licensed practical/vocational nursing is forged one day at a time – then, now, and for the foreseeable future.

## National Association for Practical Nurse Education (NAPNE)

It was not until 1959 that NAPNE formed the department of service, adding the words "and Service" to its name and becoming the National Association for Practical Nurse Education and Service, Inc. (NAPNES).

In 1940, the Ballard School of the YWCA in New York City invited the directors of the known schools of practical nursing to meet for a day at the Central Branch. By the second meeting, the increased attendance required the meeting to move from a classroom to the auditorium. The ambitious program included a full-stage demonstration of isolation technique in the home by a staff member of the Visiting Nurse Service of New York. The original objective of these conferences was to provide an opportunity for people who believed in the need for the trained practical nurse to discuss mutual problems. They were increasingly aware of the lack of opportunity for representation on the programs of national nursing organizations and faced innumerable problems involving administration, curriculum, and personnel policies.

In 1940, during the Biennial Nursing Convention in Philadelphia, Katherine Shepard, the executive director of the Household Nursing Association in Boston, invited an interested group to a luncheon conference. She presented her belief that an association to promote practical nurse education was needed – an organization with legal status capable of accomplishing more than the informal conference groups sponsored by the Ballard School. The guests included RNs Helen Gill, Etta Creech, Ella Thompson, Mrs. Charles Newhall, Lillie Young, and Hilda Torrop. With toasts, optimism, and enthusiasm the proposal was endorsed. Those were very busy years, but these torchbearers somehow found time in the midst of their multiple activities to lay the groundwork for the new organization, indeed, for the new occupation.

## The First Two Years

In 1941, during the National League for Nursing Education's convention in Chicago, 28 well-wishers participated in the meeting to organize the Association of Practical Nurse Schools. It was the unanimous desire of the group that Katherine Shepard accept the leadership of the Association. When she declined, pleading many other responsibilities, Hilda Torrop, then director of the Ballard School of Practical Nursing, was elected president. She held this office for six years. Etta Creech, director of the Family Health Association in Cleveland, was elected secretary-treasurer.

Slowly the wheels began to turn. By 1942, when the second meeting of the new association was held at the Ballard School, 35 people attended, including three practical nurses from the newly organized and first state association of practical nurses – Practical Nurses of New York. Nine new schools were identified.

At this meeting, the name of the infant association was changed to the National Association for Practical Nurse Education (NAPNE), and the policy of admitting trained practical nurses to full membership and untrained practical nurses to associate membership was adopted. This was a radical change questioned by some of the founding members.

## Boston, 1943

The third annual conference held in Boston marked a milestone for the Association. To venture abroad, to seek a larger attendance, to plan a formal program – this was progress. The treasurer's notebook shows $25 expended from association funds for the entire expense of the conference. Noting that the bank balance as of May 1, 1943, was $35.55, extensive splurging was out of order! Obviously, everyone paid his or her own expenses. During this period, the Association headquarters consisted of a corner of Etta Creech's desk in Cleveland and similar space in Hilda Torrop's office at the Ballard School in New York.

## New York, 1944

The fourth annual conference was held at the Henry Hudson Hotel in New York City. The membership rattled around in the ballroom, but attendance was definitely larger and the program showed the growing interest in the practical nurse vocation. At this meeting, the first exhibit was presented, i.e., the nationally famous obstetrical models lent by Dr. Robert Latou Dickinson from the New York Academy of Medicine. The president's report notes the lack of reliable data on any phase of practical nursing and lists the questions that could not be answered at the Washington conference, called in April by the U.S. Office of Education at the request of NAPNE.

This request was impelled, in part, by the need for trained people by NAPNE's mounting concern about the wide variations in practical nurse training courses, not only from state to state but all too frequently within the same state. The prompt acquiescence to this appeal was not without its own dramatic implications, for when Hilda Torrop presented it to the Commissioner of Education, he was quick to say that he was presently employing an untrained practical nurse in his own home.

The all-important outcome of the conference was the appointment by the U.S. Office of Education of a committee to study the practical nurse occupation. Hilda Torrop was chairperson of this Job Analysis Committee, and Arthur Wrigley directed the study.

### New York, 1945

In 1945, the fourth annual meeting was held at the headquarters of the Visiting Nurse Service of New York. This conference was especially memorable because of the inspirational address regarding the plight of the mental hospitals and their need for practical nurses.

### Accreditation Service

The NAPNE accreditation and consultation services were initiated this year, primarily as a means of giving recognition to practical nursing schools in states that were still without licensure laws and hence without state approving authority for practical nurse training. This also gave existing schools an opportunity to be identified as meeting standards above the minimum required by a state. Consultation services enabled schools about to start to have the benefit of assistance in planning facilities and curriculum and securing qualified faculty. These services were accepted on a voluntary basis by the schools.

### New York, 1946

In 1946, at the Visiting Nurse Service of New York headquarters, attendance at the annual conference topped the previous year; the quality of the speakers not only maintained previous standards but also reflected the growing national interest in the practical nurse vocation. The U.S. Office of Education's study of the practical nurse occupation was completed, and speakers from the U.S. Public Health Service and from the Children's Bureau affirmed their belief in this vocational worker. By this time most schools of practical nursing in the New York area were routinely sending students to conference sessions. Revision of the bylaws provided for group membership of alumnae associations and state organizations affiliated with NAPNE, a provision that was to bear fruit in the years ahead. At this time the American Nurses Association (ANA) was recommending that each state consider legislation leading to licensure of practical nurses.

The Board of Directors of NAPNE, although strongly endorsing this policy, also urged that practical nurse opinion and support be sought, that practical nurses be appointed to the Boards of Nurse Examiners in states where practical nurses were licensed, and that a pattern of uniformity be developed that would remove the barriers between states.

In the short life of the Association, the year that had just ended had no parallel in accomplishment. Three well-attended board meetings were held. Leadership for institutes in seven states had been provided, assistance was given in the organization of five state practical nurse associations, a representative of NAPNE had appeared on the programs of seven conventions, and requests were beginning to come in for consultation service. Hilda Torrop was instrumental in developing a public information program on practical nursing in Ohio, a project sponsored by the Family Health Association in Cleveland. This program included the organization of the Practical Nurse Association of Ohio, still in existence but now known as the Licensed Practical Nurse Association of Ohio (LPNAO), an important development in that state.

A request for funds to conduct a state demonstration of practical nurse education and service had been presented by the NAPNE to the W. K. Kellogg Foundation, the request jointly supported by the Michigan State Department of Education and the Michigan Nursing Council. Acceptance of this broadly conceived plan was announced at this convention. Three years had elapsed since the NAPNE board of directors presented their first prospectus covering this project to the National Nursing Council for War Service for approval.

Among the state practical nurse associations, NAPNE helped organize chapters in New York, Ohio, New Jersey, Colorado, Missouri, Texas, Virginia (two), and Maine. The board of directors had many problems to face and many decisions to make – not the least of these being the task of financing an organization whose only source of income was derived from membership dues and that was in dire need of a full-time staff member.

The title practical nurse, advocated steadily by NAPNE, was now accepted by the professional nursing organizations and the U.S. Office of Education and helped bring about a better understanding of the education and service of the trained worker. The publication by the U.S. Office of Education of the two-year study of the practical nurse occupation was the most reliable occupational nursing study available.

The unrelenting work of a subcommittee of the Accrediting Committee produced schedules for collecting information during a survey visit to a practical nursing school. NAPNE sought to set standards that were above the minimum outlined by state boards of nurse examiners but not impossible of accomplishment by a good school.

The Curriculum Committee revised its plan of action when the U.S. Office of Education decided to begin work on a practical nursing curriculum. It was decided to concentrate on the revision of the now obsolete "Minimum Standards for Schools of Practical Nursing" in the production of a pamphlet designed as a guide to institutions or individuals wishing to organize a school of practical nursing. From the flood of inquiries, that information interpreting the scope of the recommended practical nurse training program, faculty qualifications, space, and necessary equipment was needed as a stimulus and a way to set standards and deter those schools that did not meet such standards. A retiring officer summed it up when she said, "Seeded above timberline, without protective neighbors, with little sustenance, and under the burning sun of criticism and the strong winds of opposition, the NAPNE has had to be sturdy or die."

### Executive Director Appointed

Minutes of the Executive Committee in 1947 include this significant announcement: "The Executive Committee of the Board of Directors is glad to announce the appointment of Miss Hilda M. Torrop as the first executive director of the NAPNE, her appointment to take effect on September 1, 1947." She was NAPNE's first salaried staff member.

### The Michigan Project

The new president, Ella M. Thompson, was drafted almost immediately for active service to substitute as executive director for Hilda Torrop, who was released to organize the three-year program for training practical nurses in Michigan, under the Division of Trade and Industrial Education. This was the experimental program previously mentioned that was initiated to demonstrate the value of a statewide practical nursing program. The three participating agencies were the Michigan State Department of Education, the Michigan Nursing Council, and NAPNE. The W. K. Kellogg Foundation supplied a grant-in-aid for the project.

### Progress in 1947

NAPNE began a series of rapid forward steps with the appointment of a full-time executive director and a part-time office secretary. The headquarters office was now a small room in a suite of three, shared with the New York City Nursing Council for War Service and Nurses House.

The year 1947 was marked by the appearance of the Job Analysis of the Practical Nurse Occupation, published by the U.S. Office of Education. NAPNE and other organization representatives who participated in its preparation could hardly believe that those 144 printed pages were all there was of those grueling hours of discussion, writing, checking, and rechecking. Where was the record of those meetings of the faithful every Monday night, week after week – of the painstaking demonstrations designed to convince Arthur Wrigley, the director of the study, that "evening care" (the myriad of services provided in the home evenings and nights by the first "practicals" in the early days) was a job? (He produced indisputable proof that it was several jobs.) And, reasonably or unreasonably, the dogged NAPNE crew somehow expected that a record of the comradeship would be there, too. It was pioneer work – the first attempt by national nursing, hospital, public health, and educational organizations to agree on the duties of the practical nurse, to define the scope and limitations of those duties, and to identify the related knowledge necessary to carry them out safely and effectively.

Hard on the heels of the Job Analysis, the U.S. Office of Education set a Curriculum Committee to work on a practical nursing curriculum as a sequel and companion piece to the Analysis. During this period, the president served as chairperson of the Production Committee, in addition to her duties as acting executive director of NAPNE.

This year, 1947, saw the accrediting program, which was initiated in 1945, really start its surveys, and eight schools were soon carrying NAPNE approval.

An increasing participation in the work of other organizations is shown by NAPNE representation on the Joint Committee on Practical Nurses and Auxiliary Workers in Nursing Services, the National League for Nursing Education Curriculum Conference, the White House Conference on Child Care, and the American Vocational Association.

### Cleveland, 1948

NAPNE representation on the National Nursing Council for War Service, Inc., later the National Nursing Council, Inc., on which Hilda Torrop served, ended with the dissolution of the Council in 1948. This had been a rich, if sometimes harrowing, experience, as concern for practical nursing was not generally accepted as a desirable activity for professional nurse educators. Ella Thompson served as an alternate on the Council during the war years. Deep appreciation is recorded in the minutes of those frenetic years for the understanding support given by Elmira Wickenden, the Council's Executive Secretary, to those minority members.

### New York, 1949

This annual conference at the Hotel Statler in New York City had as its theme "Together We Weave." It was marked by the increase in attendance over the previous year and the growing number of practical nurses and practical nursing students who registered for the various sessions. An attendance of 200 is recorded at the opening business meeting. Agnes Gelinas, president of the National League for Nursing Education, and Oscar Ewing, administrator of the Federal Security Agency, appeared on the program. Ruth Bryan Rhode, former U.S. ambassador to Denmark, was the dinner speaker.

### Structure Study Requests

During 1947, 1948, and 1949, three requests were made by NAPNE for inclusion of a representative on the Structure Study Committee of the professional nursing organizations. The NAPNE board of directors believed that any overall plan for integration of nursing services and education should include practical nursing interests. These requests were refused, a decision that was deeply deplored by the NAPNE board.

The executive director was appointed in 1949 as a consultant to committees associated with important undertakings, such as the committee on training and recruitment of hospital personnel, sponsored by the Board of Education of New York City, and the Hunterdon Medical Center, Hunterdon County, New Jersey.

## *Report on Schools*

The 1949 report on schools of practical nursing, prepared by the National League for Nursing Education with assistance from the NAPNE, shows 73 approved practical nursing schools, with a total of 2,579 students enrolled in the 60 schools replying to the questionnaire. The previous year, 1,550 students had been graduated. The median school as reported in the summary of the study had the following characteristics:

- Was a hospital school.
- Did not receive public funds.
- Enrolled 32 students and graduated 15.
- Admitted students twice a year to a 12-month course.
- Was on a 44-hour week.
- Did not require pre-entrance psychometric tests.
- Accepted graduation from elementary school for admission.
- Paid a stipend of $15 per month.
- Provided full room and board.
- Employed two full-time and three part-time faculty members.

The schools were located predominantly in the northeastern and southern sections of the country.

During these growing years, the friendly support of the Public Health Relations Committee of the New York Academy of Medicine was the greatest single strength of NAPNE. Shortly after its organization, the Association asked the Public Health Relations Committee to appoint a committee on practical nursing, and this was done. By 1949, it had become a valued privilege to report biannually to this group of eminent physicians. No story of the NAPNE would be complete without mention of the debt to this famous committee and its brilliant executive director, Dr. E. H. L. Corwin. They gave NAPNE the first public endorsement of its program and continued with unfailing support.

## Saturday Evening Post Article

The year 1949 was also memorable for the *Saturday Evening Post* article written by Harold Titus on the practical nursing project in Michigan. Highlighting as it did the work of NAPNE, it focused attention on the Association and brought a flood of inquiries about both schools and NAPNE.

## NAPNE Loses Some Licensed Practical Nurse (LPN) Members

Voicing displeasure with the dominance of RNs, in this year, some LPN members of NAPNE withdrew and formed the National Federation of Licensed Practical Nurses (NFLPN).

## Grand Rapids, 1950

NAPNE achieved adult status in its annual meeting at the Hotel Pantlind by designating this meeting a convention for the first time. The records show 499 voting members. The theme was "New Designs From Traditional Patterns." The rapidly growing organization made a respectable showing in the Pantlind ballroom – a long way from the small group discreetly enclosed by screens just six years before at the Henry Hudson in New York.

The first visit to Alaska by a NAPNE representative was made in this year, at the request of the Bureau of Indian Affairs. NAPNE urged the development of a practical nursing school at Mt. Edgecumbe, and the initial planning of classrooms and curriculum was done. This was the second school under the aegis of the Bureau to be visited by a NAPNE representative. The first one, the Kiowa School of Practical Nursing, at Lawton, Oklahoma, was accredited by the Association this year.

## The First Summer School

The year 1950 saw the first NAPNE-sponsored summer school for directors and instructors in schools of practical nursing. Fifteen students enrolled at Colorado A&M College in Fort Collins. The 16-week preclinical class schedule prepared by this group was later used from coast to coast. It was pioneer work. It was the first workshop of its kind, for both instructors and students, and a new experience of contributing to a new national career that was still in the making.

## The Workshop Idea

The first workshop to interpret practical nurse education and service was held in Brookings, South Dakota, in 1950. Hilda Torrop acted as resource consultant, and the South Dakota Board of Nurse Examiners sponsored the conference.

### U.S. Office of Education Curriculum Guide

The U.S. Office of Education *Curriculum Guide* was published this year, and the NAPNE and other members of the Committee were still slightly numb, after the seemingly endless meetings – weekdays, Sundays, holidays, and vacations darkened by bulging briefcases and always the eternal wrestle with **what**, **why**, and **how**.

Correspondence during the years 1946-50 shows many requests from practical nurses for assistance in organizing state practical nurse associations. NAPNE truly served as the midwife at many births during this period, with no fatalities.

### *New York, 1951*

Mrs. Mildred Bradshaw, RN, was announced the newly elected president at the annual convention held at the Hotel Statler in New York City. This was the first of several NAPNE conventions attended by Madame Cavalcante of Rio de Janeiro, Brazil, South America, who was very much interested in practical nursing. Minutes of the meeting include a report on the initiation of the pilot study of nursing-in-the-home experience for the practical nurse student. The Accrediting Committee reported 17 practical nursing schools fully accredited by the NAPNE and nine with tentative accreditation. The pressing need for qualified faculty was recognized in a resolution urging that colleges and universities be encouraged to establish courses for the educators of practical nurses. Another resolution recommended seeking a closer relationship with the American Farm Bureau Federation and its affiliated organizations to promote the preparation of qualified practical nurses for service in rural areas.

### *On a Firm Foundation*

The wheels of progress began to spin. Funds were granted by the Milbank Memorial Fund for an initial conference and the later work of a planning committee to prepare the prospectus for a three-year study of practical nurse student home-nursing experience. The New York Academy of Medicine Public Health Relations Committee, jointly with NAPNE, sponsored a conference held at the Academy of Medicine in February, 1951 and attended by leaders in the fields of nursing, medicine and health, chronic illness, and civic welfare agencies. It was unanimously agreed that funds should be sought to support such a study.

In 1952, funds were granted by the Samuel H. Kress Foundation, and a Steering committee was appointed to develop related policies and procedures.

## *Workshop: Kansas City*

In February, 1951, a five-day workshop was held at the Medical Center in Kansas City, Kansas. At the request of the American Hospital Association, a special committee prepared an outline of information on practical nursing to be included in courses for hospital administrators.

## *Practical Nursing Launched*

For several years, NAPNE had issued a mimeographed page – later a printed bulletin – to inform members about association and school activities. In 1951, arrangements were made for an official NAPNE magazine, *Practical Nursing*, to be published bimonthly. This magazine is still circulated in the U.S. and 27 other countries under the name *Journal of Practical Nursing*.

## *First Maine Summer School*

A three-week summer course was instituted at the University of Maine, the first to be given on the Orono campus. Directors and instructors from various parts of the country attended. Ella Thompson was the instructor.

Requests for a summer school for practical nurses were increasing. In a series of conferences with the deans of education at the University of Maine and Colorado A&M College, the possibilities of waiving certain requirements, in order to make it possible to grant credit for successful completion of courses, were explored. These conferences were to bear fruit later on.

## *Colorado Springs, 1952*

A growing concern was expressed about establishing some form of instruction for licensed but untrained practical nurses that would permit them to attain a status equivalent to graduates of the approved schools. This was the shadow of the coming advent of the Education Units.

NAPNE approval of the first evening course for practical nurse training, sponsored by the Board of Education, Washington, D.C., at the Margaret Murray Washington School, was announced. At this time, there were 188 state-accredited and 38 NAPNE-accredited schools in the country.

## Colorado Summer School

A summer-school session for professional nurse instructors in schools of practical nursing was held in this year at the Colorado State College of Education in Greeley. The Army school at Fitzsimmons General Hospital presented an excellent demonstration of the situation approach in teaching nursing arts.

## NAPNE-NLN Exploring Committee

As the result of a conference requested by the National League for Nursing (NLN), NAPNE representatives were appointed to serve with NLN representatives on an exploring committee, whose objective was consideration of the feasibility of the NAPNE becoming the department of practical nursing in the NLN. Two meetings of the committee were held in 1953.

## First Summer School Courses for Practical Nurses

Acting upon the request of the Council of State Presidents presented in the previous year, the first summer courses for practical nurses were instituted at Colorado A&M College in Fort Collins and at the University of Maine in Orono.

## First NAPNE Regional Workshop

In this year, the first four-day regional workshop was held on the campus of the Texas State College for Women on the invitation of President Guinn of the Texas State College.

## Other Accomplishments

The NAPNE *Family Living Manual* and the *Clinical Teaching Guide* were published early in the year. The Curriculum Committee was restructured into three sections – nursing arts and allied subjects, home economics, and records.

The cost for the tremendous number of requests for reprints of Abraham Dobkin's article *Wayne v. Hartman*, about the court decision in favor of an enrollee in a correspondence school for practical nursing, was estimated at $40.00. The requests came from professional and practical nursing organizations, health agencies, and individuals. The executive director of the NAPNE testified at the court hearing on this case.

A grant of $25,000 from the S. H. Kress Foundation made possible the first interpretive film on practical nursing.

A constant and faithful friend of the NAPNE retired during this year, Dr. E.H.L. Corwin, executive secretary of the Public Health Relations Committee of the New York Academy of Medicine. The report of the NAPNE executive director noted,

> At a dinner honoring his many civic achievements, the list was impressively long as man after man recalled his career spent in the interest of the public's health and welfare. Dr. Corwin took a personal interest in the NAPNE over the entire life of the association. The biyearly report of the executive director of the NAPNE to the Public Health Relations Committee grew to be a cherished opportunity and privilege. In ways too numerous to mention, this brilliant committee and its secretary opened doors, gave advice, supported applications for grants, and co-sponsored conferences. We should be forever grateful to these busy, eminent men for their sympathetic understanding and belief in the Association.

### San Antonio, 1954

The 13th annual convention of the NAPNE was held in colorful San Antonio, the scene of crisis in Texas history. At the Plaza Hotel in the shadow of the Alamo, 32 states and Canada responded to the convention roll call. The theme of the convention was "Together for Community Health," and the speakers again and again emphasized the role of the practical nurse as a member of the health team and as a citizen.

A convention resolution directed a request to the ANA, asking that this organization recommend the inclusion of at least two practical nurse representatives on state boards of nurse examiners in states with practical nursing licensing laws.

### "Nurse Please"

The highlight of the convention was the premiere of the NAPNE film *Nurse Please*. It was the realization of a dream come true after many years of painful effort to produce a recruitment tool for the practical nursing schools. Produced by Trident Films, it received highly favorable mention and was shown widely through purchases and rentals as far away as Australia. It was also shown on TV circuits. The NAPNE set its sights on financing educational films for use in the practical nursing schools as part of its future program. A vote of heartfelt appreciation went to the Samuel H. Kress Foundation for the grant that made the film possible.

### Students as Future Members

Another significant development was the inauguration of the student Future Membership plan. Concerned about ways for maintaining contact with the graduates of the practical nursing schools, the way was opened to continuing contact with the NAPNE through paid-up membership at the end of the student year, continuing at the student rate for a year after graduation. This policy still remains in effect. The plan was enthusiastically received, and wholehearted thanks was given to the directors of the schools for their encouragement of this type of membership. The Board of Directors had long believed that a feeling of "belongingness" must be developed with the student group if graduates are to understand, support, and take part in the work of the NAPNE.

### Education Unit I Completed

The plan for implementing the Education Units for LP/VNs by waiver and the completed outlines for the courses were approved after review by the Curriculum Committee. The first unit was made available in October to those practical nurse associations that contributed to their preparation. Missouri was the first state to establish instruction in Unit I.

### Indianapolis, 1955

NAPNE's fourth president, Fern A. Goulding, took office at the close of this meeting. This convention was a landmark for several reasons:
- It had the largest attendance.
- The opening address was given by Dr. Norman Vincent Peale.
- There was active participation of the practical nurse delegates in all the business meetings. These nurse delegates demonstrated evidence of their desire to support NAPNE financially and strengthen it through increased membership as the organization that had made their career a living, growing entity.

This was the first convention to which students had been especially invited to a program prepared just for them. Reports of the convention repeatedly mentioned the stirring sight of seeing the meeting room packed with representatives of the schools and to hear them conduct their own sessions.

Revision of the bylaws brought several important changes:
- An increase in practical nurse representation on the NAPNE board of directors and the designation of the office of third vice president to be held by a practical nurse.
- The activation of the Council of Practical Nursing Schools.
- Provision for membership for the accredited schools.
- The establishment of the per-capita membership category for state practical nurse associations.

New Mexico and California, in a dramatic moment following the adoption of per-capita membership, came forward with their per-capita dues.

It was also at this convention that *Practical Nursing*, the NAPNE's official magazine, was introduced in its modern, enlarged form. Still a bimonthly publication at the time of theconvention, it became established as a monthly in September, 1955.

## Puerto Rico Conference

In October, NAPNE spent four action-packed days in Puerto Rico conducting conferences sponsored by NAPNE in cooperation with the Department of Vocational Education and the Puerto Rico Practical Nurse Association. Two days were devoted to all-day meetings in San Juan, in which vocational educators, professional, and practical nurses sat down together to discuss practical nurse education and service – a "first" for a meeting of this kind in Puerto Rico. The NAPNE visitors also saw two of the four practical nursing schools on the island and were impressed with the efforts made to provide adequate teaching facilities and the interest and enthusiasm of the instructional staff.

## Chicago, 1956

The 15th NAPNE convention made history for several reasons, noted below. It was by far the largest, with over 1,000 delegates and others in attendance.

### Convention Newsletter

Another **first**, the *Convention Newsletter* took a bow for its day-by-day reporting of convention highlights. This tradition is still firmly in place with the Convention *FORUM*.

### The NAPNE Will Continue

An important decision was made at this convention – a decision of great significance for the future of NAPNE, indeed affecting its very existence. In 1953, the separate boards of directors of the NLN and the NAPNE approved the appointment of a committee, composed of representatives from each organization, to explore the possibility of the NAPNE becoming the department of practical nurse education in the NLN. The NLN bylaws already provided for such a department in its organizational structure, but one had not as yet been made functional.

This Exploring Committee met four times; the last meeting was held in December, 1955. The committee reviewed the purposes and organizational structure of the NLN and the NAPNE, as outlined in their respective bylaws, in an endeavor to identify differences in policies and principles, and to determine whether or not these differences could be reconciled yet preserve the fundamental principles governing each organization.

The first report on the findings of the Exploring Committee was presented at the NAPNE convention in San Antonio in 1954. At the NAPNE convention in Indianapolis in 1955, a special session was devoted to a progress report and discussion. On each occasion, a representative of the NLN was present to explain its organization and to participate in the discussion.

## *Points of Difference*

During these explorations and discussions, several points of difference emerged. The place for practical nurse membership in the NLN presented a problem. Membership in the NLN came through its state leagues and through individuals. All members indicated the department of the NLN where their dues would be directed. It seemed logical that practicing practical nurses would check the department of nursing service. This would deflect funds from the department of practical nurse education, and NAPNE members were concerned about the effect on the income of that department. Practical nurses joining the NLN through a state or local league would be required to pay dues considerably in excess of $10.00, which were presently paid to the NAPNE, and according to NLN bylaws, only $5.00 of this amount would be paid to the NLN department of Practical Nurse Education. Many members were fearful that the program for practical nurse education would be greatly hampered by such a marked reduction in funds. On the other hand, it was explained that the resources of the NLN might be available to help support this department.

## *NAPNE's Dual Role*

The NAPNE accepted a dual obligation in the principles upon which it was founded – to set and maintain sound standards for practical nurse education and to help practical nurses improve their practice in giving safe nursing care. To these ends, NAPNE has always endorsed, in principle and practice, the belief that practical nurses should have a voice in their own affairs. Practical nurses were represented on all NAPNE committees, four practical nurses were on the board of directors, and one practical nurse was the third vice president. The structure of the NAPNE held together, in a working and promotional relationship, representatives of all groups interested in practical nurse education and service. This provided an organization with national stature to speak for practical nurse education and to sit on national committees of allied interests.

The possibility of the dissolution of NAPNE to become, in all likelihood, a small department of a large professional nursing organization created considerable apprehension within many of the state practical nurse associations. They feared they would lose the benefits won through the past years – benefits they believed were largely due to the existence of NAPNE. As it became apparent that there were definite obstacles in the way of this absorption of the organization within another, there was a growing unrest and uncertainty among potential members about joining either NAPNE or the NLN.

## Council of Presidents' Resolution

The NAPNE Council of Presidents of the State Practical Nurse Associations at their meeting in January, 1956, presented the following resolutions to the NAPNE Board of Directors:

WHEREAS, the insecurity prevalent in the state practical nurse associations regarding future of the National Association for Practical Nurse Education is a deterrent to their sound development and to the sound development of the NAPNE, and

WHEREAS, the national stability of practical nurse education leadership is retarded by the uncertainty of future planning regarding the NAPNE, be it

RESOLVED, that the Council of State Presidents request the Board of Directors of the NAPNE to table further discussion pertaining to dissolving the NAPNE and that this decision be given appropriate publicity.

## Board of Director's Action

After consideration of this resolution and of the findings of the Exploring Committee during the past three years, the Board of Directors of the NAPNE voted unanimously:

WHEREAS, the NAPNE has assumed certain responsibilities in helping to provide adequate nursing care for the people of our country, and

WHEREAS, it is the decision of the Board of Directors of the NAPNE that exploration into the possibilities of the dissolution of this organization and absorption of its functions by the NLN have not proved the desirability of the proposed actions, and

WHEREAS, the above decision is based on the obligation that the NAPNE has assumed over the years to continue, expand, and accelerate its program for the preparation of the trained practical nurse, therefore it is

RECOMMENDED that formal exploratory conferences with the NLN be terminated herewith and that we express our appreciation to the NLN for their patience and understanding and state that we urgently desire their continued joint interest in our common problems.

## NAPNE Membership Action

The above recommendation of the NAPNE Board of Directors was ratified by unanimous vote of the NAPNE membership at the opening session of the annual business meeting on May 8, 1956.

## Workshops and Conferences

The year 1956 was marked by a rapid expansion of the NAPNE program. Workshops and conferences were held in Ohio, West Virginia, Washington State, and Texas. The second conference in the Caribbean area was held in October and included Puerto Rico and the Virgin Islands. The second recruitment institute cosponsored by NAPNE and the practical nursing schools in greater New York and vicinity was conducted at the New York Academy of Medicine and was attended by a capacity audience.

## NAPNE Publications

Publications for this year included *Diversional Activities Designed to Meet the Needs of the Practical Nurse* with an accompanying teacher's guide, a set of nine record forms for schools of practical nursing, and a comprehensive brochure on NAPNE that describes its purposes, programs, and plans for the future (Archives, 1956).

## Summer School

Summer school programs for professional and practical nurses at the University of Maine and at Colorado A&M College were well attended. Scholarship funds made available to NAPNE by interested individuals and foundations made it possible to send to these sessions a number of professional and practical nurses who would otherwise not have been able to attend. Three new schools of practical nursing were able to open by securing faculty members recruited from summer school participants.

## Education Units Outlines Completed

The Education Units Committee completed the preparation of the unit outlines with the release of Unit IV in January. Twenty-three state practical nurse associations were eligible to offer the units to their members, and the number of courses in operation was increasing rapidly.

## Some 1956 Statistics

As of 1956, there were 70 NAPNE accredited schools in the United States and its possessions. The number of requests for consultation and accreditation services had never been so great. Sixteen state practical nurse associations now had per-capita membership in NAPNE – a heartening indication of the ever-widening confidence in the NAPNE program. The steady growth of the state practical nurse associations throughout the country testified to the interest of practical nurses and their ability to conduct their own affairs. *Practical Nursing*, the NAPNE magazine, had a circulation of 13,000 – a substantial gain over the previous year.

## Atlantic City, 1957

The 16th annual convention held at the Ambassador Hotel was notable for its size and enthusiasm. The student-day attendance was dramatic – many schools sent their entire student body in chartered buses. As school after school marched into the ballroom, the many-hued uniforms, the stirring music, and the sense of a new career well launched moved the audience to happy applause. This applause was many times repeated as the delegates from each school rose to be recognized.

## Publications

This was a year of important publications. The revised NAPNE handbook, *Practical Nurse Education*, demonstrated in content and size the breadth and depth of curriculum changes. *The Nurse Everybody Needs*, a promotional and interpretative pamphlet prepared by the Hospital Advisory Council, had immediate acceptance. Schools, conventions, and membership meetings reported its popularity.

## Program Expansion

This year, 1957, was a year of great expansion. The air was cleared of doubts regarding the continuance of the NAPNE, and membership increased rapidly. By December, 1957, there were 18 per-capita states and a total membership of 18,898. Discussion in the Council of Presidents indicated a desire for more emphasis on state services and recognition of the amount of financial support being given to work with the state practical nurse associations.

## A Matter of Note

The Federal Civil Service Nursing Committee recommended withdrawal of the previous recognition granted to the NAPNE 240-hour course. This allowed graduates of the course to enter Federal Civil Service at the same level as graduates of approved schools. Among the organizations approving this decision was the NFLPN. The NAPNE protest pointed out that persons with no preparation could advance to this point through tenure and that it was a fallacy to state that these experienced LPNs who had completed the 64-hour and 240-hour courses were not equivalent in nursing ability to the persons without these educational courses who had been advanced via tenure.

Executive Director Hilda Torrop spent two weeks in June attending a conference in London, England, on the assistant nurse program. It was carefully planned by the Royal College of Nursing and was most successful. Exchange visits were planned for 1959.

### Coronado, 1958

This convention saw the first meeting of the NAPNE State Services Committee. Mrs. Andrew Noe, Mr. David Neuwirth, Hilda Torrop, Adelaide Mayo, and Mrs. Mildred Smith, LPN, conferred on the implications of a new structure of NAPNE services and prepared the statement that was presented at the closing business meeting and unanimously approved.

An important decision was announced by the Curriculum Committee relative to the instruction of practical nurse students in giving medicines. It was stated as the committee's belief that sufficient evidence was available on the need for the inclusion of a thorough course in the giving of medicines. It seemed imperative for the NAPNE Accrediting Committee to give this course approval. Pilot courses were taught during the year in 22 schools of practical nursing, using the NAPNE suggested outline. This was the first offering of the current NAPNE's Pharmacology Certification. It is now offered online, available to LP/VNs from the comfort of their own home using their computer!

Symbolic of the growing strength and interest of the Hospital Advisory Council was its meeting during the convention week. It was moved that the 240-hour course brochure be mailed to the entire American Hospital Association membership, that all state and regional program committees be requested to consider practical nursing in program planning, and that postgraduate education undertaken by the individual practical nurses be encouraged.

At the closing business session, the following resolutions were presented and accepted by the membership (Archives, 1958):

WHEREAS, The National Association for Practical Nurse Education 64-hour extension course, or a course with similar content, and the 240-hour course, have been prepared at the request of the practical nurses of the country, and

WHEREAS, The National Association for Practical Nurse Education Hospital Advisory Council has endorsed and recommended the promotion of these courses, to prepare practical nurses licensed by waiver, for improved nursing service, therefore, be it

RESOLVED, that the members of the National Association for practical Nurse Education in convention assembled in Coronado, California, April, 1958, go on record as approving these courses, and urging state associations to seek financial support for these courses from funds available through vocational education.

## Publications

NAPNE publications for 1958 included a new recruitment pamphlet and the letter to hospital administrators interpreting the 240-hour course. The latter was prepared by the Hospital Advisory Council and sent to over 8,000 hospital administrators. The recruitment pamphlet was widely distributed; during a two-week period in December, 2000, inquiries were answered by the headquarters office. Mrs. Cordelia Kelly prepared an article entitled *Practical Nursing Moves Ahead*, which was published in the *New Physician* and which received wide distribution through reprints supplied by NAPNE.

## Steering Committee, Department of Service

In the interest of better service to the practical nursing schools, the Board of Directors approved a reduction in accrediting services fees to $200 a visit. The Association would underwrite the additional expense not covered by this fee.

## A Protest

At the October meeting, the Accrediting Committee reviewed the letter sent by the NLN to the schools of practical nursing and to the boards of nurse examiners announcing the increased interest of the NLN in practical nursing and in school accreditation in particular. This open letter was protested by the Accrediting Committee, the State Services Committee, the Board of Directors, and by directors of several schools of practical nursing. Both the inference that this service was needed and also the recently developed interest of the NLN in practical nursing after 18 years of pioneering by the NAPNE in the face of professional nurse opposition were protested in many letters received at the NAPNE headquarters office.

## *Ohio, 1959*

"Coming of Age" was the convention theme, highlighting the 18th birthday of NAPNE and recounting a story of accomplishment, not only for the Association but for practical nursing as well. It was marked by promise for the future and nostalgic memories of the past. Speaker after speaker emphasized the new respect for practical nurses, so hardily won, and the growing responsibilities they are proving they can handle. The grand march of students was, by all accounts, an inspiring sight, with 379 students from 41 schools in 18 states and the District of Columbia responding to the roll call.

### *Department of Education and Department of Service*

At the business meeting, action was taken to create two new departments within the NAPNE – the Department of Education and the Department of Service to State Practical Nurse Associations. The president appointed Dorothea Thompson as head of the Department of Education and Mildred Smith, LPN, as head of the Department of Service on a part-time basis.

### *Convention Resolutions*

Resolutions were adopted reaffirming the position of NAPNE that state boards of nurse examiners include practical nurses in their membership; registering opposition to the duplication of accreditation services to practical nursing schools by the NLN; and supporting the interest of the American Hospital Association in a joint accrediting service with the NLN in accrediting schools of nursing, with a request for the inclusion of the NAPNE to represent practical nurse education.

### *Hands Across the Sea*

Dorothea Thompson of the NAPNE staff spent the month of June in England, where under the auspices of the National Association of State-Enrolled Assistant Nurses (NASEAN), she visited training centers and hospitals. She met with instructors in the assistant nurse training programs and representatives of the Royal College of Nursing, the Queen's Institute of District Nursing, and many others. It was a busy but instructive four weeks, crammed with professional activities interspersed with many delightful social events planned in her honor, such as teas given by the *Nursing Mirror* and by the Council of the NASEAN.

Miss Thompson's intensely interesting report of her visit appeared in the October and November issues of *Practical Nursing*, ending with these words:

I was deeply impressed by the devoted care the state-enrolled assistant nurses gave their patients, sometimes under very adverse circumstances. . . . Nursing must always be synonymous with good patient care. Let us . . . join hands with the assistant nurses of England in putting first things first (Archives, 1959).

### A Fair Exchange

Exchange must work both ways, so in September, under NAPNE sponsorship, two of the leaders in the assistant nurse organization in Great Britain came to the United States to spend two months learning about practical nurse education and practical nurse organization. Charlotte Bentley, RN, executive secretary of the State-Enrolled Assistant Nurses (SEAN), and Muriel Butcher, chairman of the SEAN Council, visited practical nursing schools, attended NAPNE workshops and conferences for hospital administrators, and were the invited guests of the Ohio and West Virginia state practical nurse associations at their respective conventions. Upon her return to England, Miss Butcher wrote, "No one could have had a happier or more interesting 10 weeks than I have just enjoyed or gone home with so many memories of truly delightful people and many new friends as well as new ideas" (Archives, 1959).

### Hospital Administrator's Institutes

At the request of NAPNE's Hospital Advisory Council, a program of one-day institutes for hospital administrators and their nursing service directors was established. The institutes were designed as an opportunity to explore the possibilities for maximum use of the practical nurse's abilities and to provide information on current trends in the preparation and use of the practical nurse.

### NAPNE Pin

A pin for NAPNE members made its first appearance at the convention. New members received the pin without cost; it was available to other members for the infinitesimal price of one dollar. Currently, the NAPNES pin is the same design and sells for $15 and $25 for gold-filled and gold, respectively.

### From NAPNE to NAPNES

In 1959 "and Service" was added to the corporate title of the Association. The new abbreviated name "NAPNES" came into being in 1959 also. As the year ended, the necessary legal procedure to add the words "and Service" to the title of the Association was completed, thus giving official titular recognition to its function of giving service to the state practical nurse associations. So farewell to NAPNE – hail to N-A-P-N-E-S!

## Salt Lake City 1960

"Future Unlimited" was a happy choice for the theme of this 19th convention in a city founded on faith and vision by those hardy pioneers and their leader who said, looking out on the broad valley which lay at the foot of snow-capped peaks, "This is the place." As an organization that also was founded on faith and vision, NAPNES could point to battles won – for stature, for licensure, for the right of practical nurses to have a voice in her own affairs – and rise to meet the challenge of the future.

The keynoter speaker, Dr. Wilfred David, chief of the Chronic Disease Branch of the U.S. Public Health Service, praised the dedication to service to clients that has characterized practical nursing and reminded the audience of the increasing responsibility entailed for knowledge and leadership.

### Publications

The first four sections of the *Officer's Manual*, prepared by NAPNES Department of Service to State Practical Nurse Associations, were completed and made available. Part I was entitled *Human Relations and Association Leadership*; Parts II, III, and IV outlined the duties and responsibilities of association officers. Guides for preparing reports and minutes and for conducting meetings were included. Additional parts dealing with committee functions were being prepared.

### Final Note

As an interesting item on which to end the year, it is noted that in a bulletin issued as advice to contributors, the National Information Bureau included the NAPNES in a listing of 40 from among the prominent "health" agencies.

## Detroit, 1961

### Resolutions

The resolutions adopted at the closing business session stated in essence that:

I. The NAPNES urge insurance companies that provide benefits payable for nursing care to extend these benefits to include nursing care given by the licensed practical nurse.

II. The NAPNES take the appropriate steps to procure recognition of the licensed practical/vocational nurse, by employing hospitals and health agencies, as a nurse rather than as an auxiliary worker.

III. NAPNES member state practical nurse associations secure copies of state laws authorizing licensed practical/vocational nurses and practical nurse students to give medications, to be used as models for correcting such adverse situations as may exist in their respective states.

IV. The NAPNES take appropriate action in appropriate places, to reaffirm its authoritative position as an agency for accrediting practical nursing programs, by virtue of being the only national nursing organization that, for twenty years, has been solely devoted to the development and upgrading of practical nurse education and service.

V. The NAPNES send to all State Boards of Nurse Examiners a copy of this resolution, which urges all State Boards of Nurse Examiners to adopt a standard score of at least 350 as the passing score on the state practical nurse licensing examination, in order to facilitate interstate registration of practical nurses.

VI. Constituent state member organizations of the NAPNES send to their respective U.S. Senators, Congressmen and other interested parties, a copy of this resolution which urges the enactment of legislation to also include approved practical nursing schools other than those under vocational education as eligible to receive Federal funds appropriated by Congress for the expansion and improvement of practical nursing programs.

VII. The NAPNES continue to explore the possibility of unifying the efforts of the NAPNES and the NFLPN to promote the interests of practical nursing and practical nurses.

The Joint Committee of the NAPNES-NFLPN met for the first time in January in New York City.

### *Washington, DC, 1962*

The year 1962 was the year of "Educating for Leadership," and NAPNES answered the call. Throughout this year, this theme for workshops was based on the following five questions:

1. How can we, in practical nursing education, impress upon our students the requirements for good citizenship?
2. If "values determine our youth," how do our values influence our students?
3. We should ask ourselves the following questions:
   a. How much more should I know?
   b. How well prepared am I?
   c. What is our interpretation of other cultures?
   d. How can we stimulate the students to do the same?
4. If we must give attention to the quality of learning, must we not evaluate the quality of our teaching?
5. If it is important how students reveal themselves, what can we do about everyday courtesy?

The reader should keep in mind that this education is by registered nurses reflecting and worrying about their impact on students of practical nursing. This mentoring and learning is very much evident in the current processes at NAPNES. The reward for this work is the competent, caring LP/VNs of the present day.

### *Miami Beach, 1963*

In 1963, the NAPNES publication *Practical Nursing*, with new typeface, new content, new promise, and new rewards for readers, became *The Journal of Practical Nursing*. The monthly publication was a steal at the $3.00 per-year subscription rate.

### *St. Louis, 1964*

Education of LP/VNs by RNs is the long-standing tradition of NAPNES. The year 1964 saw at least 25 workshops in 20 states on a variety of subjects pertaining to nursing care. By this time, the number of LP/VNs counted 350,000 and was growing nationwide. This year, NAPNES concentrated on growing its membership from close to 33,000 at the beginning to over 38,000 by the end of the year! A healthy number to meet the awesome challenge of the devastating "1965 Proposal."

### *New York City, 1965*

In honor of the NAPNES convention, Mayor Robert F. Wagner of New York City declared Monday, April 26th, as Licensed Practical Nurse Day. And officials of the New

York World's Fair designated Thursday, April 29th, as Practical Nurse Day in recognition of the practical nurse's increasing contributions to community welfare.

In 1965, NAPNES found itself in the center of a fierce debate over the proposed title change for LP/VNs. The proposal to change the title to licensed nurse (LN) came in a letter to the editor from Mr. Henry Pfisterer, LPN. LP/VN and RN reaction rained down hundreds of letters of both praise and criticism, and an emotional debate continued over the next decade and beyond. Little did the letter writers for and against the proposed title change know that by the end of 1965, NAPNES and the country's 330,000 LP/VNs would be locked in a life and death struggle with the American Nurses' Association (ANA) for their very existence.

The "1965 Proposal," later to be dubbed the "1985 Proposal" or "entry level" because implementation was to be achieved by 1985, was published in the *American Journal of Nursing* in December, 1965. It clearly called on the nursing profession to work systematically to eliminate practical nursing programs and created the deepest and strongest division between the two levels of licensed nurses. From the six-page report, the following sentence still fills the hearts and minds of LP/VNs and LP/VN educators with hurt, anger, deep sadness, and a steely resolve and determination for survival that has never altered: "The association (ANA) therefore proposes that the nursing profession systematically work to facilitate the replacement of programs for practical nursing with programs for beginning technical nursing practice in junior and community colleges" (Archives, 1965).

### *Louisville, 1966*

The Board of Directors of the NAPNES issued a statement reproving the ANA for the published proposal that, if implemented, would have eliminated the services of over 300,000 licensed nurses providing care at the bedside. Pointing out that LP/VNs provided over 75% of the direct client care (bedside nursing), NAPNES generated opposition to the *First Position on Education for Nursing.* "All agree there is a long distance to travel from the publication of a statement to its implementation" (Archives, 1966). These were prophetic words in 1966.

In late November, the New York State Nurses' Association published the *Blueprint for the Education of Nurses in New York State.* In it, a major objective was that no new programs of practical nursing be established after January 1, 1967, in New York State.

### *Los Angeles, 1967*

Responding to the late November, 1966 publication of the *Blueprint,* NAPNES began a massive contacting of its network across the country, educating contacts of how the *Blueprint* would be used as an example in other states. NAPNES began to verify reports that several state boards of nursing were arbitrarily holding up applications for new practical nursing programs on their own initiative. NAPNES urged LP/VNs to counteract the activities of the ANA and its state constituents by fully informing legislators at the state and national level.

As debate over the now infamous proposal raged, NAPNES faced another challenge. Extended-care facilities were beginning to use LP/VNs as charge nurses. NAPNES was the first organization to request the Social Security Administration to review the regulation that prohibited LP/VNs from serving in charge-nurse capacities.

Virginia Senator Jennings Randolph summed up the tumultuous 1960s in his convention address, stating:

> There are uncertainties in the future of licensed practical nursing. Not uncertain in the future, however, is the permanence of licensed practical nursing. If the course of the future is uncertain, at least our responsibilities are not. This responsibility, which we share, is to work to deliver the best quality of health care to all of those who need it. I know that each of you will meet this beckoning challenge. Couple with your education and training the warm glow of service. (Archives, 1967)

Considered by many to be perhaps its most outstanding accomplishment was NAPNES's recognition by the Office of Education as the first agency eligible to accredit schools of practical nursing.

### Pittsburgh, 1968

In the Annual Convention Report, NAPNES (1968) stated, "The impact of licensed practical/vocational nursing on the health services area grows each year. There are now 1,149 practical nursing programs with 27,644 graduates" (Archives, 1968). Continuing its campaign to save the jobs and dedicated hard work of hundreds of thousands of direct care givers, NAPNES further stated, "The contribution of the LP/VN to patient care has received widespread recognition. The contribution of practical/vocational nursing to professional nursing seems to be wholly unexplored" (Archives, 1968).

### Dallas, 1969

The "1965 Proposal" notwithstanding, LP/VNs stepped into the limelight of another debate: whether or not they would have a role in Intensive Coronary Care Units (ICCUs) opening in healthcare facilities across the country. Not unimportant was a clarification of legal implications. Once hospital administrators were reassured of these and other points, LP/VNs were educated and assigned to ICCUs. As early as 1967, such a training program was under way. The rapidity with which LP/VNs were able to move into a role that only a year or two before was considered revolutionary for an RN is further evidence of the flexibility so characteristic of practical nursing.

The year 1969 was a very special year in the history of NAPNES. The first LPN to hold the office of president was elected this year. Mrs. Mildred Smith, an LPN from Ohio, honored by her RN and LPN colleagues, was chosen to assume the chair. Mrs. Smith holds License No. 1 in the state of Ohio. She is revered and respected by all that know her and still loved deeply by NAPNES.

All NAPNES presidents since 1969 have been LPNs. NAPNES views this statistic as evidence of the success of the RNs that mentored and guided so many nurses into leadership positions. As they take on the responsibility of leadership and management at NAPNES, LP/VNs will always remember that the organization is a gift from visionary RNs in the beginning and along the way. NAPNES is teamwork and skill building focused on one outcome: better client care by all levels in nursing.

### Atlantic City, 1970

The packed sessions at the convention heard about the promise of the coming decade to be a milestone in American medicine. Convention documents note that as the United States entered the 1970s, the professions clearly reflected the prevailing social climate of unrest, dissatisfaction, and change. The major unknowns looming on the horizon were the new concepts of Medicare and Medicaid and their eventual impact on licensed practical nursing. Also reflected in NAPNES corporate documents was the regrettable and potentially destructive element of the schism between professional and practical/vocational nursing.

The good news this year was the "striking success" accolade used to describe the experimental upgrading program in practical nursing. In this project, over 400 nurses' aides in New York City municipal hospitals completed 14 months of practical nursing education while working part-time at their regular jobs. Programs like this one represented mounting efforts to find new ways to help nursing personnel enhance their contributions to the health services. Another example was the Helene Fuld School of Nursing program, established to give interested and able LP/VNs the opportunity to enter professional nursing without unnecessary repetition of learning experiences. Several other programs became available to move LP/VNs into registered nursing in this manner. Although remaining staunchly supportive of career LP/VNs, NAPNES supported this new career ladder concept because of the strong belief that the needs of clients are best served by nurses and allied health personnel who function at their maximum capacity.

### Cincinnati, 1971

The year 1971 marked the first year that the U.S. Public Health Service included and published a comprehensive reference on LP/VNs (U.S. Department of Health, Education, and Welfare, 1971). NAPNES welcomed the publication, knowing that although, in many instances, this inventory simply reinforced what had been "educated guesses" of the practical/vocational nursing profile, sound statistical data were essential for effective planning. Future potential could be fully realized only if projections could be made based on a systematic study of past and present trends and developments.

New York Governor Rockefeller vetoed two nursing bills introduced by the New York State Nurses Association, which, if passed in their original form, would have stripped practical nursing of its identity. In the text explaining his veto, Governor Rockefeller made reference to the opposition of NAPNES and the state's medical, dental, and hospital associations.

LP/VNs at the 1971 NAPNES convention were introduced to the new program known as Health Maintenance Organizations (HMOs). Expectations were that the impact on LP/VNs would be experienced in role expansion, increased responsibilities, and new skills required, all of which underscored NAPNES's commitment to continuing education as a foundation for LP/VNs as they faced the future.

## Hot Springs, 1972

The 1970s were rapidly becoming the decade of the consumer, with predictions that many services formerly rendered by physicians could well be delegated to other health professionals. Programs for physician assistants and nurse practitioners were opening, and with much in the national literature about equal access to quality care, NAPNES launched informational programs encouraging LP/VNs to actively participate in post-licensure continuing education to prepare themselves for full participation.

## Seattle, 1973

The issue of institutional licensure was receiving growing support. The main thrust of such licensure was to replace the licensing of individual practitioners with a single license to the institution, such as a hospital or other client care facility. Supporters argued it would eliminate the rigidity and inflexibility of many nursing boards. Employing hospitals claimed the boards often hamstrung their effort to use personnel efficiently and innovatively in the best interests of clients. NAPNES stood firm against institutional licensure but warned boards of nursing that some type of licensure reform was absolutely necessary. The NAPNES executive director stated NAPNES's opposition to institutional licensure when she addressed an American Medical Association (AMA) Reference Committee at its annual convention. She reported that the "NAPNES constituency regards the proposal to license institutions, instead of the personnel employed within them, as a threat to good patient care" (Archives, 1973). At the same time, the Reference Committee was reminded of NAPNES's long-time crusade for reform of state boards of nursing so that practical nursing matters would be handled more equitably, more expeditiously, and with reduced harassment. NAPNES pushed for reform in the exclusively professional nurse makeup of boards. It believed that a combination of RNs, LPNs, and health-related professions would provide a more balanced licensing body whose broader views would be reflected in reasonable and safe standards. And long before the emphasis on consumer participation, NAPNES argued in favor of representation of public members on boards of nursing.

### Leadership or Sheepherding?

Leadership by LP/VNs was seen as crucial to the survival of this licensed group. NAPNES warned that members of LP/VN organizations intimidated from speaking out on issues vital to this dedicated group of nurses would become no more than "sheep herded" into ineffectual groups. LP/VN associations were implored to guard against the loss of their right to speak, their right to inquire, and their right to dissent. As true today as in 1973, in these rights rests the future of practical nursing as a respected voice in the healthcare family.

### Miami, 1974

Advised not to convene due to the energy crisis of 1974, the NAPNES Board met and weighed the pros and cons. Needless to say, the Miami convention boasted one of the largest turnouts ever.

This year marked the debate within NAPNES over continuing education – mandatory versus voluntary. California enacted legislation requiring continuing education for RNs and licensed vocational nurses as a condition of relicensure. NAPNES's position was one for strong support of voluntary continuing education and strove to provide opportunities for LP/VNs to demonstrate that mandating it was simply unnecessary because LP/VNs kept their knowledge and skills current voluntarily.

### New Orleans, 1975

Industrial nursing as a new place of employment for LP/VNs, the *Comprehensive Health Planning Law*, and the need to have LP/VN representation at the decision-making level of the new local and state agencies that were to implement the law, were the issues that dominated the 1975 sessions. Also on the mind of conventioneers was the Professional Standards Review Organizations (PSRO).

The 10th-year anniversary of the original "1965 Proposal," which was commonly known as the 85 Proposal, prompted renewal resolutions against the wholesale destruction of licensed practical/vocational nursing.

### *Washington, DC, 1976*

Issuing its "Statement on Practical/Vocational Nursing," NAPNES addressed the expense of nursing education, NAPNES's philosophy of promoting voluntary continuing education, and retention of licensed practical/vocational nursing as the entry level to licensed nursing.

### *Atlanta, 1977*

NAPNES launched the "Life-Long Learning Campaign" that continues in the present-day profession. The campaign developed attitudes toward acquisition of current knowledge and the ability to translate that knowledge into quality nursing care. This basic attitude took away the "burden" of continuing education and made it a challenging and meaningful quest for maintenance of competence.

### *Phoenix, 1978*

This year focused on prevention. NAPNES accepted that prevention is an approach to health care that is far-ranging and all-encompassing. It demands a change in attitude on the part of every member of the healthcare system: the client, nurse, physician, administrator, and even the researcher who is involved in combating disease when prevention fails. NAPNES concentrated on the topic from the LP/VN perspective and role in prevention and encouraged LP/VNs to prepare themselves well to become client teachers and serve the prevention efforts of the whole team.

Although the work of educating and speaking for LP/VNs was a relentlessly demanding endeavor, the underlying threat to this proud profession remained: the dreaded 85 Proposal. NAPNES practical nurse educators worked tirelessly on a campaign to help the public understand what would be lost if their graduates were phased out of the workforce. The message to the public was, "A high quality education depends upon philosophy, objectives, curriculum, and faculty, and can and is being carried out in our programs" (Archives, 1978).

### *Philadelphia, 1979*

NAPNES looked into its crystal ball and began planning education for how to move toward a healthier 21st century. Pennsylvania Senator Richard Schweiker told conventioneers, "There is one key problem facing the healthcare system today – how to keep costs down while improving the quality of patient care" (Archives, 1979). He described LP/VNs as fundamental to resolving this problem because they provide a low-cost entry into the the healthcare system. "LP/VNs can help in the effort to contain costs in other ways because they have close personal contact with patients and have the unique opportunity to promote preventive health" (Archives, 1979). He concluded with this remark: "You provide personal health care for sick people. No one can replace that. That is the key central philosophy of both your organization and your profession" (Archives, 1979).

### Houston, 1980

By this time, five states had laws requiring proof of continuing education for relicensure, many state boards of nursing anticipated similar laws, and more and more employers were requiring proof of continuing education. Recognizing these demands, NAPNES developed a new record-keeping system designed to combine LP/VN records into one computerized transcript to help keep this valuable information safe and available. This program was known as the NAPNES Continuing Education Record Keeping System (CERKS) and is still currently available to NAPNES members. The annual fee started at $5.00 and is presently $15. LP/VNs send copies of their continuing education certificates, and NAPNES enters the information into the CERKS database. Nurses can then request a computer printout of their records when they are needed.

This year brought about merger talks with the NFLPN. Proponents believed the combination of the two organizations would strengthen and unify LP/VNs in the last five years before the dreaded 1985 Proposal was to be implemented. Others from within both organizations believed the financial burden of dissolving both organizations and organizing the structure of an entirely new organization would be devastating to the entire profession. The name recognition of NAPNES since 1941, the nationally respected NAPNES Education Department, and the well-known and widely circulated *Journal of Practical Nursing* would be lost. The merger was not to be, and the two organizations currently continue separately.

### St. Louis, 1981

NAPNES spent this year consumed with issues at the National Council of State Boards of Nursing (NCSBN), the White House Conference on Aging, the American Hospital Association's National Commission on Nursing, and the *Tentative Standards for Practical Nurse Series GS-6xx and Nursing Assistant Series GS-6yy*. Although the headquarters staff worked diligently on such issues, there was a move afoot in the membership to relocate the national headquarters from New York to a "more central" location. Sparking hot debate and providing an unusual crack in the normally unified membership, this issue was to come back time and again in the following years.

## Orlando, 1982

Due to the emergence of several model nurse practice acts to be used as guidelines by state nurse organizations and governmental regulatory agencies in preparation for practice act changes, the membership directed NAPNES to prepare model guidelines covering concerns specific to practical/vocational nurse licensure. NAPNES members were not unhappy with practice acts, but the "entry-level proposal" wind carried the odor of treachery planned for the hundreds of thousands of nurses earning their living in the profession. NAPNES was ready to meet any state proposal calling for the phasing out of LP/VNs. Since the veto by Governor Rockefeller of the New York bills in 1971, proponents abandoned the overt legislative approach. The new strategy NAPNES monitored carefully was the regulatory approach. What could not be accomplished legislatively could be accomplished using regulations and pressuring the RNs on state boards of nursing to "accomplish the mission for the profession," or so the theory went.

The year 1982 was a year of numerous NAPNES orchestrated meetings that happened quietly, with no fanfare, but with matching strategy to absolutely prevent any state board of nursing from overstepping its mission of "public protection" and succumbing to the intense pressure. Meeting in homes with grandmothers manning the phones to legislators and staff, NAPNES quietly prepared to fight to the death for the profession of licensed practical/vocational nursing. Preparing for lay public sit-ins of state boards of nursing, locals prepared to make the task a very difficult one for those who would "destroy the dreams" of these hard-working bedside nurses. This was an extremely well-planned strategy that, fortunately, never had to be used.

## Cleveland, 1983

In 1983, NAPNES took a path that would prove to be disastrous for the financial stability of this proud old organization. Members voted to reorganize the 501(c)(3) NAPNES into a 501(c)(6) organization that would be incorporated as the National Association of Licensed Practical Nurses (NALPN). At the last minute, the proponents decided to keep NAPNES and form NALPN as a sister organization. The main purpose for NALPN was collective bargaining. The plan was for the two organizations to be staffed by the same people, with hours kept separately. The whole operation was extremely unsuccessful, and NALPN was eventually dissolved, but not before the destruction of NAPNES was almost complete.

## Seattle, 1984

The members rallied at this convention and, even with the 85 Proposal one year from the desired implementation date looming, began the work of getting NAPNES back on course. Executive staff was replaced, and the long debated move from New York to the Midwest became a reality. NAPNES relocated to St. Louis, Missouri, and the NAPNES "turnaround" began in earnest. Members of the St. Louis Chapter and the LeMay Chapter of the NAPNES state affiliate – the Missouri State Association for Licensed Practical Nurses (MoSALPN) – donated eight hours a day, five days a week for three months and "put Humpty Dumpty back together again." The sheer determination and selfless hard work of these LPNs was reminiscent of the founder's courage and determination. NAPNES came back stronger, and some said even better, for the experience. Nothing about NAPNES could ever be rag-tag with such will and spirit.

## St. Louis, 1985

"Still Alive in '85" took on a whole new meaning. The work of NAPNES was to rebuild, and indeed it did. Automating the office allowed NAPNES to accomplish with six staff members what had required 28 in New York. With a $5,000 grant from Shell Oil, NAPNES purchased its first McIntosh computer and began the exciting process of desktop publishing for the prestigious *Journal of Practical Nursing*.

Putting the membership database back together consumed this year of rebirth. Losing contact with thousands of members in 1984 was a setback that, short of a miracle, should have completely closed the NAPNES doors forever. The "miracles" donated hundreds of work hours, and NAPNES finished this hard year with recovery of the 30,000-member database and with much thankfulness. The 85 Proposal did not come to fruition this year, and NAPNES's resolve for maintaining support for the two licensed levels of nurse – RN and LP/VN – was alive and well. NAPNES proudly supported all nursing educational programs, even into the present.

## New Orleans, 1986

This annual convention hosted the Second NAPNES Invitational Conference. The Conference provided a national forum for discussing licensed practical/vocational nursing. The dialogue centered on the future scope, practice, and education for LP/VNs. Twelve national healthcare organizations participated, including the AMA, the NFLPN, the Federation for Accessible Nursing Education and Licensure, the NLN, the NCSBN, and the host, NAPNES.

The main objective was to discuss the retention of the one-year educational preparation for LP/VNs. The result of the conference was renewed support and determination to keep the current structure of LP/VN education.

### St. Thomas, 1987

Vocal! Vigilant! Valuable! AND Victorious! The three years following the bleak 1984 turned out to be a test of strength and courage that NAPNES passed. Operating fully in the black once again, automated and streamlined, NAPNES began cleaning house. The delegates to this 46th Annual Convention made sweeping changes in the NAPNES bylaws when they unanimously voted to combine per-capita and individual memberships. NAPNES retained constituent states, but the states no longer collected dues for NAPNES. Now, individuals sent membership dues directly to NAPNES.

NAPNES found a strong LP/VN supporter in the Virgin Islands' Governor Farrelly. Governor Farrelly stated, "The way to create a better image of nursing is in building a better work environment and working together. It defies common sense and reason to get rid of the LPN. It makes no sense!" (Archives, 1987).

### Nashville, 1988

"On the Road Again" was the theme at NAPNES this year. With NAPNES financially recovered, a change in location would lead NAPNES to its permanent home in the D.C. metropolitan area. Moving a national headquarters is not for the faint of heart, but NAPNES was recovered, members were happy, and the need to be in the nation's capitol guided members to make the relocation decision. So it was good-bye, St. Louie, and hello Beltway! When the members convened again, a new maelstrom was brewing and moving pains were short and not so unpleasant this time around.

Although each office occupied by NAPNES over the years since 1941 was a home to NAPNES, moving to the D.C. metro area was the last step in finding a permanent location. It became a task both for funding and for deciding. To facilitate this goal, the NAPNES Building Fund was created. Mr. Roy Wilson, LPN, became the poster boy for the NAPNES Building Fund, and it became a convention tradition to raise money for a permanent home.

### Washington, DC, 1989

This year brought the fierce and sometimes stinging debate over the registered care technician (RCT) proposal of the AMA. The proposal was for a care technician with two years of education, with heavy emphasis on clinical care. Regulation of this care technician would be conducted by the medical boards, not the boards of nursing. LP/VNs could have applied for and received advanced standing, completing the program in one year. All organized nursing doors began to slam shut – except for NAPNES. In a resolution passed unanimously by the membership, NAPNES agreed to keep the lines of communication open and consider the final AMA proposal fully before deciding whether to support the RCT.

NAPNES testified at the AMA house of delegates to this effect and came under immediate tremendous pressure to reverse its position. Although scorned and shamed openly by other nursing organizations in meetings, NAPNES remained open to any discussion with the AMA regarding the RCT proposal.

What actually happened in the meetings between AMA and NAPNES is not documented in writing but having been a participant, I can tell you that it simply came down to a matter of trust. From NAPNES's perspective, on the one hand, organized nursing had worked diligently since 1965 to diminish and destroy licensed practical/vocational nursing. On the other hand, the AMA simply asked that its proposal receive consideration – not just by the leaders of NAPNES, but by the membership of NAPNES as well. AMA demonstrated its respect for these valuable caregivers in word and deed. It carefully studied the programs of practical/vocational nursing and came to the conclusion that it was not necessary to throw it all away, disrupting the lives and careers of hundreds of thousands of bedside nurses to move forward with a new proposal. NAPNES was willing to listen and consider, and that was, after all, all that was asked.

When it looked as though the RCT proposal was gaining momentum, statements suddenly appeared from organized nursing that LP/VNs were now viewed as a "short-term solution" to the shortage at the bedside. LP/VNs were once again sought by nursing administration in acute care facilities. Although peace was nice in the short term, NAPNES would not be lulled into a false sense of security.

Hopefully, readers will keep in mind that NAPNES was and is privileged to have a large number of RN members who demonstrate by word and deed unflagging support and sincere interest in preparing and working with this level of bedside nurses. Never, in all the years, did the respect and harmony between the work-a-day world nurses break. They stood, as they presently do, in unity and with interest in quality client care delivered by LP/VNs. LP/VNs still enjoy the contributions they make to the profession of registered nursing when working alongside of such professionals. The RNs bent on closing these programs are a breed apart. The RNs that teach and mentor LP/VNs multiply the value of their education by sharing it so freely.

The RCT proposal did not mature to fruition, but the relationship between NAPNES and the AMA, based on mutual respect and trust, did.

*Myrtle Beach, 1990*

NAPNES began deliberations on the differentiated practice issue this year, as well as examined the LP/VN scope of practice in both acute care and long-term care.

Revisiting the history of practical/vocational nurse organizations brought old wounds to the fresh air, and NAPNES developed the posture of refusing to publicly bicker with other nursing organizations. That is not to say that NAPNES would no longer stand for its principles and standards but that whenever possible, it would avoid public arguments with other nursing organizations.

### *Indianapolis, 1991*

NAPNES turns 50 in Indiana! While celebrating its 50th birthday, NAPNES paused to salute the 900 LP/VNs who served in Desert Storm Shield. This year was the year of curriculum assessment and development. Always at the forefront of current knowledge in nursing education, the NAPNES LP/VN educators spent many hours preparing and presenting new ideas and solutions to the new world swallowing up their graduates.

The latest acronym was UAP (Unlicensed Assistive Personnel), and it denoted an unlicensed healthcare worker who did more than a nursing assistant and less than an LP/VN. Although NAPNES did not issue position statements against use of UAPs, it did use every opportunity to urge proper funding and expansion of LP/VN programs before developing and funding another level. Knowing that LP/VNs were often not used to the full extent of their scope of practice, NAPNES made every effort to publish the contributions of LP/VNs to the healthcare system.

### *Birmingham, 1992*

More and more, legal issues were coming to the front of nursing practice. Documentation was the topic of the day, and more and more types and styles of charting and documenting were emerging. LP/VNs were given lists of "red flags" to clients' lawyers when reviewing charts and educated on how to avoid legal pitfalls by competently and accurately keeping legal records of care.

Described as the "foot soldiers" in America's ongoing war against disease and human misery, LP/VNs listened to speaker after speaker describe them as the "back-bone" of the healthcare delivery system. This national discussion led to the "underpaid and overworked" issue for nurses in general, and LP/VNs were urged to actively talk with local leaders to improve the conditions many nurses were starting to find intolerable in the workplace.

### *Atlantic City, 1993*

NAPNES addresses the issues of LP/VNs in long-term care. For years, the largest employer of LP/VNs was hospitals. In 1993, the tide turned, and in several studies, the nursing home business emerged as the largest employer of LP/VNs. One such study was from the research firm FIND, projecting the nursing home business to be a $130 billion industry by the year 2000.

Resolving to work harder to increase the pay and benefits of LP/VNs, NAPNES members renewed dedication to doing so by increasing the number of educational workshops and educational conferences to build skills and expertise in bedside nursing.

### *Columbus, 1994*

Describing the shift of the healthcare system from the medical model, which focuses on curing sickness after it occurs, to the health model, which focuses on prevention and comprehensive health needs, the U.S. Deputy Secretary of Health and Human Services outlined a solid role for LP/VNs in the change. "You are invaluable to this system. Your proven track record of hard work and skill is needed today and will be badly needed tomorrow" (Archives, 1994).

NAPNES began to structure curriculum discussions among LP/VN educators to be certain that the graduates would be prepared for the change and ready to meet the newest needs of clients and families. Continuing education programs began to shift to promotion of wellness along with the standard basic nursing care still very vital to healthcare work.

### *Scottsdale, 1995*

The hotly debated decision to require five-year recertification for the NAPNES Pharmacology Certification Exam culminated in a final showdown. An overwhelming majority finally made it a reality and the work of notification and recertification began. The purpose of the original NAPNES course in the early 1960s was to meet the needs of LP/VNs whose school curriculum did not include pharmacology. Helping these nurses with employability grew into the present-day standard-setting five-year recertification program. Many employers ask LP/VNs for it by name. It is commonly known as "the NAPNES Card" and is often the competitive edge an LP/VN needs to secure the position.

### *Little Rock, 1996*

NAPNES launched the long overdue certification in long-term care. Finally, the LP/VNs who work with chronically ill clients have an opportunity to match their knowledge against a national certification exam. The current version of the exam is available online. Many LP/VNs now proudly add the designation "CLTC" – certified in long-term care – to their credentials.

This year, the Pew Commission generated the report *Reforming Healthcare Workforce Regulation: Policy Consideration for the 21st Century*. The mission of the Pew Commission was to explore how regulation protects the public's health and to propose new approaches to healthcare workforce regulation. The recommendations included closing 20% of the nation's medical schools and reducing the number of new health professionals, including nurses by 10%-25%. NAPNES adopted the open-door/open-mind approach to the report, stating that "change is necessary to meet the future" and that healthcare professionals should not automatically say no before they completely understand all ramifications.

### *Dearborn, 1997*

NAPNES's first student member elected to the board of directors! For the first time in 56 years, NAPNES's membership elected a student member for a two-year term, complete with full board privileges. Much debate and discussion preceded the necessary change in the NAPNES bylaws that would give students the right to seek election to the board of directors.

### *Birmingham, 1998*

This year saw a noticeable rise in frustration on the part of nurses, doctors, healthcare providers, and clients. Hospital closings, layoffs, and the use of managed care and price competition drastically reduced the days of hospital care after a major surgery or illness. Consequently, the growth in outpatient care, ambulatory care, and home care impacted the focus of NAPNES educational programs. LP/VNs needed different programs to cope with the workplace demands, and NAPNES spent the year making sure the necessary programs were available to its members.

### *Virginia Beach, 1999*

NAPNES's well-known certification programs in pharmacology and long-term care took a giant step from paper-and-pencil to ExPro. Currently available only at testing centers, the exams were then administered through a testing agency using the ExPro machines instead of the old-fashioned method of paper and pencil. This was a mighty step forward and only one or two back from the current online version.

### *Birmingham, 2000*

"Old Fashioned Care: The Foundation for New Millennium Nursing." Someone said,

"Stop the madness!", and that is exactly what NAPNES did this year, getting back to basics in educational programs, restructuring the internal workings of headquarters, and simply reconnecting with membership. The year was spent assessing and evaluating and NAPNES emerged centered and stable.

### *Reno, 2001*

"Every Nurse Counts!", and that sums up the 60-year history of NAPNES. From nurses' aides to UAPs, to LP/VNs and RNs, every nurse counts at NAPNES.

Finally, this year, the long-time dream of owning its own office space became a reality for NAPNES. The building fund, established in 1988 under the guidance and direction of its most dedicated advocate, Mr. Roy Wilson, was used to purchase the office condominium in Silver Spring, Maryland. Thanks to contributions from pennies to thousands, NAPNES was now a proud "home owner."

### *2002*

For the first time, NAPNES did not hold an annual convention. All efforts were concentrated on building the certification programs and increasing membership.

### *New Orleans, 2003*

This year's theme, "The Service of Nursing; A National Priority," spoke to all the issues facing nurses in this post-9/11 compounded by a severe nursing shortage era. Topics on "The Role of First Responders," "Are We Ready for Smallpox in a Bio-Terrorism Attack?", and "How to Safely Handle Mandatory Overtime" demonstrate the value of organizations that gather nurses together to share knowledge and expertise. It is much like it first began: the "invaluable invisible" must rush to the front line to serve the nation's need for competent, well-educated nurses.

### The Service of Nursing: A National Priority

Associations such as NAPNES provide student nurses with an array of human relationships. As individuals, members are focused on intervention in human life, usually under the most adverse conditions. These nurses who stand by clients and residents, whether they are drawing their first breath or last, and during every kind of human condition in between, associate for a variety of reasons. They associate to share knowledge, promote better care, socialize, and often, even if not articulated, to be valued by peers for their contribution to the welfare of fellow human beings.

Associations provide opportunities for nurses to teach and mentor other nurses. Associations offer students and practicing nurses programs such as post-licensure certification, leadership conferences, and continuing education. The pooled intellectual resource of nurses in associations serves the public in a myriad of other ways by keeping the nurse workforce current in practice and intellectually healthy.

The value of nurses educated at the next level multiplies each time they use higher education to mentor and raise the knowledge of another nurse at a different place on the pathway. The history of NAPNES is an example of how programs were developed and implemented to forge new careers for hundreds of thousands of currently licensed nurses. The ultimate measurement of success of the founders and dedicated RNs of NAPNES is demonstrated by the continuation of this old organization, in that the LP/VN beneficiaries of the hard work and dedication have matured to the point of taking over management and assuming the challenge of perpetuating the association. That is not to say NAPNES is without RN mentors who currently continue the tradition. They are a vital part of the multidisciplinary organization. RNs educate practical/vocational nursing students. It is their example that teaches LP/VNs to reach out to unlicensed nursing personnel and assist their progress in the healthcare community. It is also due to these RNs that LP/VNs recognize the need to promote the education of nurses at the associate, diploma, baccalaureate, master's, and doctoral levels as they strive to maintain their own level. LPs/VNs know firsthand the value of quality education delivered by RNs and want no less than the very best education for their teachers.

## The NAPNES Concept

The continued success of NAPNES demonstrates that the flow of shared knowledge, skills, and experience enriches all, including the final recipient of nursing care. On behalf of all participants in NAPNES for more than 60 years, I encourage readers to develop and implement projects and programs that reach and raise the knowledge level of those who practice the art and science of nursing at any level. The success of such programs is easily measured by retention of individuals in all capacities whose nursing care is exemplary, and these individuals' sense of being valued is very high because of it.

Further information about NAPNES can be obtained at their website: http://www.napnes.org. For easy access, this website is located on the CD accompanying this book. Simply launch your internet browser, put the CD-ROM in the drive, go to Chapter 43 on the CD, and then click on the website address.

## Learning Activities

1. Identify scenarios in nursing that give rise to development of a new level of healthcare giver. After exploring the scope of practice of an existing level of caregiver to determine if it can meet the new need identified, how would you lobby for creation of the new position? Why? How would you lobby against its creation? Why?
2. Design a program in which you share your knowledge and expertise by teaching a lesser prepared level of nursing. Who benefits the most – you, the student, or the recipient of care?
3. Explore the curriculum content of practical/vocational nursing and examine why you support or do not support graduates of this education as coworkers.

## References

Please note: sources of information for this chapter have been retrieved from personal knowledge on the part of the author, Helen Larsen, and archival data. This information is not accessible to the public, and is contained in corporate minutes and records.

# Chapter 44: SIGMA THETA TAU INTERNATIONAL, HONOR SOCIETY OF NURSING (STTI)

Nancy Dickenson-Hazard, BSN, MSN, RN, CPNP, FAAN, and May L. Wykle, MSN, PhD, RN, FAAN, FGSA

*Dedicated to scholarship, leadership, and excellence in nursing, Sigma Theta Tau International (STTI), Honor Society of Nursing, has the overarching goal of improved world health. Love, courage, and honor embody all that nurses would be in their provision of care and service to others. Nancy Dickenson-Hazard and Dr. May Wykle provide us with a concise overview of STTI, highlighting facets of history, membership, service, leadership, and research. – Lynn Engelmann and Linda Caputi*

## Introduction

STTI is founded in the principles of academic excellence, scholarship, and leadership. It is an organization that supports teaching and learning, including the research, education, and career and leadership experiences of faculty and their students. The prestige and honor of being recognized and supported as a scholar and leader in a global nursing community places faculty in a position to influence the scholarly careers of their students through association with the society.

### Educational Philosophy

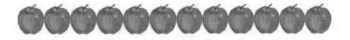

My teaching experience has occurred mostly in the patient care area, professional and career development for nurses, and staff development. Throughout these experiences, basic beliefs have been the guides, first, to help individuals grow in self-mastery and personal depth; second, to recognize and use their talents and resources to express their intellectual curiosity, third, to start where individuals are and with what they want to know during their learning journey, fourth, to offer and connect the learner to the best knowledge and resource I know of, and fifth, to share the journey with individuals, learning and growing with them. – Nancy Dickenson-Hazard

I believe in mastery learning and that education should be enjoyable, a fun process that allows all students to be successful. Teaching is a reciprocal interpersonal relationship – the teacher as a mentor guides the student to learn more so he or she can teach less. – May L. Wykle

As the only international nursing honor society, STTI is one of the most prestigious and formidable nursing organizations. Dedicated to recognizing excellence and achievement in the nursing profession, its stalwart focus on scholarship and leadership is shared and embodied in its members and chapters, which are the foundation of the society's success.

The diverse history of STTI reveals both how much and how little the society has changed over eight decades. The foci that currently engage the society – research, scholarship, preparing leaders for the future, nurturing nursing's intellect, shaping policy, and making the profession visible – are not substantially different from those that stimulated its founding. At times, organizational energies have been directed toward taking stock; getting nursing's house in order (literally, building a permanent home for nursing); and changing the governance structure to adapt to globalization demands. At other times, the society has focused outward on a troubled healthcare environment, using its influence and strength to prepare, support, and position nurses to shape and create wholesome, futuristic nursing advancement. Regardless of world, social, and national environments, STTI has clearly demonstrated the importance of scholarship, leadership, and excellence in nursing.

## History

Founded in 1922 by six nursing students of the Indiana University Training School for Nurses, STTI was envisioned as an organized way to acknowledge excellence in nursing. The founders believed that the demonstration of knowledge through academic achievement evidenced a high degree of excellence, and when this knowledge excellence was applied to practice – or service – the standard of service would be elevated, thereby improving the health of those served. The founders also adopted the Greek words of Storge (Sigma), Tharos (Theta), and Tima (Tau) as the charge of the organization in fulfilling love (Sigma), courage (Theta), and honor (Tau) as it exercised its knowledge in the service of others. Early programmatic foci were placed on identifying and inducting members, supporting research, and convening educational programs. This charge and these foci remain in place currently. Scholarship and leadership are the hallmarks and foundation of STTI.

## The 21st-Century Society

What began as six students in one chapter in the Midwest now exists as 424 chapters with 120,000 active members in 90 countries around the world. The vision of the society as reaffirmed in the year 2000 is "to create a global community of nurses who lead in using scholarship, knowledge, and technology to improve the health of the world's people" (STTI, 2000, p. 1). The society fulfills its vision through its mission to "provide leadership and scholarship in practice, education, and research . . . by supporting the learning and professional development needs of members" (STTI, 2000, p.1). Through strategic goals in the areas of membership and chapter development, global linkages, leadership, research support and scholarship, and fiscal resource development, the society strives to meet its mission.

## Governance

The organization is directed by a distinguished 12-member international board of directors, representing all facets of nursing and providing comprehensive direction through a knowledge-based policy governance model for the Honor Society (a 501 [c] 3 entity), a tax-exempt corporation as well as the subsidiary corporations of the International Honor Society of Nursing Foundation (a 501 [c] 3 entity), and the International Honor Society of Nursing Building Corporation (a 501 [c] 2 entity). The Foundation provides support to the Honor Society through active fundraising and prudent fund investment for nursing scholarship, research, and leadership. The Building Corporation is the title holding company for the Center of Nursing Scholarship and manages the real and personal property of the society. Seventy full- and part-time staff support the work of the board, its subsidiary board, committees, task forces, chapters, and members. In addition, the financial health of the organization is secure, demonstrated by its asset base and history of balanced budgets.

## Membership

Membership in the Honor Society is achieved through induction by one of the society's 424 chapters. Inductees meet the eligibility criteria, either as a basic baccalaureate – or equivalent – student, a graduate student in nursing, or as a nurse leader – one who has demonstrated excellent achievement in the profession. Honorary membership is conferred by the international board of directors upon individuals who are not nurses but who have gained national or international recognition in nursing or a field contributing to nursing.

Members of the honor society represent the following practice areas:
- Direct patient care (56%), including advanced practice nursing.
- Administrative and consulting roles (8%).
- Nurse educators (15%).
- Nurse researchers (2%).

The majority hold positions in hospitals (42%), with 13% working in ambulatory care, HMOs, home care, and nursing home settings. Fifteen percent are employed in schools of nursing. Over 50% of the membership have earned master's degrees, and 10% hold doctorate degrees.

## Chapters

Chapters of the society are organized as autonomous local groups of nurse leaders and scholars who meet specific criteria to hold a charter as a Sigma Theta Tau International chapter. These criteria include establishment in institutions of higher education that grant baccalaureate or higher nursing degrees, and accreditation or the equivalent of the nursing program by a recognized national body, such as the National League for Nursing and the America Association of Colleges of Nursing.

## Scholarship Agenda

Sigma Theta Tau International has enjoyed many firsts in nursing, including awarding the first known nursing research grant in 1936. Presently, more than $1 million dollars are awarded organization-wide to support research. Conduct of the first international capital campaign in nursing's history resulted in the founding of the Center for Nursing Scholarship. The founding of the Center Nursing Publishing in the 1960s provided the opportunity to broadcast nursing knowledge to thousands of health professionals through the following:

- *Journal of Nursing Scholarship*, the most widely circulated scholarly nursing journal globally.
- *Reflections on Nursing Leadership*, the award-winning quarterly news magazine featuring information on health topics and nursing advances around the world.
- Book publishing on diverse topics such as:
  - The art of nursing.
  - Career management.
  - Cadet nursing.
  - Making a difference in the care of clients.
  - Healthcare delivery systems.
  - Nursing and managed care.
  - Nursing theories.
- Electronic and print news briefs on excellence in nursing practice, administration, and research.

Sigma Theta Tau casts a wide web of useful knowledge for service. The society was the first to create a nursing electronic library – the Virginia Henderson International Nursing Library. This state-of-the-science library has initiated many program innovations to support nursing scholarship. Currently, the *Registry of Nursing Research*, a fully searchable database of nursing research studies, enables users to access findings, variables studied, and researchers. The conference abstract section of the library extends this search capacity for knowledge to scientific presentations and the synthesis of knowledge, readily usable for evidence-based practice nurses. This is available through the *Online Journal of Knowledge Synthesis in Nursing*. The society provides annual international research congresses and biennial research, clinical practice, and leadership conferences. On-line continuing education in evidence-based nursing practice is offered, along with over 800 annual chapter scholarly programs and community service projects.

## Leadership Agenda

As one of the first nursing organizations to offer on-line services and have a Web presence, Sigma Theta Tau International was also one of the first to establish leadership in nursing as a priority. The International Leadership Institute provides nursing with opportunities to learn and lead globally through mentoring experiences (the *Chiron* program), through career progression and mapping, through career advising and positioning, and through global think tanks that focus on professional, social, and diversity issues of importance to global health (the *Arista* series). Many of these leadership initiatives are mirrored by chapters and provide opportunity for the lived leadership experience while learning. In addition, chapter leaders reach out to nurses in many lands through exchanges, consultations, and visits to support their endeavors to enhance practice and education standards, curricula development, public health initiatives, policy formation, and nursing research. The on-line community resource of the society provides the venue for communication and learning as do multiple knowledge and talent brokering services, such as the *Media's Guide to Nurse Experts*, media education, placement on consumer organization boards, and publishing works for and about nursing in the popular press.

The *Chiron* program creates learning alliances between mentors and mentees. The mentoring relationships cross national boundaries and span diverse subjects, such as:
- Writing for publication.
- Collaborating on research.
- Establishing guidelines for evidence-based practice.
- Influencing policy.

The *Arista* series are think-tank conferences that bring together the brightest minds to examine and strategize issues germane to nursing and health care. These multidisciplinary

conferences engage respected experts representing the following:
- Healthcare professions.
- Science.
- Government.
- Media.
- Health systems.
- Healthcare policy.
- Healthcare payers.
- Research.
- Economics.

Issues such as the nursing shortage, population health needs, ethics and inequities, and nursing's preferred future have been addressed from a global and regional perspective.

## Partnerships

The society provides individuals with leadership opportunities and assumes leadership positions with other healthcare and related organizations. Partnerships between STTI and other entities have been successfully forged around such issues as the recruitment and retention of nurses and the public image of nursing (through a 40-organization coalition, Nurses for a Healthier Tomorrow). The society also addresses the need for leadership education for nurses in developing countries through collaboration with the American International Health Alliance to provide education for nurses in Central and Eastern Europe and the New Independent States. The society cooperates with the World Health Organization (WHO) World Assembly mandate to establish strategic directions for nursing and midwifery through collaboration with the Global Advisory Group for Nursing and Midwifery of the WHO and eight key organizations that contribute to the strategic directions implementation.

The faculty shortage – of both individuals and resources – is addressed through initiating and managing the International Academic Nursing Alliance. This alliance is a 23-country collaborative seeking to develop an electronic portal for all nursing academicians to share, exchange, and develop resources and standards.

The society also realizes the need for increasing the public's and nursing's access to palliative/end-of-life care resources through a multidisciplinary and consumer organization coalition to increase education about palliative care options. Additionally, chapters have assumed leadership in partnering with local affiliates of the American Cancer Society, Safe Sitters, Special Olympics, and the Alzheimer's Association to provide services for their communities.

# Recognition and Awards

Recognition of leading endeavors on the part of nurses influencing health and on the part of those not in nursing who contribute to the profession and influence the health of people is an important initiative of the society. The international awards program recognizes leaders in research, practice, education, technology, publication, heritage, professional standard setting, innovation, and creativity. Over 150 awards are bestowed biennially to nurse leaders and scholars. In addition, individuals such as Audrey Hepburn, Mrs. Rosalynn Carter, Dr. Jonas Salk, His Highness the Aga Khan, Sir George Alleyne, Aziza Hussein, and Bill and Judith Moyers have been honored with awards for lifetime achievement in advancing the health of people, for public service, and for contributions to promoting nursing and influencing world health.

Over the decades, STTI has prospered because of the visionary leadership of its elected officials. Each president establishes a biennial focus for the society, which becomes the pathway to action and the basis of rich legacies. Table 44.1 presents a list of past presidents and their visionary themes.

Table 44.1 - Past Presidents and Visionary Themes

| President | Visionary Theme |
|---|---|
| Sr. Rosemary Donley | Leadership in Action |
| Carol Lindeman | Image Makers: Richness in Diversity |
| Lucie S. Kelly | International Network of Scholars |
| Vernice D. Ferguson | Patterns of Success in Nursing: On Becoming Culture Builders |
| Angela Barron McBride | Building Career Success |
| Billye J. Brown | The Dynamics of Developing Resources: Support for Nursing in the 21$^{st}$ Century |
| Beth C. Vaughan-Wrobel | The Leadership Challenge in Nursing |
| Fay L. Bower | Leadership: Creating a New Era |
| Melanie C. Dreher | Clinical Scholarship Worldwide |
| Eleanor J. Sullivan | Avenues to the Future |
| Patricia E. Thompson | Learning and Leading Globally: Members and Chapters |
| May L. Wykle | Building Diverse Relationships |

# Summary

This chapter has presented an overview of the history, governance, membership, and chapter organization of STTI. The authors invite you to explore the rich resources available to you through STTI, which promote research and scholarly activities.

# Learning Activities

1. Design and participate in a mentoring experience.
2. Create an outline for a presentation on your area of interest and submit it to a professional society.
3. Complete media training and learn to communicate the value and contribution of nursing to reporters, interviewers, and writers for television, radio, and print.
4. Identify your talents and volunteer them to a not-for-profit organization.
5. Write the nursing story of a friend and submit for publication.
6. Develop and submit a research grant.
7. Investigate whether your alma mater or current school has a society chapter. Check membership requirements, current activities, and membership costs.

The activities listed above are available through the society and promote scholarly and leadership development of individuals. In addition to the learning activities listed above, the following are specific to opportunities provided by the society. Contact STTI at www.nursingsociety.org or 1.888.634.7575 (U.S. and Canada) or +800.634.7575.1 (International) for more detail.

1. Develop an evidence-based online case study in your area of interest.
2. Register your nursing research in the *Registry of Nursing Research*.
3. Develop your career profile and serve as a career advisor.
4. Register your expertise as a media source in the *Media Guide*.

## Contact Information

Contact STTI at www.nursingsociety.org or toll free at 888.634.7575 (U.S. and Canada) or 800.643.7575.1 (International) for more detail.

For easy launching of the STTI website, the URL is located on the CD accompanying this book. Simply launch your internet browser, put the CD-ROM in the drive, go to Chapter 44 on the CD, and then click on the website address.

### Reference

Sigma Theta Tau International [STTI], Honor Society of Nursing. (2000). *Strategic plan: 2005*. Indianapolis, IN: Center Nursing Publishing, STTI.

# Chapter 45: NATIONAL STUDENT NURSES' ASSOCIATION (NSNA): TEACHING AND LEARNING SHARED GOVERNANCE

Diane J. Mancino, MA, EdD, RN, CAE

*It is hardly prophetic to say that nursing students are nursing's future. However, with all the nursing skills, theory, critical thinking, role modeling, and a myriad of other components that go into a nursing curriculum, the notion of mentoring students to become leaders may get lost. Thank goodness for the National Student Nurses' Association to be a proud reminder of our need to educate nursing leaders.  – Linda Caputi and Lynn Engelmann*

## Introduction

The National Student Nurses' Association (NSNA) is a membership organization representing students in associate degree, diploma, baccalaureate, generic master's, and generic doctoral programs preparing students for registered nurse licensure. It is an independent student organization governed by nursing students. Since 1952, the NSNA has provided a voice for nursing students to speak out on issues related to nursing education, nursing practice, and the health needs of the public. The mission of the NSNA is to:

### Educational Philosophy

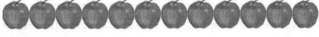

Teaching is like cultivation – all of the conditions must be right for learning: intellect, curiosity, an open mind, freedom to express ideas, and a teacher willing to acknowledge that not everything is known.

Mentorship is the special attention given to those whose potential for leadership is great – it involves recognizing and developing talents and skills, connecting people and resources, modeling professionalism, and a keen awareness that every word, action and expression convey meaning. – Diane J. Mancio

- Organize, represent, and mentor students preparing for initial licensure as registered nurses, as well as those enrolled in baccalaureate completion programs.
- Convey the standards and ethics of the nursing profession.
- Promote development of the skills that students need as responsible and accountable members of the nursing profession.
- Advocate for high-quality health care.
- Advocate for and contribute to advances in nursing education.

This chapter explores the history of shared governance in schools of nursing and introduces the reader to a contemporary method for faculty to engage students in leadership activities. The NSNA Leadership University (Leadership U), which provides a framework for learning shared governance, is also described.

## Teaching and Learning Shared Governance

Learning through real-life experience is one means of effectively transferring information and developing skills. It can shorten or even eliminate the time gap between theory and practical application. The clinical aspect of nursing education provides just such hands-on opportunity to nursing students.

Similarly, participation in the NSNA provides nursing students with structured opportunities to gain invaluable real-life leadership experiences. From serving on committees that provide community health service projects to serving on a state student nurses' association board of directors responsible for conducting an annual convention, these leadership experiences aid in the development of competent, confident future nurses. The framework that NSNA utilizes for nursing students to model real-life leadership experience is shared governance.

## Shared Governance Model
## Used at the NSNA

The primary purpose of NSNA is to develop the leadership potential of undergraduate nursing students who will be the future leaders of professional associations, healthcare organizations, and educational institutions. Generally, students have had little or no experience with shared governance, and most have never held leadership positions in voluntary organizations. They are often encouraged to participate by faculty and peers who identify leadership potential in students who may be unaware of their own potential. When students hear about NSNA, many are eager to contribute their time and talent because they believe in the association's mission. Once students are elected or appointed to leadership positions in the association, they need to hit the ground running. With peers and faculty serving as mentors and coaches, new leaders learn on-the-job, often through trial and error. Incorporating a guided method of teaching and learning shared governance into undergraduate nursing education can increase the success of fledgling leaders and lay the groundwork for future leadership roles.

The need for nurses to understand and practice shared governance has never been greater. As healthcare institutions become more competitive and the practice of nursing more complex, nursing leaders with vision are engaging their staff to design and implement effective professional nursing practice models. Thoughtful participation by all nursing staff is essential, and nurses who have learned and practiced shared governance as students are highly valued employees.

Articulate, experienced leaders are critical to the advancement of the nursing profession. Nursing faculty play a pivotal role in the identification of potential leaders. Once identified, establishing a mentor-protégé relationship with the student begins an exciting process of growing a future nurse leader.

## History of Shared Governance and the Establishment of the NSNA

Arriving at the current state of shared governance has been a slow, deliberate process. At the beginning of the 20th century, nursing leaders, influenced by the progressive education movement, introduced self-governance into training schools. These early nurse luminaries recognized the potential of bringing students into the fold of the professional community by exposing them to democratic principles during the course of their training.

The NSNA evolved after many decades of student involvement in shared governance in the nurses' residence, attendance at state and district nurses' association meetings, and observation of the democratic process at national and international conventions and congresses. After many years of nurturing by directors of nursing and faculty, state and district student nurses' associations were formed. By the mid-20th century, nursing students were well positioned for the establishment of a national organization. Currently, almost a century after the introduction of self-governance into nursing education, Leadership U offers students and faculty a practical model for teaching and learning shared governance.

The early development of shared government in nursing (referred to as **self-governance** in early literature) parallels that of the progressive education movement that encouraged children to play an active role in such affairs as student government (Morison, Commager, & Leuchtenburg, 1983). There was a shift in emphasis from subject matter to learning by experience, from education as a preparation for life to education as life itself. Many of the early nursing leaders had teaching certificates prior to entering nursing school, which may account for their affiliation with Teachers College in New York City at the end of the 19th century. It was at Teachers College that the first post-graduate course in nursing was offered in the Department of Domestic Science. Many of the leaders of the progressive education movement were at Teachers College in 1899 when the nursing course was developed. As noted by Teresa Christy (1969), nurse historian, in *Cornerstone for Nursing Education*, "Undoubtedly, the exposure to educators like Dewey, Thorndike, McMurry, and Kilpatrick augured well for the early students in the Division of Nursing Education at Teachers College, and in turn for the profession of nursing itself" (p. 110).

Articles advocating for the inclusion of democratic principles in nursing schools began to appear in the *American Journal of Nursing (AJN)*. By 1915, self-governance in schools of nursing was a topic of high interest to members of the National League of Nursing Education. In a paper presented at the New York State League of Nursing Education, F. E. Carling (1917), a nurse in New York, opened her remarks with an expanded vision for the future of training schools. Drawing from data on student government in women's colleges, Carling discussed in detail the purpose and outcomes of shared government. Carling believed that preparation of nurses should not only include proper care of the sick but also foster the ability to formulate practical solutions to social problems. Carling noted that "the whole world is turning toward democracy. . . . We must prepare our nurses to be bigger and broader and fit them to take their places in the onward march of our profession" (p. 302). An overview of the aims of student government in women's colleges included:

- To control the management of all matters concerning conduct of students in their college life that are not academic.
- To develop self-control and promote loyalty.
- To express student sentiment on matters that affect the undergraduates as a whole.
- To direct matters pertaining to the moral and social life of the college.
- To uphold individually and collectively the honor of the college.
- To prevent any form of dishonesty in academic work.
- To uphold actively the social regulations of the college.
- To preserve order and quiet in the houses (dormitories).
- To study the social needs of the college.
- To present suggestions for improved regulations.

The common structure of the shared governance organizations included an executive committee of students elected from various classes and sometimes one member of the faculty. Interpretation of rules, discussion of amendments to the constitution, and contesting questions of jurisdiction were done in "some form of conference between representatives of the students" (Carling, 1917, p. 302), and the faculty was kept informed of all actions taken by the students. Carling reported that self-governance:

has been a remarkable success, . . . a valuable asset, in bringing about a frank and candid relationship between students and the administrative force. . . . It has also tended to promote the loyalty of the students. Standards of conduct have been higher. It has increased individual responsibility. . . . It had been a good thing in the development of the students, leading them to look at their own actions and those of their fellow students from the point of view of an adult. (p. 303)

Also in 1915, extensive discussion of shared governance in reference to student discipline was recorded in the *Proceedings of the 21st Annual Convention of the National League for Nursing Education.* A paper entitled *Self Government: Its Advantages and Limitations as Applied to Schools of Nursing* was presented by Carolyn Gray (NLNE, 1915), superintendent of the New York City Hospital Training School, Blackwell's Island, New York. Gray conducted a survey of schools and colleges that had successfully adopted a system of shared governance. Her inquiry resulted in 50 letters returned from superintendents of schools of nursing throughout the country. In a summary of her results, Gray reported that

all seem ready and willing to consider the adoption of this system [of self-governance]; . . . [however,] one superintendent in a mood that one can well sympathize with claims to get good results from military discipline and asks, "Why should we experiment?" In reference to this, it might be well to ask just what we understand by discipline. If we mean better order, unthinking response to commands, implicit obedience without questioning the source of authority, then military discipline is our ideal. If, however, we understand discipline to be the orderly regulation of instincts that are struggling for expression, then a system that gives one the ability to govern one's self is our goal. (p. 194)

Gray analyzed why nursing schools did not readily adopt shared governance and commented on the "serious difficulties peculiar to our type of schools [that] confront us" (NLNE, 1915, p. 196). Difficulties cited included the dependence upon nursing students to "take their places in a scheme where their work counts and where it reflects credit or discredit on the institution and may involve questions of life and death, so far as the patients are concerned" (p. 196). She noted that for this reason mainly, military discipline retained its hold in nursing schools for it produced uniformity and prompt results. Citing another difficulty, Gray noted that nursing students are a "heterogeneous group, differing in education, nationality, and age" (p. 197).

Shared governance activities led to involvement of nursing students in district, state, and national nurses' associations. In 1922, in the *AJN*'s first *Student Nurses' Page*, Josephine Nichols explained the details of how her school selected and financed a representative to go to the national convention in Seattle and the ingenious fundraising campaigns of each class:

> The sophomore class has a Service Committee with an office and a registry. Mending, washing, sewing, pressing, facial massage, answering telephones, cleaning rooms, bed making, shoe shining, shampooing, etc. The junior class . . . socks were mended, the price varying with the size of the hole. . . . The most successful venture was a carnival given at the dormitory. Booths were erected. A cake was raffled and brought $8; the person who won it then sold the pieces for 10 cents each. . . . The fortune-telling room was well patronized, as our superintendent of nurses and educational director have enviable reputations as palmists. . . . We feel that the campaign has brought students, faculty, and alumnae into closer relationship and has helped develop a better school spirit. (p. 53)

Student government was included in a remarkable study conducted by a committee appointed by the Rockefeller Foundation in 1919. This study generated an extensive survey on nursing and nursing education in the United States. In what became known as the Goldmark (1923) report, named after Josephine Goldmark, secretary of the Committee for the Study of Nursing Education, it was reported that:

> the superintendent of nurses has an opportunity of enormous influence in creating the atmosphere and setting the tone of the nurses' home in stimulating healthy interests and in making the three years of training a broader education than that of mere technical equipment. In no case can this influence be more potently or helpfully exerted than in the matter of student government. Whether under self-government or faculty control, the aim of any modern system must be admitted to be free co-operation, not the military discipline and autocratic obedience of the old tradition. (p. 451)

Several decades later, 1,000 nursing students met several times in Atlantic City at the 1952 American Nurses Association (ANA) Convention to discuss establishing a national organization for nursing students. At the end of the convention, Miss Carolyn Kuesher, a student at the Presbyterian Hospital School of Nursing, Pittsburgh, Pennsylvania, acting chairman of the new student council, gave the following statement to the ANA House of Delegates:

> Forty-three states and two territories were represented, with more than 1,000 students in attendance. We wish to extend a vote of appreciation to the American Nurses Association, the National League of Nursing Education, and the National Organization for Public Health Nursing for the invitation and recognition we

received at the 1952 biennial nursing convention in Atlantic City, New Jersey. . . . A voting body . . . consisting of the president of each state organization and a temporary chairman of the states that do not yet have state student organizations and one representative from each territory of the United States . . . voted to form a national council of student nurses to function independently under the sponsorship of the coordinating council of the American Nurses Association and the National League for Nursing and to elect temporary officers at this time. (ANA, 1952, p. 167)

Thus began the first national association of nursing students, known currently as the NSNA. Although shared governance has been practiced in nursing schools since the turn of the 20th century, it is presently gaining renewed recognition as an important method of leadership development for undergraduate nursing students. Preparing students to participate in democratic group decision making is perhaps NSNA's greatest contribution to the preparation of future nurses.

### Present-Day Shared Governance

Shared governance is the model for group decision making commonly employed by many of the professional nursing associations. Nursing students who gain leadership experience in NSNA can easily transition to entry-level leadership positions in district nurses associations and specialty nursing organization chapters. As leaders, they bring a wealth of practical experience as well as knowledge of the tools of shared governance to the associations in which they become involved. A working knowledge of shared governance is also essential for participation as a citizen in civic affairs.

Shared governance is gaining recognition as a model for decision making in nursing practice settings. Administrators seeking ways to increase retention of nurses at the bedside and improve the quality of client care are decentralizing decision making. Savvy nurse leaders are encouraging staff nurses to have a voice in shaping their practice setting. Influencing policies, procedures, and bylaws; serving on and chairing committees; and participating on governing councils can increase the control staff nurses can have over their practice. Nurses who enter the profession with the skills needed to participate effectively in decentralized, unit-based governance are highly valued by employers. This positive empowerment of staff nurses improves morale and enhances retention. It also helps prepare staff nurses for future leadership roles as nurse managers.

Presently, many hospitals are seeking Magnet Recognition through the American Nurses Credentialing Center's Magnet Recognition Program. Practice autonomy and clear articulation of the mission, vision, and values of nursing are the hallmarks of magnetism.

The baseline document for the Magnet Program is ANA's (1996) *Scope and Standards for Nurse Administrators*. These *Standards* call for the nurse manager to facilitate participation of staff in nursing and organizational policy formulation and decision making. Institutions that have achieved Magnet status have well defined shared governance structures that ensure opportunities for nurses to influence practice policies. Although these opportunities exist, many nurses may not understand how the governance structure works and the potential positive impact that participation can have on client outcomes. Any new staff nurses who are involved as NSNA leaders in nursing school can hit the ground running in any shared governance environment. It is no wonder that new graduates who were NSNA student leaders are in search of employment at Magnet hospitals and that these institutions are eager to employ them.

## NSNA Shared Governance Model

Shared governance is a system of rules and policies that serve to engage individuals and groups to participate in decision making. The responsibility and accountability for decisions is shared by members of the group. The objective of shared governance is to afford those who are impacted when a decision is made to have an opportunity to express opinions and participate in the decision-making process. The tools of NSNA's shared governance model include:
- Local, state, and national laws and regulations.
- Articles of incorporation.
- Bylaws, policies, and procedures.
- Code of ethics (code of professional conduct; code of academic and clinical conduct).
- *Bill of Rights and Responsibilities for Students of Nursing* (NSNA, 1991) and grievance procedure guidelines.
- *Getting the Pieces to Fit* (*NSNA Handbook*, 2003).
- *NSNA Business Book* (NSNA, 2003).
- *Robert's Rules of Order Newly Revised* (Robert, 2000).
- Historical traditions.

The NSNA has a three-tier structure for decision-making by members:
- School chapter.
- State association.
- National organization.

School chapters and state associations are entitled to send representatives to the NSNA House of Delegates, which meets annually. The House of Delegates is responsible for electing the board of directors and members of the nominating and elections committees. The House of Delegates also votes on issues, usually in the form of resolutions. Having a seat at the table as a committee or board member or serving as a representative to a larger voting body (i.e., House of Delegates, senate, or council) implies commitment, interest, knowledge, and the authority to serve in the role. This form of shared governance, as practiced by members of the NSNA, is similar to governance models used by many professional associations and is similar to governance structures at colleges, universities, and healthcare delivery organizations.

One of the best methods for learning shared governance is through guided practice. NSNA provides many leadership opportunities and offers students and faculty resources to enhance learning about shared governance. Just as hospitals and community health agencies serve as sites for clinical experience, participating in NSNA shared governance serves as a practicum for gaining leadership experiences.

## NSNA Leadership University

The NSNA is a membership organization representing students in associate degree, diploma, baccalaureate, generic master's, and generic doctoral programs preparing students for registered nurse licensure. It is an independent student organization governed by nursing students. Since 1952, the NSNA has provided a voice for nursing students to speak out on issues related to nursing education, nursing practice, and the health needs of the public. The mission of the NSNA is to:

- Organize, represent, and mentor students preparing for initial licensure as registered nurses, as well as those enrolled in baccalaureate completion programs.
- Convey the standards and ethics of the nursing profession.
- Promote development of the skills that students need to be responsible and accountable members of the nursing profession.
- Advocate for high quality health care.
- Advocate for and contribute to advances in nursing education.

In 1999, NSNA conducted a Participatory Forum on Leadership at the 47th Annual NSNA Convention. At the Forum, students and faculty participated in focus groups. When asked, "What is the value of NSNA on leadership development?", participants responded as follows:

- Participation in NSNA shared governance fosters the development of leadership attributes and management skills needed in integrated health systems; skills learned in

NSNA are transferable to other settings.

- Leadership and management skills are learned and practiced in an organization that involves students in democratic decision making.
- Learning and practicing leadership skills beyond the boundaries of classrooms and campuses accelerates the development of leadership in students and broadens their perspective of the nursing profession.
- Opportunities to examine issues facing the nursing profession prior to graduation prepares nurses for greater involvement in professional organizations.

When the students and faculty were asked why students were or were not involved in NSNA, "lack of faculty support" was identified as the greatest barrier to NSNA participation. The schools with the most participation attributed their success to "supportive deans or directors, faculty, and administrators." At the Participatory Forum, three nursing programs were identified as outstanding examples of how students are recognized for the learning that takes place when they participate in NSNA. The nursing programs, Valencia Community College (Orlando, Florida), Golden West College (Huntington Beach, California), and Grand View College (Des Moines, Iowa), all link participation in NSNA shared governance activities to academic content through structured leadership experiences. Students who participate are eligible to receive academic credit. One school, Grand View College, integrates NSNA participation throughout the four-year curriculum.

The Participatory Forum on Leadership led to the development of Leadership U. The objective of Leadership U is to communicate the value of NSNA as a practicum in leadership development. Students and faculty are provided with resources to assist them to integrate NSNA activities into undergraduate nursing education, and faculty are encouraged to offer academic credit to students who meet the Leadership U learning objectives. Examples of how faculty may offer academic recognition for NSNA involvement include:

- Establishing a one-to-three-credit NSNA Leadership U course (this may also serve as an excellent bridge course for students waiting entry into upper division nursing programs).
- Adding NSNA Leadership U participation to course fulfillment options for projects or service-learning activities.
- Providing independent study credit.
- Establishing a leadership and management internship or preceptorship.
- Adding points to grades for serving in leadership roles or participating on committees.
- Link appropriate course syllabus to NSNA's program areas (e.g., community health, legislation education, and Breakthrough to Nursing recruitment into nursing project).
- Including the hours for participation in NSNA community service projects to count toward college- or university-wide community service graduation requirements.

NSNA programs and activities that develop leadership and management skills take place at the school, state, and national levels of the NSNA. Participation teaches students how to work in cooperative relationships with peers, faculty, and students in other disciplines and with the public. Following are several examples.

## *School Chapter Level*

### *Breakthrough to Nursing Project*

Created in 1965, the goal of this program is to increase the number of nurses from underrepresented populations in nursing. Breakthrough to Nursing committee members participate in career days and visit elementary, junior-high, and high-school students and guidance counselors to inform them about nursing careers. Providing services that help to retain students in nursing school is also part of the Breakthrough to Nursing Project. Many nursing schools have adopted NSNA's Breakthrough to Nursing Project as their college or university nursing student recruitment programs.

### *Community Health Projects.*

This NSNA program engages students in the development and implementation of community-centered activities based on a public health needs assessment. For example, students may provide health screenings for medically under-served populations, conduct food and clothing drives, or sponsor health fairs. Community projects often extend beyond the boundaries of the college or university. Involvement in national and international projects helps students to see the big picture of global health care. Many faculty include involvement in NSNA's community health program for community service credit and as one option for partial fulfillment of public health-course requirements.

### *Legislative/Public Policy Education*

This program provides opportunities for students to learn about and address health- and nursing-related legislative and regulatory issues. Examples of activities include:
- Writing resolutions for presentation at the annual NSNA House of Delegates.
- Visiting the state capitol for nurse lobby day.
- Participating in voter registration and get-out-the-vote activities.
- Letter-writing campaigns to increase funding for nursing education and nursing research.

### State Chapter Level

Serving in an elected position on the state board of directors offers students opportunities to build on the learning that takes place at the school chapter level. For example, many state organizations have positions for Breakthrough to Nursing, community health, and legislation education committees. Team skills that are learned during school chapter involvement are practiced and enhanced when students from various schools and types of educational programs learn how to work together to accomplish goals. For example, one of the responsibilities of a state board of directors is to plan and implement an annual convention. Other examples of annual convention activities that teach leadership and management skills include:

- Planning workshops and seminars.
- Marketing the convention.
- Writing, presenting, and defending resolutions.
- Conducting and participating in the annual state association membership meeting and the election of officers.
- Celebrating accomplishments at the awards banquet.

### National Level

Students who participate in the House of Delegates and who serve in leadership positions at the national level of NSNA are introduced to the big picture of shared governance. They build on school and state governance experiences and work with NSNA's management team to accomplish the mission of the association (see Figure 45.1, Leadership Skills Developed during the NSNA Resolutions Process).

Shared governance is the framework that provides the structure needed to implement involvement at the school, state, and national levels. Examples of shared governance activities include:

- Preparing agendas and conducting meetings.
- Recording minutes.
- Learning the fiduciary responsibilities associated with dues and fund raising.
- Conducting and participating in a membership meeting using parliamentary procedure.
- Representing student interests on faculty committees.
- Publishing a newsletter or a website.
- Organizing a workshop.
- Writing, presenting, and defending resolutions.

NSNA members who participate in shared governance develop:

- Increased leadership and management skills and the self confidence to practice those

skills.
- Enhanced relationships with peers and faculty.
- Awareness of professional values.
- Loyalty to the nursing profession.
- Informed perspective of the issues facing the nursing profession and an ability to articulate personal views and ideas on these issues.
- Awareness of the many opportunities that professional nursing has to offer.
- Networking skills and mentor-protégé relationships.

Leadership U provides an opportunity for students to be recognized for the skills they develop by virtue of their participation in NSNA's programs and activities. From the school chapter level to the state and national levels, nursing students learn how to work in cooperative relationships and to develop esprit de corps. Figure 45.2 provides examples of competencies developed by students participating in Leadership U.

Figure 45.1 - Leadership Skills Developed During the NSNA Resolutions Process

---

Competencies learned and practiced are in **bold** type. See Figure 45.2 *Attributes and Competencies Needed by Future Nurse Leaders and Managers* (NSNA, 2003)

Outcome: Develop and master the leadership skills needed to participate in the democratic process.

Stage I

- Identify a topic/issue **(enhance intellectual and analytical capacity).**
- Determine relevance to nursing students, nursing education, nursing practice **(develop systems thinking; identify global, national, and local trends).**
- Investigate what has been done, if anything, on this topic/issue in past (i.e., does NSNA already have a position on this topic?) **(enhance intellectual and analytical capacity).**
- Investigate whether other nursing organizations have positions on this topic/issue (if so, what are their positions or policies?) **(develop systems thinking; identify global, national, and local trends).**
- Before taking a position, compile a list of the pros and cons for topic/issue **(develop systems thinking; identify global, national, and local trends).**

Stage II

- Once topic/issue has been established as viable and appropriate for a resolution:
  - Decide position (support or oppose) **(enhance intellectual and analytical capacity).**
  - Use the literature to support the decision and to document "whereas" statements **(enhance intellectual and analytical capacity; enhance writing skills).**

---

Figure 45.1 - Leadership Skills Developed During the NSNA Resolutions Process cont.

- Determine what is the appropriate action that the organization can take within the human and financial resources available and write the "resolved" statements **(develop understanding of strategic/tactical planning, implementation, and outcome evaluation; enhance writing skills).**
- Using the correct format as provided by the organization, submit the resolution, documentation, and other requested information **(enhance intellectual and analytical capacity).**
- Inform others about the resolution and seek their support **(develop effective interpersonal and communication skills, critical thinking, and listening skills; empower others; motivate others to participate in decision making).**
- Speak with people who have opposing views about the resolution as well as those who support it so that all sides of the issue are understood; attempt to counter opposition with facts **(manage conflict and master conflict resolution; treat others with respect and acceptance; enhance intellectual and analytical capacity; develops critical-thinking ability; enhance interpersonal and communication skills).**

Stage III

- Learn parliamentary procedure and understand how a resolution is presented in the House of Delegates **(understand and master democratic process, *Robert's Rules of Order*, play by prescribed rules and regulations).**
- Meet with resolutions committee to review the resolution; take the committee's comments and suggestions under consideration **(manage conflict and master conflict resolution; treat others with respect and acceptance; enhance intellectual and analytical capacity; develop critical-thinking ability; enhance interpersonal and communication skills).**
- Attend resolutions hearings to hear debate; be prepared to answer questions and to defend position **(develop effective interpersonal and communication skills, critical thinking, and listening skills; enhance interpersonal and communication skills; motivate others to participate in decision making).**
- If needed, compromise and resolve concerns about the resolution **(learn to adapt quickly to new situations; develop effective interpersonal and communication skills, critical thinking, and listening skills; motivate others to participate in decision making; treat others with respect and acceptance).**
- Speak to resolution at the House of Delegates **(develop effective interpersonal and communication skills, public speaking, parliamentary procedure, and debate skills).**
- If action fails, analyze why **(develop intellectual and analytical capacity).**
- If action carries, communicate this at school and state levels **(develop effective interpersonal and communication skills, public speaking, and writing skills).**

Stage IV

- Build on this process by participating in similar policy development in professional organizations as a Registered Nurse (e.g., American Nurses' Association, State Nurses' Association, District Nurses' Association, and specialty nursing organizations) and as a citizen (e.g., state legislative and Congressional bills).

Figure 45.1 - Leadership Skills Developed During the NSNA Resolutions Process cont.

---

**For further information visit:**
**www.nsnaleadershipu.org**

---

Figure 45.2 - Attributes and Competencies Needed by Future Nurse Leaders and Managers*

- Intellectual and analytical capacity
- Critical-thinking ability
- Systems thinking
- Ability to comprehend interdisciplinary models
- Effective interpersonal and communication skills
- Empathetic/active listening skills
- Ability to adapt quickly to new situations
- Ability to identify global, national, and local trends
- Ability to accept high moral and ethical standards
- Ability to manage conflict and master conflict resolution
- Ability to facilitate collaboration and group process
- Ability to motivate others to participate in decision making
- Capacity to interchange leadership/followership roles
- Ability to mentor future leaders
- Ability to empower others
- Ability to be a team player
- Capacity to understand strategic/tactical planning, implementation, and outcome evaluation
- Ability to treat all human beings with respect and acceptance
- Capacity to strive for an inclusive society
- Ability to balance professional responsibilities and personal life
- Ability to accept responsibility and accountability for decisions
- Ability to demonstrate a commitment to lifelong learning
- Ability to practice the spirit of cooperation
- Ability to balance high tech with high touch
- Ability to solve problems creatively
- Capacity for deep introspection and reflection
- Capacity to connect with the spiritual nature of human beings

*These competencies and attributes are developed during participation in NSNA's leadership activities at the school, state, and national levels of the association.

© National Student Nurses' Association, Inc., 1999-2003, compiled by Dr. Diane J. Mancino

The rewards of participation in Leadership U are many. One tangible reward is a personalized certificate that is presented to both students and faculty at the Annual Awards Ceremony that takes place at the NSNA Convention. Both students who receive academic recognition and the faculty who offer that recognition receive Leadership U certificates.

## Conclusion

Shared governance, with all its rules, regulations, bylaws, and procedures, is not an exact science. It is ripe for both qualitative and quantitative research studies. By documenting the value of teaching undergraduate nursing students shared governance, the framework for teaching and learning shared governance is thus based on scientific investigation rather than empirical evidence alone. Faculty who are interested in conducting such research are encouraged to contact the NSNA.

The education of leaders who are prepared to take on the enormous challenges facing health care is the shared responsibility of educators, practicing nurses, managers, executives, and leaders in professional nursing organizations. NSNA serves as the entry point for future nurse leaders. Nurse educators can play a critical role in preparing nurse leaders by endorsing the NSNA Leadership U and by encouraging students to learn and practice shared governance. The learning that takes place in real-life experiences adds value to nursing education and makes a valuable contribution to the future leadership of the nursing profession.

## Websites

Following is a list of websites that may be helpful in learning more about NSNA. For easy launching, these are also located on the CD accompanying this book. Simply launch your internet browser, put the CD-ROM in the drive, go to Chapter 45 on the CD, and then click on the website address.

- National NSNA (hosted by Delmar Thomson Learning): http://www.nsna.org
- NSNA Leadership University (hosted by Decision Critical, Inc.): http://www.nsnaleadershipu.org

Additional sites:

- American Association of Colleges of Nursing: http://www.aacn.nche.edu/
- American Nurses Credentialing Center: http://nursingworld.org/ancc/

- American Nurses Association: http://www.nursingworld.org/
- American Organization of Nurse Executives: http://www.hospitalconnect. com/
- Center for Civic Education: http://www.civiced.org/
- Center for Nursing Leadership: http://www.cnl.org/the_learning_community. htm
- Cultural Competence: http://cecp.air.org/cultural/default.htm
- Educators for Community Engagement: http://www.e4ce.org/
- Grand View College: http://www.gvc.edu/academics/nursing/other.html
- Leader to Leader Institute (Drucker Foundation): http://www.pfdf.org/
- National League for Nursing: http://www.nln.org/

The following NSNA shared governance resources are available on http:www.nsna.org and www.nsnaleadershipu.org websites:

- *Getting the Pieces to Fit* (published annually)

- *NSNA Guidelines Booklets* (Consultants and Advisors; Budget and Finance; Image of Nursing; Community Health Projects; Legislation Education Activities, and Get out the Vote; Policies, Procedures, and Bylaws, Recording and Corresponding Secretaries; Writing Resolutions; Breakthrough to Nursing Projects; Planning Meetings and Conventions)

- *Bill of Rights and Responsibilities for Students of Nursing and Grievance Procedure Guidelines*

## Photographs

Student photographs from the 2003 NSNA Convention may be viewed on the CD-ROM accompanying this book.

## Learning Activities

1. Design a syllabus for undergraduate nursing students to learn shared governance at the school NSNA chapter level. As you develop the syllabus, consider the following:
   - Level of learner (e.g., entry-level leader with minimal leadership experience).
   - How active is the NSNA chapter at your school?
   - If there is no active chapter, design the syllabus so that the students plan and implement an NSNA chapter.

- Include leadership theory readings and references.
- Include reflective journaling as a requirement.

2. Develop a sample learning contract for students to use as part of the requirements for an independent study project to learn NSNA shared governance.

3. Conduct a facilitated group exercise for professional development. Follwing are some ideas for presenting professionalism and leadership to groups of students:
   - Begin by introducing yourself, and then ask all students to introduce themselves and say who they are, where they go to school, why they want to be nurses, and what they plan to do after graduation, if they know. If there are too many people and not enough time, just ask for names and schools and one sentence addressing "why do you want to be a nurse?" This helps create networking and also helps you know who is in the audience. Then break the students into groups (no more than 10 per group). Separate friends and schools so that the students meet new people. Each small group gets 10 minutes, which can be adjusted according to how much time you have. You can modify this plan in any way.
   - Pose the question: What is the difference between a job and a professional career? Students have 10 minutes to come up with:
     1. A one-sentence description answering "What is a profession?"
     2. Three differences between a job and a professional career.
     One person reports for the group. Look for themes in the responses and then point them out and encourage students to talk about them.
   - Ask students to come up with at least five characteristics of a profession (e.g., specialized body of knowledge; education; credential; code of ethics) and discuss this for 10 minutes. Then have a different person come up and report three of the five. Again, look for themes and point them out (or ask them to think about the themes). Usually **leadership** emerges during the reports, which provides a perfect segue into a short discussion of what leadership is. (e.g., Leadership is a verb – an action word that means that being a leader is about doing something – what is that something?) Ask them to come up with a one-sentence definition of what a leader is. Use the same reporting method – having a different student from the group give the report.
   - The next and final small group assignment is: "What are the characteristics or attributes of leaders?" Come up with at least 10 characteristics and then select the three most important ones to report. This is the fun one, and it helps to segue into NSNA and professional organization involvement.

Before they give their reports, hand out NSNA's (2003) *Attributes and Competencies Needed by Future Nurse Leaders and Managers*, and ask them to check them off as the reports are given. Again, another person gives the report.

Then, make the connection between what they reported and how NSNA involvement helps to develop these competencies. Give an example from the list of what they learned by doing this exercise (from group collaboration to speaking in front of an audience, etc.). Generally, nursing's core values come out during the discussion (e.g., caring, compassion, competency, commitment, responsibility, respect, etc.) Talk briefly about how the core values attract people to nursing and how these are universal values that every nurse in the world shares. Use the example of being at an international meeting such as the International Council of Nurses with students and nurses from other lands and feeling connected to them – it is these core values that connect us to each other, to our clients, and to our profession.

Close with the importance of student involvement in NSNA, and by that time, they understand the role of professional involvement. End with a quote that captures the essence of nursing.

## References

American Nurses Association [ANA]. (1952, June 16-20). Proceedings (Vol. I). House of Delegates, 38th Convention, Washington, D.C.

Carling, F. E. (1917). The possibility of introducing self-government into schools of nursing. *American Journal of Nursing, 17*(4), 299-306.

Christy, T. E. (1969). *Cornerstone for nursing education.* New York: Teachers College Press.

Goldmark, J. (1923). *Nursing and nursing education in the United States: Report of the committee for the study of nursing education and a report of a survey.*New York: MacMillian Company.

Morison, S. E., Commager, H. S., & Leuchtenberg, W. E. (1983). *A concise history of the American republic.* New York: Oxford University Press.

Nichols, J. (1922). How we sent a representative to Seattle. *American Journal of Nursing, 22*(10), 53.

National Student Nurses' Association. (1915, June 21-25). *Proceedings of the 21st Annual Convention of the National League of Nursing Education.* Baltimore, MD: Williams & Wilkins.

Robert, H. M. (2000). *Robert's rules of order* (newly rev. 10th ed.). Cambridge, MA: Perseus Publishing.

*NSNA Guidelines Booklets* (Consultants and Advisors; Budget and Finance; Image of Nursing; Community Health Projects; Legislation Education Activities and Get out the Vote; Policies, procedures and Bylaws; Recording and Corresponding Secretaries; Writing Resolutions; Breakthrough to Nursing Projects; Planning Meetings and Conventions).

NSNA (2001). *Bill of Rights and Responsibilities for Students of Nursing and Grievance Procedure Guidelines.*

# Bibliography

## Nursing

Andersen, C.A. (1999) *Nursing student to nursing leader: The critical path to leadership development.* Albany: Delmar Thompson Learning. This is considered required reading for the NSNA Leadership University.

Bolman, Lee G., & Deal, Terrence. (1995). *Leading with soul: An uncommon journey of spirit.* San Francisco: Jossey-Bass Publishers.

Chitty, K. K. (2001). *Professional nursing: concepts and challenges.* Philadelphia: W. B. Saunders Company.

De Pree, M. (1997) *Leading without power: Finding hope in serving community.* San Francisco: Jossey-Bass.

Ellis, J. R.,& Hartley, C. L. (1998). *Nursing in today's world: Challenges, issues and trends.* Philadelphia: Lippincott-Raven.

Gardner, H. (1995). *Leading minds: An anatomy of leadership.* New York: Basic Books.

Guilini, R. W. (2002) *Leadership.* New York: Hyperion Miramax Books.

Henzi, S. (2001, Feb./March). Leadership development and NSNA. *Imprint.* 37 & 44.

Hesselbein, F., Goldsmith, M., & Beckhard, R. (1996). *The leader of the future.* New York: Drucker Foundation Future Series.

Hesselbein, F., Goldsmith, M., & Beckhard, R. (1997). *The organization of the future.* New York: Drucker Foundation Series.

Huber, D. (1996). *Leadership and nursing care management.* Philadelphia: W. B. Saunders Company.

Kelly, L Y., & Joel, L. (1999). *Dimensions of professional nursing.* New York: McGraw-Hill.

Lancaster, J. (1999). *Nursing issues in leading and managing change.* St. Louis: Mosby.

Logan, J. & Franzen, D. (2001). Leadership and empowerment: The value of the National Student Nurses Association for Beginning Students. *Nurse Educator, 26*(4), 198-200.

Mancino, D. J. (1995). *The role of the National Student Nurses' Association in addressing social and political issues that contributed to student unrest from 1960-1975*, Doctoral Dissertation, Teachers College, Columbia University, NY.

Mancino, D. J. (2002). *Fifty years of the National Student Nurses Association.* New York: NSNA. (Call 718 210-0705 for ordering information).

Mason, D. J., Leavitt, J., & Chaffe, M. W. *(2002). Policy and politics in nursing and health care.* St. Louis: Saunders.

Mindell, P. (1995). *A woman's guide to the language of success: Communicating with confidence and power.* New Jersey: Prentice Hall.

Phillips, J., Watkins, K., & Marsick, V. (1996). *Creating the learning organization.* Virginia: American Society for Training and Development.

Quigley, J. (1993). *Vision: How leaders develop it, share it, and sustain it.* New York: McGraw-Hill.

Roberts, J., & Group, T. M. (1990). *Feminism and nursing: An historical perspective on power, status, and political activism in the nursing profession.* Connecticut: Praeger.

Schwarz, R. (1994). *The skilled facilitator: Practical wisdom for developing effective groups.* San Francisco: Jossey-Bass.

Vance, C., & Olson, R.K. (1998). *The mentor connection in nursing.* New York: Springer

## Non-nursing literature:

Bolman, Lee G., & Deal, Terrence. (1995). *Leading with soul: An uncommon journey of spirit.* San Francisco: Jossey-Bass Publishers.

De Pree, M. (1997) *Leading without power: Finding hope in serving community* San Francisco: Jossey-Bass.

Gardner, H. (1995). Leading minds*: An anatomy of leadership.* New York: Basic Books.

Hesselbein, F., Goldsmith, M., & Beckhard, R. (1996). *The leader of the future.* New York: Drucker Foundation Future Series.

Hesselbein, F., Goldsmith, M., & Beckhard, R. (1997). *The organization of the future.* New York: Drucker Foundation Future Series.

Mindell, P. (1995). *A woman's guide to the language of success: Communicating with confidence and power.* New Jersey: Prentice Hall.

Phillips, J., Watkins, K., & Marsick, V. (1996). *Creating the learning organization.* Virginia: American Society for Training and Development.

Quigley, J. (1993). *Vision: How leaders develop it, share it, and sustain it.* New York: McGraw-Hill.

Schwarz, R. (1994). *The skilled facilitator: Practical wisdom for developing effective groups.* San Francisco: Jossey-Bass.

Journals:

*Harvard Business Review,* Boston, MA.
*Leader to Leader*, New York: Peter F. Drucker Foundation.

**Videos:**

For information about the following videos, Call (718) 210-0705 or write to receptionist@nsna.org

*To Advance We Must Unite: 100 Years of the American Nurses Association.* (1996). Foundation of the National Student Nurses Association, NY. Uses a socio-political framework to trace the development of the American Nurses Association. Includes *Teaching Guide.*

*Not for Ourselves But for Others.* (2002). National Student Nurses Association, NY Uses a socio-political framework to trace the development of the National Student Nurses Association. Used as a companion teaching tool with *Fifty Years of the NSNA*, by Diane J. Mancino.

*Nursing: The Ultimate Adventure* (2000). National Student Nurses Association, Inc. Fast-paced, high energy video for recruitment of teens into nursing.

# Faculty Support and Development

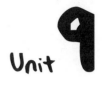

Unit 9

# Chapter 46: FINDING SUCCESS IN THE FACULTY ROLE

### Jane M. Kirkpatrick, BS, MSN, RNC, and Juanita M. Valley, BSN, MSN, RN, ANP

*As a new teacher, my focus was on teaching – being the best teacher I could be. At that time, I had a very narrow focus – teaching was what I did in the classroom. I soon realized that teaching, like nursing, requires ongoing education and discovery, then sharing with colleagues all that I learned. Now teaching **really** got exciting.*

*This chapter discusses those scholarly activities that contribute to the growth of an educator. It has been my experience that these activities are to be embraced and celebrated. These activities are the scholarly works that become operationalized in each and every interaction with our students. – Linda Caputi*

## Introduction

Becoming an effective and scholarly faculty member is an ongoing process that encompasses an entire career. All faculty, whether new or seasoned, need to assume a proactive stance and take charge of their own academic careers. Learning how to achieve and document scholarly professional growth is an essential part of the process of achieving success in the faculty role.

## Educational Philosophy

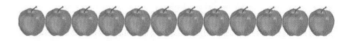

I believe that teaching and learning is an active process with faculty and students each accepting responsibility for the outcomes. The cornerstone of this collaborative venture is honesty and mutual respect. The ultimate goal of learning is beyond the short-term exams and papers. The real final exam is the nursing care provided for our clients. – Jane M. Kirkpatrick

I believe learning is a life long process and the role of the faculty is one of facilitating the learning process through cognitive, affective, and psychosocial domains. I also believe the transference of knowledge and understanding to the novice can be creative and enjoyable and that there should be mutual respect between the person teaching and the person learning. – Juanita M. Valley

# Defining Scholarship

What is scholarship? In many institutions, the traditional model used to demonstrate scholarship is the classic triad of:

1. Research.
2. Teaching.
3. Service.

In this model, the category of research includes the discovery of new knowledge in the discipline. This knowledge is communicated to others through publication and presentations. The research component of this three-pronged model is usually the most visible to others for the purposes of evaluation.

Teaching is considered the process of facilitating student learning. For nursing faculty, this process occurs in both the classroom and the clinical setting. Documenting excellence in teaching is challenging, as it is unusual to have peer colleagues view you in this role.

Service can be demonstrated in various settings. For example, participation on committees is an example of service to the school/university. Holding office in professional organizations is one example of service to the profession. Faculty practice and/or the process of recognizing and acting on community needs, where your professional expertise can facilitate improvement, are examples of service to the public.

In institutions where this traditional triad is the model for promotion and tenure, the interpretation of scholarship primarily emphasizes research. For a practice discipline like nursing, where a large number of hours are spent in teaching and service, this traditional model presents challenges to successful promotion of nursing faculty in the larger university community.

Today many institutions are reconsidering and redefining the scholarly role of faculty. Boyer (1990) and Rice (1991) challenged professional schools in all disciplines to reevaluate the scope of academic work and move beyond the traditional interpretation of research as the only way to increase the knowledge of the discipline and as the only means for incentive and compensation of the academic professional.

The American Association of Colleges of Nursing (AACN) elaborated on the works of Boyer (1990), Diamond & Adam (1995), Donaldson & Crowly (1978), and Stevenson (1988). The AACN (1995, 1997a, 1997b, 1998) also incorporated statements from interdisciplinary collaboration of their research, faculty practice, and education workgroups to define four scholarships that represent the scholarly work of faculty in schools of nursing. The scholarships are:

1. Discovery (Acquisition of new knowledge).
2. Teaching (Sharing knowledge).
3. Application (Clinical practice).

4. Integration (Ideas from nursing and other disciplines).

Each of the four scholarships supports values and beliefs of the nursing profession and emphasizes both the art and science of nursing. See Figure 46.1 for a scholarship model that represents traditional and AACN scholarship categories.

Figure 46.1 - Scholarship Model

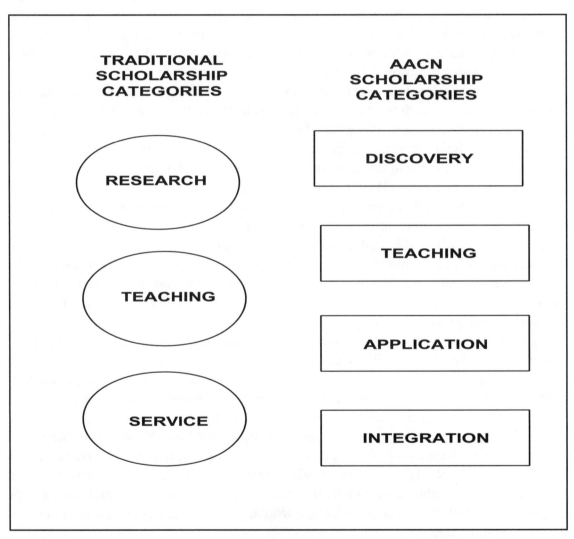

From, Kirkpatrick, J., Schafer, K., Schmeiser, D., Richardson, C., Valley, J., & Yehle, K. (2001). Building a Case for the Promotion of Clinical Faculty. Nurse Educator, 26, pp. 178-181. Adapted with permission, Lippincott, Williams, & Wilkins.

## The Scholarship of Discovery

This scholarship is similar to what academia has always recognized as **research**. It is acquiring new knowledge and presenting this knowledge in a peer-reviewed format. Empirical research (the collection of information data to answer questions), methodological research (generating knowledge by testing new or revised methods of inquiry), and philosophical inquiry are all processes faculty may use to demonstrate the scholarship of discovery (AACN, 1999).

## The Scholarship of Teaching

Scholarly teaching takes the teaching and learning process to a higher level. Scholarly teachers apply educational research findings to facilitate learning in all domains (cognitive, affective, and psychomotor). They also spend time creating an environment for learning that supports a variety of learners and learning styles. Innovations in teaching and the evaluation of the effectiveness of these innovations are examples of scholarly teaching (Schoffner, Davis, & Bowens, 1994).

## The Scholarship of Application

This scholarship is much like the **service** component of the traditional triad. Scholarly work in **application** includes clinical nursing research and building the knowledge base for management of clinical issues. Promoting strategies to apply new knowledge to practice is also a part of this scholarship. The scholarship of application is also referred to as **practice scholarship** or, in the traditional term, as **service**. Boyer (1990) described **service** as a scholarship directly impacting faculty of a clinical specialty or professional development activity.

## The Scholarship of Integration

The scholarship of integration combines nursing knowledge with that of other disciplines within the context of health care. For example, if issues relating to diabetes are researched by a team representing the disciplines of nursing, medicine, pharmacy, nutrition, and health promotions, the synergy created by sharing the insights from the various disciplinary groups could result in new insights and new paradigms that might not have occurred if researched by only one discipline (AACN, 1999).

# Defining Scholarly Performance

To better identify the criteria for scholarship, the AACN (1999) position paper on scholarship for the discipline of nursing listed the following characteristics:
- Demonstrates significance to the profession.
- Needs to be creative.
- Can be documented.
- Can be replicated or elaborated.
- Can be peer-reviewed.

Not every activity in the day-to-day life of a faculty member will meet the criteria; however, it is important to remember that in the larger view of promotion and tenure, scholarly activity provides strong evidence of effectiveness in all the faculty roles.

# Developing a Strategy for Success

Ideally, the criteria for merit will match the criteria for promotion and tenure. In some institutions the emphasis may be heavier in one area than in the other areas. To be successful in achieving merit and promotion, faculty must learn the system that is in place at their college or university.

## *Clinical Track versus Academic Track*

Many institutions have a two-track system. The expectations for success on each track differ. Clinical track faculty frequently carry heavy teaching loads and the reward system will emphasize teaching and service in the traditional model and teaching and application in the AACN model. Clinical track faculty typically do not hold tenure-earning positions. However, clinical track has the opportunity for promotion.

Academic track faculty need to explore the expectations for promotion, and tenure at the institution where they work. Typically, an academic track faculty member has six years to meet the tenure criteria. Academic track faculty may be assigned in such a way that time for research is considered part of their workload.

No matter which track faculty are on, it is important to investigate the culture of the institution. Faculty are encouraged to take a close look at the strategic plan and institutional goals. These help discern the institutional values and help faculty set their trajectory. Faculty need to find out what behaviors have been rewarded in the past. It is also helpful to identify other faculty who have recently been through the process and ask them to share their wisdom. Speaking with the Head or Dean of the program to discuss personal plans and progress is also essential to the process.

It is important that you know how the institution where you are employed views the merit, promotion, and tenure process. You need to ask the following questions in order to plan ahead:

- What is the time-table for promotion?
- How many years do you have to meet tenure?
- Is there a probationary period? What happens at the end of the probationary time?
- What is the practice for pre-tenure review at your institution?
- How do you know if your progress is on track?
- What is the process of decision-making on promotion and/or tenure decisions?
- What resources and/or resource people are available to guide and mentor new faculty?
- What supporting documentation will you need to build your case for merit, promotion, and tenure

Once you have identified your strengths and passions, develop a systematic plan. This plan will serve as a lens for you to evaluate opportunities and help you decide where to spend your time. Set goals and divide them into workable units. Be realistic; if this is your first experience in teaching, be sure to allow time to learn the skills needed to become a good teacher. Becoming an excellent faculty member has its own learning curve and takes time.

### *Demonstrating the Scholarship of Discovery*

The scholarship of discovery is familiar to most faculty, as research has long been associated with scholarship. Nursing research easily represents all five criteria AACN describes for scholarly work.

### *Issues Associated with Discovery*

Probably the biggest concerns for faculty involved with research include time, funding, support, and resources. In the process of starting a program of research, time must be devoted to the background work. This time may appear to have little evidence of scholarly output, yet it is critical to the eventual outcome of the research project. Educators can ask the Dean, as well as someone who has been successfully promoted on the basis of their research, the following questions as they develop their research plans:

- Does the program and/or institution value research?
- How does the institution reward research activities?
- Is research time considered a part of the faculty workload, and if so, how much time is provided?

- What other scholarly work does the program value?
- What is the time span for tenure?
- What role on a research team will I be expected to fulfill? Principle investigator or member of a research team?
- Who at the institution is willing to serve as a mentor for others in the research role?
- What resources and funding are available?

### *Demonstrating the Scholarship of Teaching*

In general, teaching is not highly visible to peers and is not chronicled in a documented format. Many faculty develop a teaching portfolio as a way to document their teaching.

Because teaching is a private activity, it is more challenging to demonstrate the scholarship of teaching. There are three main data sources available to build the case for excellence in teaching. These data sources are:

1. The faculty member.
2. Peers.
3. Students.

### *Data from the Faculty Member*

Faculty members should write out their personal philosophy of teaching. The process of writing out a philosophy can help one examine the tenets of one's belief structure. These beliefs can be used as criteria for critiquing the strategies faculty employ in their teaching. For example, if one identifies independent thinking on the part of the learner as a part of the teaching-learning process that one highly values, then one can examine the strategies employed to determine if those strategies support independent thinking.

Faculty members should document the faculty development activities they undertake. Do they attend conferences or workshops that build their teaching skills? Are they keeping up-to-date on educational research and applying it to their teaching practice? What teaching innovations have they implemented? How did they evaluate the effectiveness of those innovations? Are they considered as mentors for new teachers?

Evidence of an educator's work can include the following:

- Course outlines.
- Syllabi.
- Course policies and expectations.
- Student assignments.
- Learning experiences he or she designed.
- Evaluation tools he or she developed:
  - Exams.

- Assignments.
- Care plans.
• Creative projects he or she developed (such as videotapes, computer simulations, and case studies).

***Issues associated with self-evaluation.*** One of the biggest challenges in the process of self-evaluation is taking the time to do it. Self-evaluation requires time for reflection. Attending faculty development activities takes time. Keeping good documentation takes time, but with a little initial organization, educators can easily develop a storage system. It is highly likely that they will not submit everything they have collected for a promotion document, but it is also likely that if they do not keep good records, relevant items will be missed that could support excellence in teaching.

For the purpose of tenure or promotion, educators need to know if their school values a process or end-product portfolio. With a tenure clock ticking, they can begin with a process-oriented portfolio. This means that they keep evidence of their teaching successes as well as those that were less than successful. They should document revisions and the outcomes of those revisions. This information is useful in demonstrating their interest in the learning outcomes and documenting efforts to improve their teaching effectiveness. By keeping this documentation up-to-date, they will have the evidence they need to support the development of a promotion document.

It is common in nursing education for courses to be team-taught. This may mean that the syllabus, course assignments, etc., are a reflection of the team's work. Educators need to document their role as team members with the various teaching activities. At some point, they will need to show evidence of their own work – a lecture, a unit, or an assignment they developed independently.

Maintaining objectivity about one's own teaching is difficult. When educators are assessing their own work, they must use the eyes of a researcher and take an unbiased look. They need to keep in mind that self-evaluation is not the only source of data available to demonstrate one's teaching ability.

### Data from Peers

Documentation of peer evaluation may be accomplished through special forms designed by a given institution or by anecdotal reports. If an external peer review was solicited, then that reviewer's report form can be submitted.

Teaching awards for which peers select the winner are another possible source of documentation of teaching excellence. These awards may be conducted within the institution or outside the institution. Some professional nursing organizations have excellence-in-education awards that serve as evidence of peer evaluation.

The award of a grant to support the development and/or evaluation of a teaching innovation is another source of peer recognition. Because grants go through a review process and are competitive in nature, peer review is established. The criteria used by the granting institution should be documented.

*Issues associated with peer evaluation.* Few faculty are eager to be a peer evaluator or have a peer evaluation completed. Most likely, this dislike of peer evaluation is related to a problem with the validity and reliability of the evaluation and its perceived value and use.

For peer evaluation to be a relevant activity for both participants, the purpose should be clarified prior to the evaluation. Possible purposes include:

- Effectiveness of the teaching.
- Content expertise of the teacher.
- Classroom/clinical management skills.
- Quality of teaching materials developed.
- Ability of faculty to maintain the integrity of the curriculum.

Obviously, the purpose of the peer evaluation helps to determine who the peer will be. If the purpose is to evaluate content expertise, then the peer must be knowledgeable of the content area. Some institutions seek a peer from outside the institution for this kind of evaluation. If the classroom management or effectiveness of teaching strategies is the focus of the evaluation, then a peer from another department may be asked to objectively evaluate the work.

Once the decision is made regarding **who** the peer will be, the next question is, how many times is the teaching to be evaluated? If peer evaluation is a sampling of teaching effectiveness, how many samples will it take to determine saturation? Is attending one class adequate? Will the teacher being evaluated determine which class will be evaluated, or will it be a surprise? Will the evaluator attend at various times during the term?

### Data from Students

As recipients of the instruction, students experience the teacher in action. Students are qualified to reflect on the experience and the learning environment. However, they are not able to evaluate content expertise in the way a peer evaluator can.

Every institution has some mechanism for obtaining evaluation from students. It is important for faculty to know the process. There should be a standardized process that addresses issues such as timing, confidentiality for both students and faculty, processing of the data, and the distribution of the results.

Formal evidence can be collected using computer-based forms, short-answer narratives, small-group discussion, and student performance on national exams.

Many schools use a computerized evaluation conducted at the end of a course. This can provide the faculty with a normative-referenced score. Short-answer narrative can be combined with this process to solicit more detailed information.

One technique called Small Group Instructional Diagnoses (SGID) uses an outside evaluator discussing specific issues with students in the absence of the faculty. If the faculty has no specific issue they wish discussed, the facilitator seeks consensus on three questions:

1. What do you like best about this class (instructor behaviors that facilitate your learning)?
2. What do you like least about this class (instructor behaviors that interfere with your learning)?
3. What suggestion do you have that would improve this course (instruction)?

The facilitator shares the students' discussion both in written and verbal form with the faculty.

Informal evidence of teaching effectiveness is usually brief and limited to a specific issue. This may be as informal as conversation with students. This evidence is typically used for formative evaluation. For example, an assessment technique such as asking students at the end of the class to turn in a paper listing the aspect of the class they found most confusing would serve as informal evidence of the effectiveness of the class. This information can help the faculty modify and improve the instruction.

Other evidence of student evaluation includes:
- Exit interviews.
- Unsolicited notes from students.
- Employer feedback.
- Graduate follow-up.
- Teaching awards from student groups.

***Issues related to student evaluation.*** As faculty, it is important to know how the data collected from students is used in the faculty evaluation process. Some schools have required processes that must be followed.

The purpose for collecting evaluation data varies with the timing of the evaluation. Many schools require evaluation at the end of the course, providing a summative evaluation of the course and faculty. Certainly exit interviews, graduate follow-up, and employer feedback are summative in nature. Summative evaluation provides information about the instruction after it is complete. Changes in teaching resulting from the feedback can be used with subsequent classes.

Formative evaluation data is data collected while the course is ongoing. The data can be used to revise teaching methods used with students currently enrolled in the class. It is advantageous to collect some formative feedback to improve teaching. Midterm is a good time for this type of evaluation. Results from the evaluation can positively influence the remainder of the instruction provided for the term. A short-answer narrative or the SGID can be useful techniques for formative evaluation.

Evaluation results can vary between required and elective courses. It is assumed that in large, required courses – especially when these classes are not specifically related to the nursing major – some students are not as excited about the course as those who are enrolled in elective courses. This attitude could be a variable influencing the students' satisfaction with the course and faculty.

It is important not to limit the evaluation of teaching to just the data from the students. Multiple sources of data are required to demonstrate scholarly teaching. This data can help build a case when demonstrating one's abilities in teaching.

## Demonstrating the Scholarship of Application

Historically, nursing faculty spend many hours providing service to others. The challenge in this new paradigm is to demonstrate how this service is scholarly.

When considering the application aspect of the faculty role, faculty must recognize the opportunities available for scholarship in this role. They may be involved in faculty practice, which provides awareness of practice issues that need to be improved. They may develop solutions to clinical problems. If they take the scholarly approach, they will also evaluate and share with others the knowledge they have gained.

Another example of making community service more scholarly is sharing professional expertise through a community education program. The educational event itself may not fully meet the criteria for scholarship; however, it can be expanded to incorporate a follow-up event. Perhaps the insights gained by working with this group could stimulate a larger intervention project and add to the body of nursing research.

Professional service is another avenue for application. Perhaps as experts, educators can initiate educational activities for other professionals to share knowledge. Faculty may serve as mentors or write articles or book chapters in their area of expertise. They must keep in mind that service to both the community and the profession can become scholarly endeavors. The biggest issue for most faculty is deciding how much time to devote to these activities. This decision can be based on both personal and institutional reward structures.

## Demonstrating the Scholarship of Integration

This scholarship adds another dimension to the traditional triad of research, teaching, and service. The best fit for the scholarship of integration may be with research in the traditional triad; however, it also overlaps into teaching and service. The scholarship of integration places nursing knowledge in a larger context of health care, where nursing knowledge becomes more comprehensive when combined with another discipline than if performed separately. Teaming up with other disciplines such as health promotion, education, technology, medicine, pharmacy, nutrition, or others can provide a more comprehensive approach to needs of special populations. For example, improving the outcome for clients with Type II diabetes involves multiple disciplines.

This scholarship emphasizes the relationship of thoughts and conveys new insight into the innovative ideas and research. Two primary methodologies are used – critical analysis and interpretation – but interdisciplinary work can be accomplished through any of the previous scholarships.

Original work from a variety of disciplines offers new paradigms and insights. By combining knowledge and responding to both intellectual questions and human problems, comprehensive approaches to health-related issues can evolve. Development of educational programs, review of literature, analysis of health policies, service projects, and interdisciplinary research provides many illustrations of the scholarship of integration.

Establishing relationships with other professionals in one's area of interest is a major issue in developing the scholarly role of integration. It is helpful to network with colleagues in the college who are knowledgeable and work in the same area of interest. Educators need to remember that the scholarship of integration is not limited to clinical care issues but includes a broader scope such as health policy, ethics, etc.

Other issues associated with working with a multidisciplinary team include:
- The composition of the team.
- Who will take on the leadership role.
- Clearly defined roles and responsibilities for all team members.
- Time frames and deadlines.
- Authorship – best to establish this early in the process.
- If securing a grant is part of the process, the decision of how the proposal is to be developed and the resources allocated.

## Summary

If one has never taken the time or is new in the faculty role, it is important to seriously consider the choices one is making. Educators must honor the professional activities that flow from their strengths and interests. It is more important that they match their strengths and passions for nursing with their development as scholarly faculty than it is to take on tasks solely to enhance their chances of promotion. The winning combination is a match in both personal preference and professional growth.

Keep these key points in mind:

- Know the culture of the institution.
- Multiple sources of data are important to establish evidence of effectiveness in the faculty roles and to demonstrate the criteria for scholarship.
- Keep good records.
- Be proactive.

Table 46.1 is a self-assessment worksheet that can be used to help develop a strategy for success. Possible activities and documentation examples for each scholarship are provided, along with a column to encourage the development of personal goals. This tool may be duplicated for use and appears on the CD-ROM accompanying this book.

Table 46.1 - Self-Assessment Worksheet

| Activity | Documentation (Examples of possible activities that demonstrate scholarship) | Future Goal |
|---|---|---|
| **Scholarship of Discovery**<br>Types of Research Studies:<br>• Experimental<br>• Descriptive<br>• Exploratory<br>• Case studies<br><br>Roles in Research:<br>• Principle investigator<br>• Member of a research team<br>• Committee member<br>• Mentoring junior colleagues | • Peer reviewed publications and/or presentations of research, theory, or philosophical essays<br>• Grants awarded in support of research or scholarship<br>• State, Regional, national, or international recognition as a scholar<br>• Other evidence of peer evaluation of the work | |

Table 46.1 - Self-Assessment Worksheet cont.

| | | |
|---|---|---|
| **Scholarship of Teaching**<br>Possible teaching environments<br>• Clinical<br>• Classroom<br>• Community<br><br>Learning theory<br>• Integrating existing theory into practice<br>• Developing research questions<br><br>Mentorship of new teachers<br><br>Sources of data<br>• Self-assessment<br>• Peer-review<br>• Student-assessment | • Peer-reviewed publications and/or presentations of research focused on the teaching and learning process<br>• Peer-reviewed publications of teaching innovations<br>• Creative projects you developed (such as videotapes, computer simulations, case studies)<br>• Local, state, regional, national, international recognition as a master teacher<br>• Grants awarded in support of teaching scholarship<br>• Published evaluation tools<br>Other outcome measures that provide evidence of teaching effectiveness (program outcomes, board results, employer interviews, etc.) | |
| **Scholarship of Application**<br>Faculty practice that emphasizes scholarly approaches to improving client outcomes and care delivery<br><br>Professional development to improve clinical practice skills<br><br>Research and clinical demonstration projects in the area of clinical expertise<br><br>Development of practice standards<br><br>Mentoring students, colleagues<br><br>Community education in area of expertise | • Peer-reviewed publications/ presentations of clinical research, application of clinical skills, client outcomes to demonstrate the effectiveness of nursing care delivery, case studies<br>• Professional certifications, degrees, and other specialty credentials<br>• Consultation outcome reports<br>• Reports of practice innovations and their outcomes<br>• Development of products (patents, licenses, copyrights)<br>• Peer reviews of practice<br>• Grant awards relating to practice (such as improved access to health care, new care delivery strategies, new intervention strategies, etc)<br>• State, regional, national, international, recognition as a master practitioner<br>Policy papers related to clinical nursing practice | |

Table 46.1 - Self-Assessment Worksheet cont.

| | | |
|---|---|---|
| **Scholarship of Integration**<br>Expanding on ways available knowledge in various disciplines can come together to improve the well-being of individuals and populations<br><br>Developing educational programs<br><br>Interdisciplinary service projects<br><br>Interdisciplinary research | • Peer-reviewed publications/ presentations that may include analysis of prior research focused on healthcare issue, critique of healthcare policy, reviews of literature that integrate multi-disciplinary issues<br>• Reports of interdisciplinary educational programs or service projects<br>• Interdisciplinary grant awards<br>• Author or co-author of policy papers designed to make recommendations for organizations or governments<br>•Other evidence of peer evaluations of contributions to integrative scholarship (selection as expert witness, selection to advisory board on healthcare issues in area of expertise, etc) | |
| **Scholarship of Discovery**<br>Types of Research Studies:<br>• Experimental<br>• Descriptive<br>• Exploratory<br>• Case studies<br><br>Roles in Research:<br>• Principle investigator<br>• Member of a research team<br>• Committee member<br>• Mentoring junior colleagues | • Peer reviewed publications and/or presentations of research, theory, or philosophical essays<br>• Grants awarded in support of research or scholarship<br>• State, Regional, national, or international recognition as a scholar<br>• Other evidence of peer evaluation of the work | |

Table 46.1 - Self-Assessment Worksheet cont.

| | | |
|---|---|---|
| **Scholarship of Teaching**<br>Possible teaching environments<br>• Clinical<br>• Classroom<br>• Community<br><br>Learning theory<br>• Integrating existing theory into practice<br>• Developing research questions<br><br>Mentoring new teachers<br><br>Sources of data<br>• Self-assessment<br>• Peer-review<br>• Student assessment | • Peer-reviewed publications and/or presentations of research focused on the teaching and learning process<br>• Peer-reviewed publications of teaching innovations<br>• Creative projects you developed (such as videotapes, computer simulations, case studies)<br>•Local, state, regional, national, international recognition as a master teacher<br>• Grants awarded in support of teaching scholarship<br>• Published evaluation tools<br>• Other outcome measures that provide evidence of teaching effectiveness (program outcomes, board results, employer interviews, etc.) | |

## Learning Activities

1. Write your personal philosophy of the teaching and learning process.
2. How would you assess the way your teaching practice honors your personal philosophy?
3. Research the mission and goals of the nursing program where you are currently employed or where you would like to be employed.
4. Interview the dean or department head of a school of nursing to determine the criteria currently used for tenure, promotion, and merit. Compare and contrast the merit criteria and the promotion criteria.
5. Develop an outline for a promotion portfolio, including the documentation you would provide to demonstrate each criteria.
6. As a class, determine the goals of a peer review if you were a junior faculty member (you can choose to develop a formative or summative evaluation). After completing this activity, analyze the points of agreement and disagreement that evolved in the discussion.
7. Develop a five-year plan to achieve success as a scholarly faculty that exploits your personal strengths and interests.

# References

American Association of Colleges of Nursing [AACN]. (1995). *Interdisciplinary education and practice*. Washington, DC: Author.

American Association of Colleges of Nursing [AACN]. (1997a). *A vision of baccalaureate and graduate nursing education: The next decade*. Washington DC: Author.

American Association of Colleges of Nursing [AACN]. (1997b, Feb 20-22). *Faculty practice: Old questions, new answers*. Proceedings of the AACN's 1997 Faculty Practice Conference, Phoenix, AZ: Author.

American Association of Colleges of Nursing [AACN]. (1998). *Position statement on nursing research*. Washington DC: Author.

American Association of Colleges of Nursing [AACN]. (1999). *Position statement on defining scholarship for the discipline of nursing*. Washington, DC: Author.

Boyer, E. L. (1990). *Scholarship reconsidered: Priorities for the professoriate*. Princeton, NJ: Carnegie Foundation for the Advancement of Teaching.

Diamond, R. M., & Adam, B. E. (1993). *Recognizing faculty work: Reward systems for the year 2000*. San Francisco, CA: Jossey-Bass.

Donaldson, S. K., & Crowley, D. M. (1978). The discipline of nursing. *Nursing Outlook, 26* (2), 113-120.

Rice, E. R. (1991). The new American scholar. Scholarship and the purposes of the university: *Metropolitan Universities, 1* (4), 7-18.

Schoffner, D. H., Davis, M. W., & Bowens, S. M. (1994). A model for clinical teaching as a scholarly endeavor. *IMAGE: Journal of Nursing Scholarship, 16*, 181-184.

Stevenson, J. S. (1988). Nursing knowledge development: Into Era II. *Journal of Professional Nursing, 4*, 152-162.

# Bibliography

Applegate, M. (1998). Educational program evaluation. In D. M. Billings & J. A. Halstead (Eds.), *Teaching in nursing: A guide for faculty* (pp. 179-208). Philadelphia, PA: W. B. Saunders.

Arreola, R. A. (2000). *Developing a comprehensive faculty evaluation system* (2nd ed.). Boston, MA: Anker.

Bartels, J. E. (1997). Understanding teaching scholarship: Beyond the dichotomization. *Journal of Professional Nursing, 13*(5), 278.

Boyer, E. L. (1996). From scholarship reconsidered to scholarship assessed. *QUEST, 48*, 129-139.

Costello, J., Pateman, B., Pusey, H., & Longshaw, K. (2001). Peer review of classroom teaching: An interim report. *Nurse Education Today, 21*, 444-454.

Edgerton, R. (1991). *Higher education white paper*. Washington, DC: Pew Charitable Trusts.

Glassick, C.E., Huber, M.T., & Maeroff, G.I. (1997). *Scholarship assessed: Evaluation of the professoriate*. San Francisco, CA: Jossey-Bass.

Kirkpatrick, J., Schafer, K., Schmeiser, D., Richardson, C., Valley, J., & Yehle, K. (2001). Building a case for the promotion of clinical faculty. *Nurse Educator, 26*, 178-181.

Nidou, V. R. (2000). Faculty service activities. In L. Scheetz (Ed.), *Nursing faculty secrets* (pp. 53-56). Philadelphia, PA: Hanley & Belfus, Inc.

Phillips, N., & Ducke, M. (2001). The questioning skills of clinical teachers and preceptors: A comparative study. *Journal of Advanced Nursing, 33*, 523-529.

Ryan, K. E. (2000). *Evaluating teaching in higher education: A vision for the future*. San Francisco, CA: Jossey-Bass.

Seldin, P. (1997). *The teaching portfolio: A practical guide to improved performance and promotion/tenure decisions* (2nd ed.). Boston, MA: Anker.

Seldin, P. (1999). *Changing practices in evaluating teaching*. Boston, MA: Anker.

Starck, P. L. (1996). Boyer's multidimensional nature of scholarship: A new framework for schools of nursing. *Journal of Professional Nursing, 12,* 268-276.

Sullivan, E. J. (1996). Expanding the definition of scholarship. *Journal of Professional Nursing, 12,* 4.

Zahorski, K. J., & Cognard, R. (1999). *Reconsidering faculty roles and rewards: Promising practices for institutional transformation and enhanced learning*. Washington, DC: CIC.

# Chapter 47: SELF-DEVELOPMENT AND SELF-APPRAISAL

Russell Watson, MA, EdD

*Self-appraisal is a trait of a professional. As with all aspects of a professional position, research yields new approaches, and self-appraisal is no exception. Dr. Watson has conducted research in the field of self-development and self-appraisal for more than 20 years. He has designed self-development and self-appraisal instruments for use with both educational and healthcare professionals. In this chapter, Dr. Watson shares his personal perspective as well as some intriguing instruments for this highly important professional and personal activity. – Linda Caputi and Lynn Engelmann*

## Background and Introduction

### *A Variety of Processes and Procedures Available*

All nursing students, professors of nursing, or healthcare professionals have been exposed to a variety of self-appraisal models during their academic and working careers. This concept is not new. However, with the growth of a variety of management and organizational models, several newer designs have made some important progress in the healthcare arena. A few of those are explained in this chapter.

## Educational Philosophy

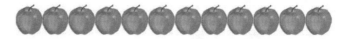

We remember best the things we do ourselves. Therefore, I believe that students of any age need to be active agents in the learning process. The more personal and meaningful we can make each session, the easier for all participants to recall later. I use small group discussions, group quizzes, and worksheets, as well as individual surveys and checklists, to help make the material come alive for participants in sessions. – Russell Watson

Healthcare professionals and nursing faculty are busy people. Not only do they perform in a working environment with enormous pressure, but they are also expected to keep current in a variety of related areas and to be able to apply their new learning rapidly and accurately. Time for self-development and objective self-appraisal is sometimes scarce. This becomes a classic problematic situation, sometimes even a double-bind: busy healthcare professionals need to maintain academic currency and also need to attend to their own self-development. Rarely is there time to do it all, but they need to try, for their own sake, for the sake of their professional teams, for the sake of the students, and for the sake of the clients.

Newer types of self-development instruments tend to be less of a one-shot, one-event situation and more of an ongoing process and series of activities. This methodology tracks with many of the continuous-improvement models currently active in many educational and healthcare settings. These include healthcare and education-related versions of Baldridge online criteria, as well as a variety of quality models available through organizational improvement organizations. Improvement is a process, a journey, and not a clearly defined end or destination. In continuous improvement, getting a little bit better at what one does (or what a team does) with each cycle means that self-development and self-appraisal can assist greatly in that continuous-improvement process.

Many hospitals, medical clinics, and colleges have written their own types of self-development and self-appraisal instruments. Although they are not nationally standardized, they do not have to be. They are themselves of enormous value and importance in beginning a dialogue about improvement. In addition to an improvement dimension, there also needs to be a strengths-based dimension upon which to base the appraisal. When learning how to improve, learners also need to be affirmed in those things they are good at doing. It is the opinion of this author that professional nursing faculty should spend 80% of their personal development time and effort working on amplifying their strengths and only 20% of their time working on areas for improvement, the reason being that if they hone those strengths, they become even stronger. Working on areas of limitations or weaknesses much more than 20% of one's development time may be getting into an area of diminishing returns.

### *A Development and Appraisal Perspective*

Some quite recent trends emerging in leadership and management initiatives are centered on a strengths-based model. This design is based upon illuminating one's strengths and positive attributes and focusing most attention in honing these areas, with secondary emphasis on overcoming limitations and weaknesses. The idea, in part, is one that says people are motivated by those things that make them strong and successful, and those traits should be supported and not hidden. In the midst of honing strengths, taking note and improving some areas of limitations becomes a more easily accomplished endeavor.

With regard to overcoming limitations and working on areas for continuous improvement, these items are prominent in many performance appraisals and can become especially critical in the healthcare profession. It becomes mission-critical to be certain that essential skills and behaviors are maintained at optimal levels of performance. For nursing professionals, there is a high degree of responsibility for individual and team development processes.

What emerges from this initial exploration is a variety of methods and reasons to employ self-appraisal and self-development designs. The results are a variety of opportunities: to amplify strengths, to appraise interactions with others on the teaching team, and to demonstrate continuous improvement. All of these activities are critical to individual success, and the success of the teams in which nursing professionals work.

### *A Personal Development Perspective*

Nursing professionals need to embrace a commitment to professional growth and development. Self-appraisal and planning are important aspects in the development of such perspective. In particular, personal designs should amplify strengths, promote effective performance, reflect an understanding of the job culture, and build goals for the future. This perspective should also provide for reflective feedback on accomplishments, performance, and areas for improvement. The following sections will address this self-appraisal process.

### *Building One's Own Self-Appraisal Worksheet and Process*

The following steps are offered as a means to develop a self-appraisal worksheet.
1. A period – 30 days, 60 days, etc. – is chosen for the self-appraisal.
2. This process allows opportunity for reflection and discussion with manager, mentor, or peers.
3. A personal development file or folder is begun now, whether it is early or later in one's career. The folder is used to collect short notes, memos, and reminders about one's own career and development (e.g., a half-day workshop attended; a book or article read; or a job-related skill learned. A brief note should be included about what each item was, the date it occurred, and a brief sentence or phrase about learning and growth as a result.) In a six-month or year's period of time, nursing faculty are frequently amazed at the large number of **little things** that have merged into a substantial amount of additional career development activity.
4. Peers can be encouraged to use the same process. Once or twice per year, professionals can share information learned with others in a **Personal Development Debrief Lunch** by offering a summary of what has been learned and new topics and important issues that

have been explored recently. This can be done as an informal collegial lunch or brown bag lunch to share learning or to discuss areas in which members are strong and feeling good about their activity, as well as one item or area in which each is working to improve. This activity can be done between regular performance reviews with one's manager, and can be discussed in a **safe** manner with peers or mentors.

## *Purposes of a Self-Appraisal Worksheet*

- To increase professional and personal growth and development.
- To amplify strengths one offers the college, hospital, clinic, or healthcare team.
- To create clear goals and goal setting.
- To improve understanding of one's job culture.
- To encourage personal reflection and regular discussion between peers and managers regarding performance, goals, and expectations.
- To set future goals and objectives.

## *A Sample Self-Appraisal Worksheet*

Figure 47.1 provides a sample worksheet that can be redesigned for the reader's own use or printed from the CD accompanying this book to use as is. For each of the competency areas, one may insert any of the suggested competency areas listed below, establish one's own, or select those in the area important to the reader's work environment.

## *Examples of Competencies*

In the list below are some general team-related competencies common in educational settings. These do not include the additional professional and licensure competencies required in specialty areas of hospitals or healthcare environments.
- Accountability.
- Adaptability/flexibility.
- Achievement orientation.
- Analytical and systems thinking.
- Communication.
- Conflict management.
- Helping others.
- Intellectual curiosity.
- Interpersonal skills.
- Positive contributions to the work environment.
- Problem solving.

Figure 47.1- Sample Self-Appraisal Worksheet

Name _____ Date _____

Department _____

The key to the column codes:
- CCE = Clearly and consistently exceeds established goals or expectations.
- RMSE = Regularly meets and sometimes exceeds established goals, etc.
- CM = Consistently meets the goals established for the healthcare position.
- DNCM = Does not consistently meet the established goals or expectations.

| | Self-Rating | | | |
| | 4 | 3 | 2 | 1 |
| **Competency** (choose job-related items) | CCE | RMSE | CM | DNCM |
| Item:<br>Supporting example: | | | | |
| Item:<br>Supporting example: | | | | |
| Item:<br>Supporting example: | | | | |
| Item:<br>Supporting example: | | | | |
| Item:<br>Supporting example: | | | | |
| Item:<br>Supporting example: | | | | |
| Item:<br>Supporting example: | | | | |
| Item:<br>Supporting example: | | | | |

(Permission to photocopy this worksheet is granted.)

- Project management.
- Technology.
- Valuing diversity.

## An Alternative Method: The Self-Appraisal Journal

This approach is more a narrative than an objective checklist method (see Figure 47.2). It can be recorded as a monthly notation from one's own perspective regarding performance, events, training, and specific situations during the past month. The narrative need not be extensive, but a paragraph describing job-related skills, requirements, and behaviors can provide substantial anecdotal information to assist with the formal appraisal process. This method allows one to be better prepared for the evaluation conference than walking in **cold**. Stating the narrative in specific job-related behaviors and specific competency areas maintains focus of the narrative on topics relevant to the evaluation session.

Figure 47.2- Sample Self-Appraisal

---

**A Sample Self-Appraisal Journal**

Name _____ Date _____

Department _____

For (time period, month, etc.) _____

During the past month or two, describe specific job-related behaviors, skills, competencies, situations, and events that demonstrate some of the strengths you bring to the job. Also note areas for professional growth or opportunities for improvement of competencies or skills and ideas for action plans for support.

---

(The above text and format may be photocopied and reproduced for use.)

## A Third Alternative: A Structured Self-Appraisal Form

The example provided below (see Figure 47.3) is a hybrid between the objective checklist and the free-form narrative. It tends to be a popular option for many in the healthcare profession. A primary reason for its popularity may be that the form provides a series of prompts to which a person responds. This method is also useful as a discussion starter among peers during a "mentoring lunch bunch" session. This mentoring and peer-

Figure 47.3 - Sample Structured Self-Appraisal Form

**Structured Narrative Self-Appraisal Form**

Name _____ Date _____

Department _____

1.  Some of the aspects of my job that I like best include:

2.  Some aspects of my job that I like least include:

3.  Some of the most important skills and abilities that my job requires include:

4.  Some of my major accomplishments during the past year include:

5.  In what ways are my superiors rewarding me or praising me when I exceed expectations?

6.  In what ways are my superiors coaching and guiding me to do my job more effectively?

7.  In what aspects of my job do I need additional training and professional development?

8.  In what ways have I been an active agent in my own personal or professional development? What do I need to do in the next year in this area?

9.  What changes could be made in the job culture or environment that could improve my effectiveness?

10.  How can my capabilities be better utilized in my present job responsibilities?

11.  What type of work do I see myself doing in three years? What am I doing now to prepare for this work?

12.  How is my present job preparing me for my role in the future?

Figure 47.3 - Sample Structured Self-Appraisal Form cont.

---

13. Other:

14. Other:

15. Other:

---

(Permission to photocopy this form is granted.)

sharing process also encourages a culture of mutual support, personal development, and respect.

A series of suggested prompts are offered, as well as areas to insert one's own items and prompts. The author of this chapter strongly suggests that the reader complete the form and encourage peers to do the same. When completed, a discussion gathering can be hosted so that peers can share the information in small groups of four to six people. Each person may suggest additional items to include in the Structured Self-Appraisal Form for group discussion and sharing.

### *A Manager's or Supervisor's Perspective*

An important part of the role of a manager or supervisor is to provide feedback, guidance, and coaching to staff on their strengths, progress toward goals, and areas for continued development. School-of-nursing administrators are busy people with enormous responsibility but sometimes are given limited authority without obtaining higher approval for many actions for which they carry the responsibility. As a result of the busy activities, the healthcare culture, and the wide scope of responsibilities, performance appraisals sometimes fall to the lower items on one's to-do list. It is hoped that some of the ideas and tools offered here may assist in making the process more efficient and effective for both oneself, and their direct reports.

Certainly a primary goal of appraisal is to provide professional staff with feedback on their performance during the past year or assigned time period. This feedback should amplify the strengths that the teacher has demonstrated and also provide guidance and areas for improvement. Through this interaction, the teachers should also increase their understanding of both their job responsibilities as well as the manager's expectations of those roles. In addition, the evaluation discussion should include goals and opportunities for the upcoming year or season, as well as additional competencies that may be needed from the faculty.

# A Three-Dimensional View of Development and Appraisal

Taking self-development and self-appraisal one level deeper reveals three layers of this extended perspective:

1. **How** professionals do what they do, i.e., behavioral style.
2. **Why** professsionals do what they do, i.e., values and drives.
3. The **context** in which professonals work, i.e., the job culture.

This author has worked for the past 30 years as a behavioral scientist, and the instruments shared herein may be used for the reader's self-appraisal in the work environment. The instruments produced for this text are proprietary and are reprinted with permission.

For a more in-depth examination of one's behavioral style, values drives, and job culture, and for a courtesy report on these dimensions, the reader is asked to explore the website http://www.activeprofiles.com, where the reader can find information specific to these instruments. By contacting the author at: russell.watson@activeprofiles.com and including the reader's name, organization, and Purchase Order Number for this book, the reader will receive access codes to receive courtesy reports based on these dimensions. The standard fee for these reports is over $100, but the reports will be written for the reader as a courtesy from the author. The code can be used as a one-time response to obtain a custom report for the reader of this book. Go to Chapter 47 on the CD accompanying this book, for information on contacting the author.

## *How Professionals Do What They Do: Behavioral Style*

Many behavioral models are in use in the healthcare profession, and the one described herein is one of the more popular models in use. It is based on the DISC model, which has origins with Dr. Carl Jung (1971) and Dr. William M. Marston (1979). The DISC design is in the public domain, and as such, there are many derivatives from a variety of companies, and many nursing schools, hospitals, and clinics use one of these models (see Figure 47.4).

Briefly, the DISC concept identifies four different styles of behavior across the following dimensions:

1. **Dominance**: Approach to problem solving and obtaining results.
2. **Influence**: Approach to interacting with people.
3. **Steadiness**: Approach to the pace of the work environment.
4. **Cautiousness**: Approach to following procedures and standards.

An individual may score high or low in each of those four dimensions, and each person brings a certain amount of **elasticity** within each area. Figure 47.4 explains the primary

Figure 47.4 - Four Dimensions of Behavior

**Four Dimensions of Behavior**

As an initial self-development tool, circle High or Low for your own self-perception in each of these categories. Remember that "High" doesn't mean 'good,' and "Low" doesn't mean 'bad.' Each of the positions describes a preferred 'comfort zone' of our behavior.

Name: _____ Date of response:_____

| | |
|---|---|
| **P R O B L E M S** | **"D" – Dominance: Approach to obtaining results & problem-solving.**<br><br>**High D:** Tends to solve **new** problems quickly, directly, takes an active approach to results, and gets to the bottom line.<br><br>**Low D:** Tends to solve **new** problems in a controlled, organized, and calculated manner. |
| **P E O P L E** | **"I" – Influence: Approach to interacting with people, and emoting.**<br><br>**High I:** Tends to meet **new** people in an outgoing, gregarious, socially assertive manner. Tends to be emotional, talkative, and reactive.<br><br>**Low I:** Tends to meet **new** people in a more quiet, reserved, controlled manner. Prefers logic over emotions. |
| **P A C E** | **"S" – Steadiness: Approach to the pace of the work environment.**<br><br>**High S:** Tends to prefer a controlled, deliberate, predictable environment. Values disciplined behavior and security of the situation.<br><br>**Low S:** Tends to prefer a flexible, dynamic, unstructured environment. Values freedom of expression and ability to change quickly. |
| **P R O C E D U R E S** | **"C" – Cautious: Adherence to established standards, and protocols.**<br><br>**High C:** Tends to adhere to established rules. Likes things to be done the correct way. Says, "Rules are made to be followed."<br><br>**Low C:** Tends to operate more independently from the protocols, develops a variety of strategies. Says, "Rules are only guidelines." |

definitions of each of the four dimensions and both high and low scores. The reader may note that there are strengths to each style and strengths to both high and low scores. Therefore, **high** does not mean good, and **low** does not mean bad. Some practical examples of healthcare profession situations appear below. Readers may compare their own *QuickDISC* responses to the abbreviated descriptions herein (see Figures 47.5-47.7).

In the educational and healthcare arenas, all four styles are needed, both high and low. These styles represent **comfort zones** of one's behavior. At any time, and depending on the circumstances, any person can choose to behave through any one of the four styles. For some, shifting style is more of a stretch than for others, but the most important concept to understand is that these styles are no more than **comfort zones** in behavior. This DISC model is not intended to pigeonhole anyone or to be used as an arbitrary labeling system. It is designed to add a greater dimension to understanding the normal aspects of human behavior on the job. In a school of nursing, and with a faculty team, each of the behavioral styles brings value and strengths to the institution.

- The High D style may offer a new teaching method or experiment.
- The Low D style demonstrates expertise at a specialty.
- The High I style encourages others, both staff and students in the class.
- The Low I style contributes a sense of reflection and control.
- The High S style brings a sense of patience with students and a high sincerity factor.
- The Low S style brings a high sense of urgency and openness to change or to try out new teaching techniques.
- The High C style offers a high sense of quality control, detail orientation, and a strong knowledge base in the subject matter.
- The Low C style challenges current thought, sets new precedents, and takes calculated risks.

If one examines the above list, one finds that each role is both valuable and needed in a healthcare educational setting. These styles are essentially descriptive of how one performs job requirements and tasks.

Many people make the mistake of assigning the term **personality test** to these results. This model is not a personality test and the term **personality** should not enter into discussion regarding job tasks and behaviors. Healthcare professionals know that personality is a complex term covering a wide variety of behaviors and thought patterns that are not necessarily job-related. There are a variety of objective and projective clinical personality tests that are used in the diagnosis and treatment of psychological disorders. This DISC model does not fit into that category; it is designed to identify job-related behaviors and how one completes job responsibilities.

Figure 47.5 - QuickDISC.

| Quick DISC | | | | |
|---|---|---|---|---|

Name _____ Date of response _____

In each of the following groups of four words, rank order each of the groups of words from highest (4) to lowest (1).  That is: 4 = MOST like you, down to 1 = LEAST like you, as you see yourself <u>ON  THE  JOB</u>.

*Rank order each*

| | D | I | S | C |
|---|---|---|---|---|
| **1. Rank order each of the following groups of words from highest to lowest.  4 = Most like you down to 1 = Least like you.** | | | | |
| **Bold** | | | | |
| **Charming** | | | | |
| **Controlled** | | | | |
| **Gentle** | | | | |
| **2.**      **4=Highest… 1= Lowest** *Rank Order Each* | | | | |
| **Adventurous** | | | | |
| **Entertaining** | | | | |
| **Humble** | | | | |
| **Sympathetic** | | | | |
| **3.**      **4=Highest… 1= Lowest** *Rank Order Each* | | | | |
| **Cooperative** | | | | |
| **Determined** | | | | |
| **Helpful** | | | | |
| **Sociable** | | | | |
| **4.**      **4=Highest… 1= Lowest** *Rank Order Each* | | | | |
| **Considerate** | | | | |
| **Jovial** | | | | |
| **Outspoken** | | | | |
| **Restrained** | | | | |
| **5.**      **4=Highest… 1= Lowest** *Rank Order Each* | | | | |
| **Good mixer** | | | | |
| **Obedient** | | | | |
| **Orderly** | | | | |
| **Strong-willed** | | | | |
| **Add the numbers in each column and insert TOTALS here:** | **D** | **I** | **S** | **C** |

**Transfer the totals above onto the graph on the next page (Figure 47.6).**

Figure 47.5.  QuickDISC. (Copyright © 1984-2002 Target Consultants, Inc., Oswego, IL. All rights reserved. Reproduced with permission.)

Figure 47.6 - Scoring the QuickDISC Work Style

---

**Determining your "QuickDISC" Work Style**

In the graph below, place an "X" in each column corresponding to the **totals** for each letter: D, I, S, and C from the previous page. Once you have placed the "Xs" in the spaces, then connect the "Xs" to form a graph.

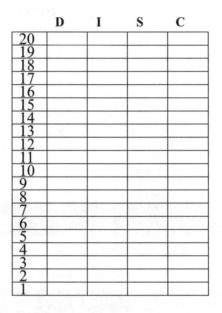

Look at your highest score and circle the letter at the top of the graph. If two are tied for your highest, then circle BOTH letters. If your highest score was:

**D:** You tend to be decisive, solve problems quickly, and see the big picture easily and communicate it to others (about 10-15% of the population).

**I:** You tend to be talkative, outgoing, like working with people, enjoy parties, and show a sincere interest in others (about 30-35% of the population).

**S:** You tend to enjoy a steady, predictable pace of the workday; show a high degree of support to projects and tasks, and high follow-through (about 40-45% of the population).

**C:** You tend to adhere to rules, procedures, and protocol; demonstrate high quality control, and high process and procedure knowledge (about 20-30% of the population).

---

Figure 47.7 - DISC Examples

| High D | Decisive, rapid solutions to problems, competitive, sometimes egocentric, sometimes impatient. Motivated by power, authority, new experiences, and challenges. For increased effectiveness, may need challenging assignments, awareness of sanctions, and clarification of authority. |
|---|---|
| Low D | Cautious, conservative, detail-oriented, makes deliberate decisions, sometimes slow in deciding. Motivated by specialized work, has ability to weigh pros and cons, prefers a predictable work environment. For increased effectiveness, may need to accept change more readily, make quicker decisions. |
| High I | Talkative, people-oriented, optimistic, emotional, trusting, sometimes impulsive. Motivated by friendly working conditions, contact with people, and social recognition. For increased effectiveness, may need increased objectivity, increased control of emotion, and time management skills. |
| Low I | Reflective, reserved in meeting new people, emotionally controlled, works effectively alone, sometimes pessimistic. Motivated by sincere environment, time to react to change, and scheduled events. For increased effectiveness, may need increased spontaneity and wider involvement with people. |
| High S | High degree of patience with people, good listener/coach/counselor type, sometimes possessive. Motivated by clear responsibilities, little conflict, and secure situations. For increased effectiveness may need time to adjust to change, streamlined methods, and increased sense of urgency. |
| Low S | Change-oriented, spontaneous, has high sense of urgency, many activities, sometimes fault-finding. Motivated by wide involvement, freedom from control, new activities. For increased effectiveness, may need better listening skills, increased patience, and increased consistency. |
| High C | Accurate, precise, high detail-orientation, controlled, well-prepared, sometimes overly sensitive. Motivated by high-quality standards, doing things the "right" way. For increased effectiveness, may need to see things in a wider perspective, spend less time on details, and develop ability to delegate. |
| Low C | Independent, opinionated, persistent, rebellious, sometimes sarcastic. Motivated by opportunities for new methods and ideas, varied activities, and freedom from controls. For increased effectiveness, may need to pace self, less arbitrary change, more identification with a group. |

## *Something Deeper than Behavioral Style and Preferences*

As one who has worked in the healthcare arena and higher education, this researcher has overheard many conversations of nurses and other healthcare professionals as they have discussed interpersonal conflicts. Many of those conversations have mentioned a **personality conflict** between two or more people on the team. The nature of these conflicts tends not to be about personality, and they really do not surface as DISC-related preferences. What frequently emerges from these conflicts is a values-related misunderstanding. Once these value differences are clarified, many times the source of the conflict is eliminated or reduced.

### *Why Professionals Do What They Do: Values Drives*

- "I didn't get along with my nursing manager; it was a 'personality conflict.'"
- "Our teaching team wasn't effective because there were too many 'personality conflicts.'"
- "I don't believe in personality testing because I have three nurses with very different personalities who are all doing very well in their jobs."
- "Of the hospitals I've talked with, only 30% are happy with their pre-hire personality screening tests."

These are statements possibly heard throughout professional careers, statements that are symptoms of underlying issues. One of those issues is the use and understanding of the term **personality**. The word itself is complex and nebulous and describes the unique constellation of one's consistent behavioral tendencies. Personality can be explored in both normal and clinical settings, and from that stems a frequent avoidance of the term **personality** when referring to behavioral instruments used in the workplace. Terms used instead of **personality** include **type**; **behavioral style**; **preferences**; **traits**; and **temperament**, among others. All these terms more closely describe work behaviors and attempt to illuminate one or more aspects of **how** one does the job or goes about normal day-to-day activities.

### *The Importance of Understanding Values*

With research that began in 1979 related to on-the-job conflicts in a variety of healthcare organizations, it was quickly discovered that behavioral style or type was not the principal cause of **personality conflicts**. Professionals with similar behavioral styles either worked effectively together or not, and those of very different styles either got along or not. The bottom line was: behavioral style did not seem to be the only predictor of success in professional working teams. Some other dynamic was at work here. The operative dynamic that clearly emerged as critical to a team's success was the dynamic of **values**. Although behavioral style describes **how** one does a job, **values** illuminate **why** one does the job, i.e., one's wins, drives, and intrinsic motivators when performing duties.

When **values** are understood, appreciated, and respected, a substantial reduction in on-the-job conflicts between people and between teams becomes evident. Interestingly, this process does not involve any members of the team necessarily changing what they do, or the team changing its methods or direction. This remarkable reduction in perceived conflict is achieved through an awareness of what **drives** individual behavior. Those behavioral drive factors are one's **values**, and six values clearly emerge as common across a variety of healthcare dimensions:

| *Workplace Value* | *The Drive to:* |
|---|---|
| • **Theoretical** | Acquire knowledge. |
| • **Economic** | Acquire money and materials. |
| • **Individualistic** | Be seen as a unique contributor. |
| • **Altruistic** | Help others. |
| • **Political** | Acquire power and control. |
| • **Regulatory** | Establish routine, order, and structure. |

Values are sometimes called the **hidden motivators**, not because of hidden agendas but because one's values may not be readily observed by others except in spending considerable time together. When school-of-nursing faculty in conflict realize that the conflict may well have emerged because of different **beliefs** about the job or how it should be done, then many of those conflicts dissolve. Values are beliefs held so strongly that they influence the behavior of an individual or an organization. Values initiate and guide one's behavioral style. Everything we do is:

- Values dependent – Through the values-base against which we determine our behavioral choices.
- Values rooted – Through our deeply held beliefs established and supported throughout our lifelong development.
- Values perceived – Through an internal evaluation, judgment, and information-filtering process.
- Values guided – Through our internal decision-making process in determining our next words or actions.

### Values Driven Teams

Across many faculties, successful teams contain a variety of behavioral styles and values drives. However, winning teams demonstrate at least two (and sometimes three) values drives in common among their members. What this says is that members of winning teams have certain values that they can agree upon, at least in part. Those areas of values differences are usually neutralized upon the identification or understanding of the values position, pending the acceptance of a few points:

- One's values come from deeply held beliefs.
- Behavioral style changes more easily and frequently than one's values.
- All values positions are positions deserving of respect.
- There are no **right** or **wrong** values positions (in the six listed above), there are simply **different** positions.

### *An Instrumented Solution: Obtaining a Values "Pulse"*

The *Pro-Active Values* instrument model demonstrates the values drives and strengths offered by each member of the teaching team. In addition, enormous insight within a healthcare organization or school of nursing can be obtained by exploring the collective values of specific teams, then rolled upward into organizational norms by aggregating team data. This information is of critical importance and insight when healthcare organizations examine their mission, vision, and goal statements in light of their collective values. No one is asked to change their behavioral style or their values, but they are asked to agree on certain values, at least in part, and accept that other values positions differ.

When all individuals on the teaching team feel free to amplify their own strengths and allow enough space for the others on the team with different strengths to amplify theirs, therein is found successful people, successful teams, successful schools, and successful healthcare organizations (see Figure 47.8 for an overview of potential situations and outcomes when taking a values **pulse**.). It is to that end that the *Pro-Active Values* model was developed. Written between 1979 and 1984 and based upon values research that began in 1930, the *Pro-Active Values* model was introduced in 1984, with continual upgrades to the report program and a most recent revision and release in 2002. Readers are invited to complete the *Pro-Active Values* instrument online and receive a complimentary report on their results by contacting the author at russell.watson@activeprofiles.com and providing their name, organization, and Purchase Order Number for this book. Access codes will be sent via return e-mail, and the reader may obtain a courtesy *Pro-active Values* report.

Go to Chapter 47 on the CD accompanying this book, for more information on obtaining a courtesy *Pro-active Values* report.

Figure 47.8 - Obtaining a Values "Pulse": Initial Situations in Recap

| Situation | Outcome |
|---|---|
| "A personality conflict with my nursing manager." | The manager had a lower theoretical value and preferred the bottom line. The employee had a higher theoretical score and misread the manager's need for the "bottom-line" as disinterest, which it was not. When each understood the other's values, each realized that the necessity of each other's strengths. |
| "An ineffective teaching team with too many personality conflicts." | The team's ineffectiveness was rooted in the fact that there were a variety of different values espoused. This was okay, once they each agreed in part on the values that were important to the functioning of their team. |
| "I don't use personality testing because I have three very different people who are all doing very well on the job." | The success of the three different styles of people on similar jobs is in part due to the fact that they believe the same things. They share similar values across three of the six values areas and agree that those are key areas for job success. |
| "Only 30% of hospitals I've talked to are happy with their pre-hire testing." | That may be in large part because one's behavioral style or type accounts for only about 30% of one's success on the job. A much larger portion of the success factor is measured by one's values drives. |

(Copyright © 1984-2002 Target Consultants, Inc., Oswego, IL. All rights reserved. produced with permission.)

## A Brief Pulse of Our Values Drives

The statements in Figure 47.9 are summary statements related to each of the values drives. The values themes are indicated along with a high or low scoring parameter. **High** does not mean **good**, and **low** does not mean **bad**; they are indicators of the relative importance of each of the values drives. For the purposes of this brief review, most readers should choose three **high** indicators and three **low** indicators for these values statements. (When the *Pro-Active Values* instrument is completed online, there may be different indicators that emerge because of the detailed nature of the instrument and scoring.)

Figure 47.9 - Leadership Values in Healthcare

| Leadership Values in Healthcare: Our Drives & Motivators |
| --- |
| *Choose three "high" and three "low" areas among the six values descriptors listed.* |
| **Theoretical: The Drive for Knowledge**<br>  **High:** Shows a high degree of curiosity in a variety of areas; enjoys learning for learning's sake; high technical competence beyond the basics.<br>  **Low:** Wants to learn enough to be practical or get successful results; does not need to go beyond necessities; likes quick implementation of ideas; likes the big picture. |
| **Economic: The Drive for Money and Materials**<br>  **High:** Competitive and bottom-line oriented; wants practical solutions; high achiever when money is the motivator.<br>  **Low:** Frequently service-driven or support-driven; enjoys helping others; puts others before self; tends to be nonpolitical; not motivated just by money. |
| **Individualistic: The Drive to Be Unique and Independent**<br>  **High:** Enjoys demonstrating personal freedom; self-reliant; trendsetter; pacesetter; an active, independent agent; brings unique solutions to the table.<br>  **Low:** Enjoys working with others in time situations; supportive of the goals and project; excellent follow-through; doesn't require the limelight of attention. |
| **Altruistic: The Drive to Help Others**<br>  **High:** Shows generosity in sharing time and talent with others; genuine concern for others; a willing teacher and coach.<br>  **Low:** Will not be taken advantage of; maintains a business guard on giving away time and talent; takes care of own needs. |
| **Political: The Drive for Power and Control**<br>  **High:** Likes to take charge of projects; enjoys being a leader; competitive; willing to take the credit or the blame.<br>  **Low:** Very good team player; supports the project or cause; no hidden agendas; good stabilizing force on a project. |
| **Regulatory: The Drive for Order, Routine, and Structure**<br>  **High:** High degree of respect for rules, procedures, and tradition; well-disciplined; detailed problem-solver; prefers order and structure in the work environment.<br>  **Low:** Very adaptable to new projects; sets new precedent when necessary; sees the big picture and communicates it; a flexible problem-solver. |

The list of values drives identified above is not an exhaustive list but rather tends to be a list of enduring values that emerge in most educational settings. Taking this list one level deeper, readers may examine the mission, vision, and goal statements for their school, hospital, clinic, or practice and determine values themes that emerge from those statements. Finally, they may ask the self-appraisal or system-appraisal question: Are the values expressed in the mission statement visible in the day-to-day operations of our teams of professionals?

Strengths and areas for improvement for each of the six values themes are listed in Figure 47.10. For each of the themes, the first two items are areas of primary strengths and the third item is an area for improvement. For each of the three values themes that were selected on the previous page as **high** areas, readers should place a check mark in front of each of the strengths and areas for improvement where there is agreement with the item.

Figure 47.10 - Strengths and Areas for Improvement.

---

**High Theoretical**
\_\_\_\_1. Asks active questions, has an appetite for learning even for its own sake.
\_\_\_\_2. High process and procedure knowledge; high product knowledge.
\_\_\_\_3. May sometimes bog down in too many details.

**High Economic**
\_\_\_\_1. Competitive player, keeps an ear to the revenue clock.
\_\_\_\_2. 'Return on Investment' oriented, financial/business orientation.
\_\_\_\_3. May tend to be a workaholic at times.

**High Individualistic**
\_\_\_\_1. Stands up for own rights; brings unique solutions to problems.
\_\_\_\_2. Projects confidence to others; high creativity factor.
\_\_\_\_3. May sometimes be a nonconformist on certain issues.

**High Altruistic**
\_\_\_\_1. High desire to be helpful; ready to assist others on the team.
\_\_\_\_2. A generous teacher and coach to others; good listener.
\_\_\_\_3. May seldom say **no** to requests for help from others.

**High Political**
\_\_\_\_1. Strong ambitions and goals; sets high standards for self and others.
\_\_\_\_2. Shows a "buck stops here" attitude; willing to take the credit or blame.
\_\_\_\_3. May be somewhat impatient when situations are not in their favor.

**High Regulatory**
\_\_\_\_1. Follows and enforces protocol and quality procedures.
\_\_\_\_2. Precise time and organization management skills.
\_\_\_\_3. May be overly rigid at times.

---

A knowledge and awareness of the values drives that provide an intrinsic motivation, along with an appreciation of various behavioral styles and preferences, can be of enormous benefit to teams and individuals in the process of self-appraisal and self-development. Knowing about **how** individuals do what they do (DISC behavioral preferences) and **why** they do what they do (workplace values) can assist in focusing professional development and amplifying strengths.

## The Job Culture Analysis

The third and final dimension of this appraisal process is for each professional in the teaching profession to examine the job **culture** or environment in which the work is performed. This chapter has explored several facets of self-appraisal and self-development for nursing professionals:

- Objective appraisal.
- Journalizing appraisal.
- Structured appraisal worksheets.
- Behavioral preferences (DISC).
- Workplace values themes.

One item frequently omitted in many appraisal models is an exploration of the "job culture" or work environment in which the professional functions are completed. The final application in this chapter explores the job culture of workplace environments.

In exploring the DISC model for individual behavioral preferences, a **language** has been established to take the DISC model one level higher to the organizational culture level. In this premise, high or low "D" style cultures are identified, as are the "I," "S," and "C" style preferences, as the pulse or tempo of the work environment. It is interesting to note that within a hospital or clinic, nearly a full spectrum of highs and lows across each of the DISC dimensions can be observed. The Emergency Department for example, is a High D and Low S work culture: quick reactions, original thinking, immediate results, and a high sense of urgency are some of the environmental cultural attributes that contribute to the success of an emergency procedure. Conversely, on the oncology unit, one observes a comparatively more predictable environment, standardized policies, and a more steady and stable sense of urgency. Both environments are needed and both are successful. Both depend on the pulse or tempo of the immediate situations.

Figure 47.11 illustrates the degree of change from one job culture to another across the DISC model. Readers are encouraged to circle the descriptor group that most identifies their current work environment to obtain a perspective of that culture across the DISC model.

Figure 47.11. The Job Culture Interpretation of a Workplace Environment

| | "D" Job Expectations | "I" Job Expectations | "S" Job Expectations | "C" Job Expectations |
|---|---|---|---|---|
| **Very High** | • Immediate results<br>• Rapid decisions<br>• Quick reactions<br>• Demanding pace<br>• Original thinking | • Optimistic spirit<br>• Persuasive approach<br>• High people contact<br>• Verbal expression<br>• Inspirational attitude | • Very high patience<br>• Gather facts and information<br>• Routine procedures<br>• Sensitivity to others<br>• Systematic approach | • Very high quality<br>• High detail orientation<br>• High concentration<br>• Precise problem solving<br>• Cautious decisions |
| **High** | • Firm decisions<br>• Rapid achievements<br>• Creative ideas<br>• Use of authority<br>• Rapid pace | • Contact with people<br>• Counseling approach<br>• Open door for others<br>• Sociable relationships<br>• Friendly atmosphere | • High follow-through<br>• Solo & team efforts<br>• Established methods<br>• Deliberate pace<br>• Completion of projects | • Standard Operating Procedures<br>• Clear expectations<br>• Quality standards<br>• Detailed tasks<br>• Gathering data and information |
| **Low** | • Careful delegation<br>• Leading by example<br>• Cautious decisions<br>• Stable pace<br>• Time to weigh pro/con | • Sincere in helping<br>• Meeting deadlines<br>• Some tasks alone<br>• Individual reflection<br>• Facts before emotions | • Moderate urgency<br>• Some multi-tasking<br>• Flexible solutions<br>• Some mobility<br>• Some changes | • Independence in tasks<br>• Individualistic solutions<br>• Bottom-line approach<br>• Some new precedent<br>• Firm decisions |
| **Very Low** | • Standardized controls<br>• Conservative decisions<br>• Predictable events<br>• Calculated risks<br>• Stable procedures | • Many tasks done alone<br>• Controlled environs<br>• Logic comes first<br>• Time for reflection<br>• Specialized tasks | • Very high urgency<br>• Many tasks<br>• High mobility<br>• Substantial changes<br>• Very active pace | • New ideas needed<br>• Act w/out precedent<br>• Freedom from controls<br>• Many activities<br>• No routine work |

In reviewing the job culture interpretation, it is important to note that within each nursing school and nursing education department, a variety of roles are needed, and those roles may change from stable to urgent, sometimes moment by moment. An awareness of the differences within specific departments in a healthcare organization can be of enormous benefit to the teaching professionals as they educate their nursing students. It is also essential to note that one's own behavioral style preferences, as indicated by the DISC model do not need to match point-by-point the job culture interpretation. The reason for this is that all styles of teaching professionals are needed throughout the educational environment.

## Conclusion

This chapter has attempted to expand the envelope of self-development and self-appraisal by going beyond the traditional checklists provided for readers' self-reflection and appraisal. This chapter has also provided some open-ended tools that can be modified for the readers' use. Finally, no effective self-development and self-appraisal process is complete without looking at the **context** of the job environment, namely, the three dimensions of:

- Behavioral preferences (DISC).
- Values drives.
- Job culture.

If readers want to explore these later dimensions in more detail, the author has provided the opportunity to receive a courtesy report on both behavioral preferences and values drives. These reports may be accessed on a one-time courtesy basis by contacting the author at russellwatson@activeprofiles.com and supplying reader's name, organization, and purchase order number for this book. Access codes will be provided to take the assessments on a pro-bono basis. Go to Chapter 47 on the CD accompanying this book, for more information on obtaining an access code for a courtesy report. These reports are provided as a courtesy from the author and the website principals as a way of saying "thanks" to the many nursing faculty and future nursing faculty who may read this valuable, useful, and practical textbook.

## Websites

Following is a list of websites that may be helpful in learning more about self-development and self-appraisal. For easy launching, these are also located on the

CD accompanying this book. Simply launch your internet browser, put the CD-ROM in the drive, go to Chapter 47 on the CD, and then click on the website address.

activeprofiles.com: Various instruments and assessments used for self-development and self-awareness, as well as research background and statistics provided. Available at: http://www.activeprofiles.com (access here for complimentary reports as described in the chapter).

Baldridge National Quality Program: Many resources for educational institutions in establishing quality programs. Available at: http://baldridge.org

Center for Creative Leadership: Resources for leadership development. Available at: http://www.ccl.org

Drucker Foundation (for nonprofit organizations): A variety of resources for educational institutions and education professionals. Available at: http://pfdf.org

## Learning Activities

1. Compare the results from any of the checklists or assessments in this chapter with peers. Discuss similarities, differences, and strengths as you prepare for your chosen field.
2. Explore some of the websites listed above and others especially dealing with nursing and nursing education. Share your findings with your peers.

### References

Jung, C. J. (1971). *Psychological types*. Princeton, New Jersey: Princeton University Press.

Marston, W. M. (1979). *The emotions of normal people*. Minneapolis Minnesota: Persona Press.

Target Consultants, Inc. (1984-2002). *Various forms, instruments, and tables* (reprinted with permission) [online]. Available: http://www.targetconsultantsinc.com

# Chapter 48: PERSONAL POWER AND CONFLICT RESOLUTION

Sandy Forrest, MSN, MEd, PhD, RN

*Power in nursing is an extremely interesting concept. The nurse is empowered by education but so many times feels powerless. Power often brings conflict, especially in the many stressful situations nurses, faculty, and students seem to encounter on a regular basis. Dr. Forrest looks at power as a positive and energizing force. From this perspective, faculty can teach students to deal with both power and conflict throughout the nursing program so newly graduated nurses will be prepared to cope with the current climate in health care. – Linda Caputi and Lynn Engelmann*

## Introduction

Nurse educators can assist their students to differentiate external power – the outer capacity for action – from internal power – the inner capacity for reflection. Moreover, application of these power constructs can enable nurses to demonstrate an enhanced capability of dealing with personal and environmental sources of conflict.

This chapter explores the positive and negative relationships between power and conflict and the various outcomes that can occur when they come into contact with one another. Moreover, it affords readers an opportunity to assess their degree or stage of personal power and how this sense of power influences their ability to manage conflict.

### Educational Philosophy

I believe that it is a privilege to teach, as it affords me an opportunity to perfect my artistic skills. My craft is to encourage curiosity, critical thinking, and caring of one individual for another. I choose to promote this wisdom in an atmosphere that fosters cooperative activity as well as independent effort. Moreover, it is an opportunity to instill, within each student, a holistic perspective that will heighten the ability to critically assess the well-being of all individuals placed in their care. – Sandy Forrest

# Issues that Create Conflict

There are numerous empirical studies of the effects of, experience with, and methods for resolving conflict among professional nurses and nursing students. Issues that create conflict reported by nurses in various countries include the following:

- American nurses expressed concern about colleagues withholding information and breaking rules (Gold, Chamabers, & McQuaid, 1995) and their inability to be client advocates (Riley & Fry, 2000). Nurses who perceived themselves as having a low status in hierarchical, bureaucratic organizations described conflict relative to time constraints, lack of staff, scarce resources, and a demand for increased effectiveness, all of which initiated feelings of powerlessness in terms of providing quality care (Chambliss, 1996).
- Dutch nurses experienced conflict when colleagues treated them aggressively, behaved in incompetent and unauthorized ways, were indecisive, sedated clients for convenience, had insufficient knowledge, discriminated against clients, kept silent about errors, and administered treatment against clients' wishes (Van der Arend & Remmers-van den Hurk, 1999).
- Israeli nurses reported that 4 out of 10 most frequent and problematic ethical dilemmas were an inability to treat patients due to staff shortages, indecision about reporting an incompetent nurse or physician, offensive behavior toward a client, and treatment perceived as mistaken or wrong (Wagner & Ronen, 1996).
- Korean nursing students experienced conflict when nursing staff deviated from principles, made a medication error due to negligence, did not report a medication error, failed to use aseptic technique, withheld information about a colleague's drug abuse, and clashed over differing educational levels (Han & Ahn, 2000).

## *What is Power?*

*An open mind brings compassion. Compassion builds power.*
*Such power is natural. Tao 16*

Some define power as the ability to influence and change the behavior of others in order to achieve a specified end and the possession of authority to control or command others (Random House, 2001). Why the emphasis on **the behavior of others**? Can one person control the behavior of another? Perhaps a better way to understand power is to examine it as a personal trait or quality. Thus, the definition becomes that of personal power. Power can be further characterized with some positive descriptors, such as eloquence, energy, greatness, privilege, talent, and strength. Now the word power – personal power – takes on a different flavor, especially when compared to more negative descriptors of authoritativeness, control, governance, and impulse.

## *What is Conflict?*

Again, referencing Random House (2001), conflict is defined as a clash or disagreement between opposing elements or ideas and a mental struggle arising from incompatible demands. Within this framework, conflict emerges when there are unclear expectations, poor communications, lack of clear jurisdiction, differences in attitudes, and changes. Essentially, descriptors such as contention, disaccord, hostility, and psychological stress provide a rather negative connotation to the experience of conflict. Experts, however, assert that conflict is inherently neither positive nor negative but rather an inevitable consequence of the natural process of change and growth (Crum, 1987; Fisher, Ury, & Patton, 1991).

Power is what an individual wants it to be. What power is depends on how it is used when interacting with others. When the negative aspects of power are allowed to influence one's actions, others may choose to back away, relinquishing their needs and desires and forfeiting their power. However, if handled in a positive manner, the resulting conflict can encourage growth in both the individual and the relationship among the people involved in the conflict.

## Power

According to French and Raven (1959), individuals may influence and be influenced by other persons, depending on their relationship. Power derives from multiple sources that may be operating simultaneously. These available sources are all available and their planned use is referred to as a power strategy. Specifically, five sources of power are recognized, depending on one's belief:

- Reward: An individual can provide desired or positive sanctions that are won only through compliance (i.e., money or compliments).
- Coercive: This is the opposite of reward – it involves threats of punishment. This is the most visible form of power, and its strength centers on the magnitude of the forms of punishment available.
- Legitimate: An individual has a right to exert power based on a role, position, or office. The perception of power is based on internalized values implying that people in specific positions have a right to demand specific behaviors from other individuals.
- Expert: An individual is perceived to possess compelling knowledge or information in a specific domain.
- Referent: An individual is attractive and influential because that individual belongs to a desirable group or has personal characteristics that another wishes to emulate.

This is a subtle form of power.

Personal power can also derive from an individual's ability to create a perception of power (Haddock, 2002; Hagberg, 1984). Perception alone is often enough to give the individual actual power in a situation. The wizard in *The Wizard of Oz* is an example of an individual granted perceived power. Some helpful descriptors include vision, realization, consciousness, mindfulness, astuteness, discernment, and insight.

When individuals recognize their personal power and are comfortable using it, life can be easier and more enjoyable. This is an important trait to pass on to nursing students when socializing them into the role of the nurse. Students must learn about personal power and how to use it constructively when working with clients and families

*It is the eternal struggle between these two principles – right and wrong.*
*They are the two principles that have stood face to face from the beginning*
*of time and will ever continue to struggle. It is the same spirit that says,*
*"You work and toil and earn bread, and I'll eat it." Abraham Lincoln*

### Power Over

"Power over" implies a dependency relationship associated with forcefulness in which people take on superior and subordinate roles (French & Raven, 1959). It is an interpersonal construct that develops early in life. Humans are always struggling to rise from an inferior to a superior position, from one of weakness to one of strength. Individuals endorsing this style of dealing with others do so by:
- Commanding or encouraging dependent relations.
- Demanding authority affording them control of events or behaviors.
- Exhibiting prestige as a result of struggling for dominance.
- Rising from a position of weakness to one of strength.

*Power will intoxicate the best hearts, as wine the strongest heads.*
*No man is wise enough nor good enough to be trusted with unlimited power*
*Charles Caleb Colton*

### Power To

"Power to" is a process that relates to a capacity (the role) and the ability (the competence) to use direct, rational tactics when faced with conflict (French & Raven, 1959). The intent of "power to" is to achieve objectives (i.e., prestige, esteem, legitimacy) through interpersonal processes. The means to achieve these objectives are mutually established and all people work toward achieving these goals. Individuals with "power to" possess the following:

- Ability, strength, might, or force to do or act.
- Capacity to inspire others to formulate goals.
- Processes available to assist in achieving these goals.

Environmental factors that encourage this form of interaction include trust, caring, concern, knowledge, and good communication processes.

*Meeting conflict with force overcomes opposition, but never the conflict.*
*Blame and attack, rage and resentment perpetuate cycles of violence and pain.*
*The wise leader seeks real solutions, resolving conflict*
*with understanding and wisdom. Tao, 79*

### *The Power Model*

The Power Model is described by Hagberg (1984). The following explanations of six stages of power are adapted, with permission of the author, from *Real Power* (Hagberg, 1984). According to this model, people move from stages of external power to internal power. External power is developed in Stages 1 through 3. External power then becomes integrated with internal power in Stages 4 through 6. Personal power increases as people develop both external and internal power and when they lead from their souls rather than from positions of authority.

Hagberg (1984) defines external power – Stages 1 through 3 – as the capacity to act with confidence, competence, and expertise; it is represented by titles, success, degrees, stature, money, recognition, and self-esteem. In Stages 4 through 6, external power is integrated with internal power and is characterized by the capacity to reflect. Internal power emerges from one's inner self, soul, and deeper values. Internal power reflects who the person really is and the person's life purpose. A description of each of the six stages follows.

### *Stage 1: Powerlessness*

- Description: Feels stuck with no relief in sight; feels manipulated and controlled by others.
- Characteristics: Is dependent, uninformed, confused, learned helplessness.
- Catalyst: The will to change and knowledge to build coalitions.
- Deterrent: Fear of punishment, failing, and finding out what can be done to change the situation.
- How to handle conflict: A person in Stage 1 handles conflict in a rather passive

manner. It would be acceptable for the other individual to **win**. The sense of **loss** will likely be felt as manipulation and control, associated with a sense of helplessness.

- Ways to move: Build self-esteem; find allies; confront, appreciate, and share self.
- Activity to encourage movement: People in Stage 1 needs to identify five things that they like about themselves and share these with a friend or colleague. They should plan something to do within 10 days that demonstrates appreciation for themselves and share this plan with their peers. P.S. They must carry the plan out!!

*To know what you prefer, instead of humbly saying "Amen" to what the world tells you you ought to prefer, is to have kept your soul alive.*
*Robert Louis Stevenson*

### Stage 2: Power by Association

- Description: Identifies with a role model or more powerful people; views power as elusive; believes that certain people have influential power that will take care of, lead, and nurture them.
- Characteristics: Has a sense of belonging; is dependent on leader as main source of information; is beginning self-exploration to identify strengths and weaknesses.
- Catalyst: Lack of self-confidence and need for security; likes others to pave the way; can push self or stay stuck.
- Deterrent: Not aware of being stuck.
- How to handle conflict: A person in Stage 2 would still handle conflict in a passive manner, depending on the issue. At times, it would be desirable for the other individual to "lose." Winning will be attributed to associations that are considered valuable and powerful.
- Ways to move: Develop a network and find a mentor; take risks and get involved.
- Activity to encourage movement: People in Stage 2 need to identify three things that they like and dislike about their life at this point in time. They can then explore how to capitalize on the likes and work around the dislikes.

*You must be the change you wish to see in the world. Mahatma Gandhi*

### Stage 3: Power by Achievement

- Description: Has learned to play the game; is oriented to winning and self-promotion; appreciates symbols that are external and recognizable (i.e. degrees, awards for competence) and that represent a prize that makes the person feel more worthwhile.
- Characteristics: Is egocentric, competitive, charismatic, and ambitious; has accumu-

lated knowledge or expertise, which offers sense of control but still lacks influence.

- Catalyst: Beginning to question self-integrity.
- Deterrent: Not being aware of being stuck.
- How to handle conflict: A person in Stage 3 would handle conflict in a forceful style, depending on the issue. Winning is important, especially when the issue at hand is related to this individual's symbol of power. Losing is connected to an inability or to limited knowledge of how to **play the game** correctly.
- Ways to move: Being alone and reflecting on self; concentrating on the present; thinking differently and experiencing new things.
- Activity to encourage movement: People in Stage 3 need to make a list of five things that their parents wanted them to do with their life and circle the items that they did not want to do, asking themselves, "Have I done them?" They should explore the implications of doing things to please others.

*I can only please one person per day. Today is not your day.*
*Tomorrow isn't looking good either. Dilbert*

### Stage 4: Power by Reflection

- Description: Is compelled to act or influence others.
- Characteristics: Is confused yet competent in collaboration, strong and comfortable with personal style; skilled at mentoring and leading.
- Catalyst: Letting go of one's ego and facing fears.
- Deterrent: Being unsure of life purpose; poor ego control.
- How to handle conflict: To a person in Stage 4, winning, regardless of the issue, is becoming less important. This person chooses to enter a confrontation yet is able to relinquish a need for control. The person may even search for opportunities that allow others to win.
- Activity to encourage movement: People in Stage 4 need to sit still and listen for the small voice inside. They must begin to hear it. It can only be heard when the noise of the mind quiets down.

*Some things arrive in their own mysterious hour, on their own terms,*
*and not yours, to be seized or relinquished forever. Gail Godwin*

### Stage 5: Power by Purpose

- Description: Is guided by inner intuitive voice; has a life purpose that extends beyond self; believes that the more power given away the better as it will come back full circle, even if not in the same form in which it was given; sees self as insignificant and also recognizes, in the larger scheme of things, that the importance of self.

- Characteristics: Is self-accepting and content with personal situation in life; has a sense of internal calm; is courageous yet humble; is able to empower others.
- Catalyst: Trying to understand the cosmos and that no longer does the individual matter in the larger scheme of things and yet the individual is all that matters.
- Deterrent: Lack of faith; too much to lose.
- Ways to move: Developing deep understanding of self-motivation; developing individual path.
- How to handle conflict: A person in Stage 5 does not view conflict as a win-or-lose situation as there are advantages to either position. Time and energy is devoted to understanding the self.
- Activity to encourage movement: People in Stage 5 need to reflect on their mission in life. What do they need to let go of? How can they learn a healthy way of approaching life? They must get in touch with themselves – their souls.

*All good work should have an edge of life and death to it, if not immediately apparent, then to be found by ardently exploring its greater context. Absent the edge, we drown in numbness. David Whyte*

## Stage 6: Power by Wisdom

- Description: Understands life beyond a situation; asks questions on a higher level; has an inner well of calm, of quiet strength.
- Characteristics: Is content for things to be ambiguous and abstract; needs little tangible power; has high integrity and sense of moral justice; knows that there will always be conflict and understands that the richness of life emerges from within.
- Catalyst: Becoming more than human and struggling with an inability to tap the inner source of power.
- Deterrent: Human constraints; inability to challenge, enlarge their vision, and give wisdom.
- How to handle conflict: A person in Stage 6 is comfortable being viewed as powerless. Conflict is an experience that the person would choose to avoid.
- Activity to encourage movement: People in Stage 6 need to identify three significant events in their life. How do these events relate to one another? Do these individuals see these events as separate occurrences or as part of a process?

*Even if I knew that tomorrow the world would go to pieces,*
*I would still plant my apple tree.  Martin Luther King*

## Conflict Behavior

Conflict behavior is a person's reaction to the perception that one's own and another person's current aspirations can not be achieved simultaneously (Rubin, Pruitt, & Kim, 1994). A person's reactions to conflict are characterized by a number of integrative and distributive activities (Van de Vilert & Euwema, 1994).

- Integrative activities: Generally viewed as positive. These activities assist individuals to find a common ground and exhibit concern for the interests of all parties.
- Distributive activities: Generally viewed as negative. These are activities in which the focus or concern is mainly on oneself.

Individual responses to conflict are considered effective if the issue becomes less serious or even resolved and/or if the shared relationship of the disgruntled parties has improved (Thomas, 1992; Tjosvold, 1991).

*What you do speaks too loud*
*that I cannot hear what you say. Ralph Waldo Emerson*

### *Conflict Resolution*

Weeks (1994) explored conflict resolution as a process, explaining that it is a process that empowers people to build mutually beneficial relationships and to resolve conflict effectively. This mutually beneficial relationship, or partnership process, is based on five principles:

1. Think **we**, rather than **I versus you**; working together helps solve conflicts.
2. Try to keep in mind the long-term relationship.
3. Good conflict resolution will improve the relationship.
4. Good conflict resolution benefits both parties.
5. Conflict resolution and relationship building go hand in hand.

This process to resolve conflict effectively includes eight steps:
1. Create an effective atmosphere.
2. Clarify perceptions.
3. Focus on individual and shared needs.
4. Build shared positive power.

5. Look to the future, then learn from the past.

6. Generate options.

7. Develop aptitudes.

8. Make mutual benefit agreements.

In a conflict, language is used to exchange information on both a content and relational level (Watzlawick, Beavin, & Jackson, 1967). Individuals in conflict are less likely to remain in conflict if their interactions shift from a blaming orientation to one that is more relationship oriented. For example, the use of the pronoun **we** can indicate closeness, intimacy, or acceptance and can increase the amount of inclusion of the other as each person talks.

Addressing the other and the self with **we** instead of **you** and **I** can be seen as symbolizations of a common identity. If parties come to believe that their interests are joined, they may identify with each other in a sense of communality leading to a more effective conclusion (Burke, 1962; Giles & Fitzpatirck, 1985).

Conflict is likely to have a negative consequence when one or both parties address the dispute with **win-lose** tactics. These tactics rarely provide a final resolution of the dispute because conflict resolved by subjugation tends to breed new conflict. Effective conflict resolution occurs when each party collaborates to create solutions that sufficiently meet the needs of all parties. Thus the key element in effective conflict resolution is a willingness to engage in mutual collaboration (Fisher et al., 1991). Moreover, the way the parties address each other and the conflict issue can have positive effects on the outcome.

*Everyone wishes to have truth on his side, but not everyone wishes to be on the side of truth.  Richard Whately*

### Conflict Resolution Styles

Conflict resolution styles refers to a patterned response to conflict involving the repeated use of the same tactics to resolve disputes (Hocker & Wilmot, 1991). Just as power and conflict have positive and negative connotations, so does the style or behaviors used in resolving a dispute. Typically, the method(s) used to deal with opposing elements or desires are categorized as either assertive (positive) or nonassertive (negative) (Rahim, 1983).

Assertive or positive styles include:

- Collaborating or integrating: These styles seek a resolution that maximally meets the needs of both parties. They attempt to sort out where each person stands and identify all plausible options. The parties search for a true win-win solution that maximizes benefits for both parties. Win-win solutions may include concurring and cooperating or yielding and acquiescing. To be a true win-win solution, the party that yields or acquiesces must be happy with that solution. If the person is not happy with yielding in an effort to end the conflict, this solution may produce resentment. This would not be a win-win situation (Caputi, 1999).

- Accommodating or obliging: These styles combine high concern for others with low concern for self and tend to readily accede to demands of the other party. Equalizing, conforming, reconciling, and modifying are examples of this conflict resolution style.

- Compromising: This conflict resolution style shows concern for self and others. Individuals offer solutions at a midpoint between their respective positions without seeking a solution that maximizes both of their gains. All involved make a few concessions – eager to end the conflict as soon as a minimally satisfactory solution for both parties is found, even if a more mutually beneficial solution could be reached with further effort. Acknowledging, reconciling, giving way, changing, and making concessions further illustrate this conflict resolution style.

Nonassertive or negative styles include:

- Competing or dominating: In this conflict resolution style, individuals pursue their own needs with determination, regardless of the other person's concerns. This technique is characterized by grappling with, fighting against, contending with, and striving against.

- Avoiding: This style involves aversion to engaging in discussion about conflict and thus evidences low concern about meeting either self's or others' needs. This style downplays the seriousness of the problem and suggests that further attention to the situation is a waste of time. Abstaining, pulling back, retreating, denying oneself, and evading characterize this style.

### *The Pinch Theory*

The Pinch Theory (Sherwood & Glidewell, 1973) details a model for clarifying and resolving conflict issues though problem-solving (see Figure 48. 1). In brief, these theorists propose that when working with others, people typically share information about each other's expectations. They then clarify and agree to roles and responsibilities hopefully to achieve stability and productivity. Conflict develops when individuals:

- Experience frustration due to being blocked from satisfying a goal or alleviating a concern.
- Conceptualize and perceive others are to blame for the dissatisfaction.
- Act on these perceptions escalating the discord.

Figure 48.1 - The Pinch Theory

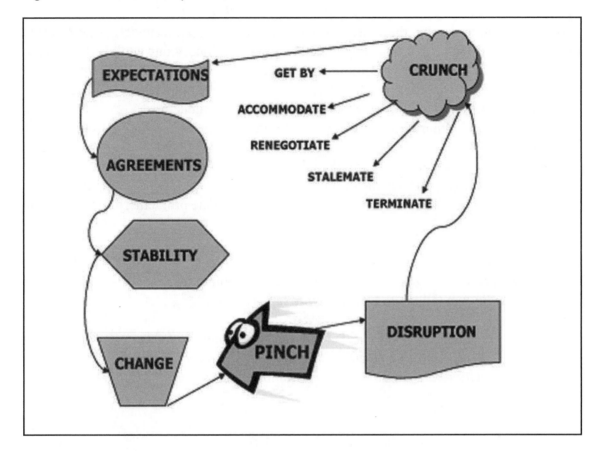

This leads to a **pinch**. The individual can choose to (a) respond to the pinch through negotiation and achieve stability and productivity; or, (b) ignore the pinch and endure **disruption**, distinguished by ambiguity, uneasiness, anxiety, blaming, guilt, and resentment.

When negotiation is used, requisites include delineating:

• The issues – acknowledging one another's point of view and feelings.
• Each person's needs – identifying, clarifying, and agreeing upon each person's needs.
• Creative options to address these needs.
• Modifications of options allowing for solutions that satisfy everyone.

Pinches are managed by sharing feedback on the negotiation and addressing the change successfully.

*People change and forget to tell each other. Lillian Hellman*

If still unable to resolve the **issue**, the individuals are forced to undergo the **crunch**. Physiological responses to a crunch include increased respiratory rate and heart rate, fear, a desire to go away, anger, sweating, immobilization, and tears. When the issues are not solved, negative consequences occur. These consequences are not desirable and include:

- Accommodation: returning to what used to be or accommodating.
- Renegotiation: ignoring emotions and submitting to power or renegotiating under duress.
- On-the-job retirement: retiring on the job; performing the minimum to get by.
- Stalemate: entering a stalemate or power struggle.
- Termination: resentful termination without insight into the problems, almost ensuring reoccurrence.

A possible outcome of a crunch is lose-lose, where the goal is set aside and all parties **let it go**. More beneficial conclusions are resolving the conflict through win-lose (someone gives in) and win-win (all individuals go away satisfied).

*He who makes another powerful ruins himself, for he*
*makes the other so either by shrewdness or force, and both*
*these qualities are feared by the one who becomes powerful. Machiavelli*

## Cognitive Analysis

Cognitive analysis is a systematic methodology for analyzing and resolving conflict situations that proposes that cognitive differences among individuals are capable of producing conflict (Al-Tabtabai, 2001). It is based on social judgment theory, which suggests that the nature of human judgment provides a prime source of conflict, as often disagreements flow from the exercise of human judgment. Consequently, interpersonal conflict persists even when self-serving motives are eliminated.

Cognitive analysis, as a resolution technique, is based on the assumption that human judgment is a reflective process (Hammond, Stewart, Brehmer, & Steinman, 1975; Stewart, 1988). In this process, an individual comes to a conclusion or makes a judgment about an uncertain event. Although specifics about the event are unclear, environmental cues are available that are perceived as representing a potential for conflict. The cues, however, are perceived differently by various individuals and thus become the source of the conflict. Through discussion, judgment differences are communicated and people are encouraged to understand the viewpoints of others and to reduce, if not eliminate, the conflict that exists among them. Once these judgments are voiced, the individuals are encouraged to revise their conclusion about the conflict issue by reducing the differences in their thinking rather than by focusing on the differences in outcomes.

## Websites

Following is a list of websites that may be helpful in learning more about personal power and conflict resolution. For easy internet launching, these are also located on the CD accompanying this book. Simply launch your Internet browser, put the CD-ROM in the drive, go to Chapter 48 on the CD, and then click on the website address.

- CRInfo, About Conflict Resolution: www.crinfo.org
- Rahim Organization Conflict Inventory: www.ag.arizona.edu
- Taking Conflict Personally Scale: www.humanlinks.com
- The Building Tool Room: www.newhorizons.org/trm_johnson
- The Power Orientation Test: www.humanlinks.com
- Thomas-Kilmann Conflict Mode Instrument: www.career-lifeskills.com

## Conclusion

Why is it difficult for nurses to accept power, not as a tool that corrupts or destroys, but as a compelling basis for establishing change? Power is a positive and energizing force that can assist nurses to become more effective leaders. There are many nurses who, if they were to actualize it, have the legitimate power that offers a more commanding role in the healthcare environment, which is teeming with conflict. Learning about and applying positive conflict resolution styles further empowers nurses. Of course, this requires nurses to take action and accept risks – to be responsible and accountable for the results. If not now, when?

*Those who want power, seek it.*
*Those who have power, wield it.*
*Those who keep power, understand it. Joan Kyes*

Please note: The website for the quotes used throughout this chapter is: www.ntlf.com/html/lib/quotes.htm. This is "The National Teaching and Learning Forum".

# Learning Activities

1. Review the definitions for power and conflict. What would you add to the definitions? What other descriptors do you think should be considered when discussing these two concepts?
2. Explore why personal power and conflict resolution are important issues for nursing.
3. Complete the questionnaire profile evaluating stages of personal power. In which stage did you score the highest? Are you ready to move to a higher stage?
4. Explain why collaborating, accommodating, and compromising are considered assertive ways of dealing with conflict.
5. Analyze why competing and avoiding are considered nonassertive ways of dealing with conflict.
6. Analyze the positive aspects of employing win-lose, lose-lose, and win-win approaches when resolving conflict.
7. Explore how nurses "get caught" in situations that bring out assertive or nonassertive methods of resolving conflict.
8. Examine where nursing is in achieving a sense of "power over" others.
9. Examine a recent conflict. How does it fit the pinch theory? Could the results have been different, more satisfying, for those involved?
10. How can you teach students to resolve conflict using assertive techniques?
11. Based on the information given for each stage of power, identify a potential method for handling conflict. Develop an activity for yourself and potential students that encourages movement to the next stage.

# References

Al-Tabtabai, H. (2001). Conflict resolution using cognitive analysis approach. *Project Management Journal, 2,* 4-17.

Burke, K. (1962). *A grammar of motives and a rhetoric of motives.* New York: World.

Caputi, L. (1999). *Conflict resolution.* Glen Ellyn, IL: College of DuPage.

Chambliss, D. E. (1996). *Beyond caring: Hospitals, nurses, and the social organization of ethics.* Chicago: University of Chicago.

Crum, T. F. (1987). *The magic of conflict.* New York: Touchstone.

Fisher, R., Ury, W., & Patton, B. (1991). *Getting to yes: Negotiating agreement without giving in.* New York: Penguin.

French, R. P., & Raven, B. (1959). The basis of social power. In D. Cartwright (Ed.), *Studies in social power* Ann Arbor, MI: University of Michigan.

Giles, H., & Fitzpatrick, M. A. (1985). Personal, group, and couple identities: Towards a relational context for the study of language attitudes and linguistic forms. In D. Schiffrin (Ed.), *Meaning, form, and use on contest: Linguistic applications.* Washington, DC: Georgetown University.

Gold, C., Chambers, J., & McQuaid, D. E. M. (1995). Ethical dilemmas in the lived experience of nursing practice. *Nursing Ethics, 2*, 131-142.

Haddock, P. (2002). Communicating personal power. *Supervision, 1*, 13.

Hagberg, J. O. (1984). *Real power: Stages of personal power in organizations*. Minneapolis, MN: Winston.

Hammond, K. R., Stewart, T. R., Brehmer, B., & Steinman, D. O. (1975). Social judgment theory. In M. Kaplan & S. Schwartz (Eds.), *Human judgment and decision processes* New York: Praeger.

Han, S. S., & Ahn, S. H. (2000). An analysis and evaluation of student nurses' participation in ethical decision making. *Nursing Ethics, 7*, 113-123.

Hocker, J.L. & Wilmot, W.W. (1991). *Interpersonal conflict*. IA: Brown.

Rahim, M. A. (1983). Measurement of organizational conflict. *Journal of General Psychology, 2*, 189-199.

Random House. (2001). *Webster's college dictionary*. New York: Author.

Riley, J. M., & Fry, S. T. (2000). Nurses report widespread ethical conflicts. *Reflections on Nursing Leadership, 2*, 35-36.

Rubin, J. A., Pruitt, D. G., & Kim, S. H. (1994). *Social conflict: Escalation, stalemate, and settlement*. New York: McGraw-Hill.

Sherwood, J., & Glidewill, J. (1973). Planned renegotiation. In J. E. Jones & J. W. Pfeiffer (Eds.), *The 1973 annual handbook for group facilitators*. San Diego, CA: University Associates.

Stewart, T. R. (1988). Judgment analysis: Procedures. In B. Brehmer & C. R. B. Joyce (Eds.), *Human judgment*. Amsterdam, Holland: North-Holland.

Thomas, K. W. (1992). Conflict and negotiating processes in organizations, In M. D. Dunnette & L. M. Hough (Eds.), *Handbook of industrial and organizational psychology*. Palo Alto, CA: Consulting Psychologists Press.

Tjosvold, D. (1991). *The conflict-positive organization: Stimulate diversity and create unity*. Reading, MA: Addison-Wesley.

Van de Vilert, E., & Euwema, M. C. (1994). Agreeableness and activeness as components of conflict behaviors. *Journal of Personality and Social Psychology, 66*, 674-687.

Van der Arend, A. J. G., & Remmers-van den Hurk, C. H. M. (1999). Moral problems among Dutch nurses: A survey. *Nursing Ethics, 6*, 468-482.

Wagner, N., & Ronen, I. (1996). Ethical dilemmas experienced by hospital and community nurses: An Israeli survey. *Nursing Ethics, 3*, 294-304.

Watzlawick, R., Beavin, J. H., & Jackson, D. D. (1967). *Pragmatics of human communication: A study of interactional patterns, pathologies, and paradoxes*. New York: Norton.

Weeks, D. (1994). *The eight essential steps to conflict resolution*. New York: Penguin.

## Bibliography

Brewster, B.M. (1992). *Journey to wholeness*. Portland, OR: Four Winds.

Campbell, J. (1991). *Reflections on the art of living*. New York: Harper Collins.

Cohen, A. R., & Bradford, D. L. (1991). *Influence without authority*. New York: John Wiley.

Goldberg, P. (1983). *The intuitive edge*. Los Angeles: Jeremy P. Tarcher.

Grudin, R. (1982). *Time and the art of living*. New York: Ticknor & Fields.

Halpern, S. (1993). *Migrations to solitude*. New York: Vintage.

Moss, R. (1981). *The I that is we*. Berkley, CA: Celestial Arts.

Rilke, R. M. (1984). *Letters to a young poet*. New York: Vintage.

Sarton, M. (1978). *A reckoning*. New York: W. W. Norton.

Satir, V. (1972). *Peoplemaking*. Palo Alto, CA: Science and Behavior.

Singer, J. (1990). *Seeing through the visible world*. San Francisco, CA: Harper.

Sullivan, T. J. (1998). Collaboration: A healthcare imperative. New York: McGraw Hill.

Von Post, I. (1996). Exploring ethical dilemmas in perioperative nursing practice through critical incidents. *Nursing Ethics, 3*, 236-249.

Weeks, D. (1994). *The eight essential steps to conflict resolution*. New York: Penguin.

Whyte, D. (2001). *Crossing the unknown sea: Work as a pilgrimage of identity*. New York: Riverhead.

# Chapter 49: MENTORING NEW FACULTY

Marilyn Herbert-Ashton, BSN, MS, RN, BC

*The average age of a registered nurse in the United States is 45.2 years. Approximately half of the 2.7 million registered nurses will reach retirement age within 15 years. Nurses in their 40s outnumber nurses in their 20s by a 4:1 ratio. Nursing faculty, typically older than other college professors, are reaching retirement age at a time when the number of nurses entering academia is declining. With this large exodus of experienced nurses and nursing faculty, it is imperative that these nurses pass on their knowledge, experience, and skills and serve as role models to inspire the next generation of nurses.*

*This chapter explores mentoring and why it is important to nursing. It also looks at the characteristics and roles of the mentor and the steps in creating a mentoring-mentality environment. The chapter concludes by offering some words of wisdom to the protégé.*
*– Linda Caputi and Lynn Engelmann*

## Introduction

The Department of Labor (2001) estimates that by the year 2010, the United States will need one million additional nurses. To achieve this, strong nursing faculty and staff development educators are essential to educate future nurses. The literature abounds as to how mentoring can facilitate personal growth and satisfaction for both the mentor and the mentee. The reader is encouraged to explore some of the ideas, presented in this chapter, to facilitate or develop mentoring relationships.

### Educational Philosophy

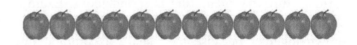

As teachers, we are mentors and role models to our students, colleagues, and clients. We must create a caring, open, and active learning environment. We must continuously challenge our students to strive for excellence and to seek knowledge. – Marilyn Herbert-Ashton

Mentoring can promote career commitment and career satisfaction – both important for retention of nurses. Business and industry have long used mentoring as a successful strategy for recruitment, development, and retention. Although the nursing profession has also employed mentoring programs, predominantly female professions such as nursing have not used mentoring to its potential to promote job satisfaction. The time is now to revisit and implement effective mentoring programs to more effectively recruit, nurture, and retain nurses in all areas of the nursing profession.

## What is a Mentor?

Some believe the term **mentor** derived from Greek mythology. In *The Odyssey*, Homer wrote that around 1200 BC, the goddess Athene assumed the identity of a mentor to guide and teach Telemachus, son of Odysseus. The word mentor appeared in 1750 in the *Oxford English Dictionary* as a noun. Since that time, mentoring has been defined in many ways. Following is a sample of these definitions:

- Huang and Lynch (1995) defined mentoring as "a two-way circular dance that provides opportunities for us to experience both giving and receiving each other's gifts without limitations and fears" (p. Preface xii).
- Murray (2001) defined mentoring as "a deliberate pairing of a more skilled person with a less skilled or less experienced one, with the mutually agreed goal of having the less skilled person grow and develop specific competencies" (p. Preface xiii).
- Merriam-Webster's Dictionary (2002) defines mentor as a "trusted counselor or guide."
- Vance and Olson (1998) defined mentoring as a "developmental, empowering, and nurturing relationship extending over time in which mutual sharing, learning, and growth occur in an atmosphere of respect, collegiality, and affirmation" (p. 5).

Mentoring takes on specific characteristics. For example, mentoring focuses on a relationship with one individual or group of individuals. Mentoring can be informal or formal. Informal mentoring is spontaneous. Examples of informal mentoring include an expert-novice, preceptor-student, or teacher-learner relationship. Individuals are often drawn together because they share a common interest or goal. Frequently there is a "chemistry" that draws the mentor and protégé together.

A formal mentoring program is a structured and planned version of an informal relationship. A mentor may be matched with a protégé based on factors such as a goal, need, or specialty area. Formal mentoring takes on a more structured and organized format. Formal mentoring has also been termed facilitated mentoring (Murray, 2001). Facilitated mentoring "is a structure and series of processes designed to create effective mentoring relationships; guide the desired behavior change of those involved; and evaluate results for the protégé, the mentors, and the organization" (p. 5).

## Mentoring in Nursing Education

In nursing education, there are a growing number of formal mentoring programs. Many nursing education programs involve alumni and faculty in developing and implementing mentoring programs.

Student nurses realize the value of mentoring. In 1996, the National Student Nurses Association (NSNA) passed a resolution in "support of the promotion, awareness, and development of mentorship programs" (p. 1). This resolution encouraged the development of mentorship programs in schools of nursing.

Sigma Theta Tau International, the honor society of nursing, also values mentoring. A 12-month program called The Chiron: The Mentor-Fellow Forum offers members the chance to work in a formalized fellowship program with a mentor to develop leadership skills. Nurses looking for development in a specific leadership area are guided by experienced mentors. Mentors can assist nurses to improve and advance their professional practice in all fields of nursing.

## Mentoring Characteristics

Often the terms **role model**, **sponsor**, **preceptor**, or **coach** have been confused with mentoring.

- A role model may have skills that are respected at a distance or who influences others in a positive way. In many cases this occurs without knowledge of the relationship from the role model.
- A sponsor may be an advocate for a group of people but the sponsored people may not know who is sponsoring them. For example, a sponsor could establish a fund to develop a mentoring program, but the individuals being sponsored might not be aware of the identity of the sponsor. The relationship is informal and may continue indefinitely.
- Preceptors are usually assigned to teach or assist learners in an organized program. An example is the nursing preceptor programs that are available in many clinical settings for newly graduated nurses.
- Although coaching is usually a characteristic of a mentor, mentoring is somewhat different. A coach can work with an individual or a group with a variety of skills/experiences at the same time. The relationship with the coach is frequently short term.

Although a mentor may have the characteristics of a role model, sponsor, preceptor, or coach, the role of the contemporary mentor is different. Currently the mentoring relationship takes on the form of a partnership rather than a patriarchy. Mentors develop a powerful, personalized, intense, long-term partnership with the protégé, which provides for challenges as well as give and take between the mentor and protégé.

As the essence of nursing is caring and nurturing others, mentors in all areas of nursing must convey a caring and nurturing attitude. Mentors see the best in others. They support and encourage even as they offer challenges. Because mentors believe the protégés will be successful, they are committed to the protégés and motivated to maintain a relationship with them. Excellent interpersonal skills, especially listening skills, are extremely important. Mentors are positive and open-minded and provide varying perspectives on the protégé's performance.

As team members, mentors collaborate and share their knowledge and expertise. They are experts in their field and professionally involved. The mentor ultimately sets the tone of the relationship, remembering what it was like to be a protégé.

## Roles of the Mentor

When considering the roles of the mentor, it is important to realize that the relationship with the protégé is reciprocal – both are responsible for maintaining the relationship. Ultimately, the mentor provides for guidance, direction, growth, and support. To meet these objectives, the mentor serves in the following roles:

- Coach: Mentors serve as coaches in demonstrating how to carry out a task or activity.
- Facilitator: Mentors are facilitators creating opportunities for protégés to use new skills.
- Advisor/counselor: Mentors serve as advisors or counselors, assisting protégés to explore the consequences of potential decisions.
- Liaison: Mentors network with other experts when their own experience is insufficient to meet protégés' needs.

Mentors serve in these roles by challenging the protégés' views, sharing various perspectives, and encouraging the protégés to examine various ideas and ways of thinking.

## Creating a Mentoring Mentality

It has been noted that mentoring promotes all of the following: career advancement, work satisfaction, improved productivity, increased self-worth, preparation for leadership positions, and strengthening of the profession. Mentoring is important for the transition from student to novice, as well as for enhancing career development. Vance (2000) stated that healthcare professionals must "adopt a 'mentoring mentality' wherever we find ourselves" (p. 2). It is critical that a mentoring mentality environment be created. The following are mentoring mentality strategies that can be incorporated in all areas of nursing, including the classroom and clinical setting.

## *Mentoring Attitude*

Being an effective mentor begins with the mentor. A mentor should take the time to examine and inventory strengths, talents, areas of expertise, and areas for growth. Mentors should ask themselves the following questions:

- Have I shared my talents and skills with others? If not, why?
- Are there areas in which I can improve?
- Do I have a mentor? Mentors need mentors to help them grow and develop professionally.

Individually, mentors can engage in the following to promote professional growth:

- Participating in programs that promote personal development.
- Becoming involved in professional and community organizations.
- Continuing to learn about other cultures; travel and meet people outside of the profession to enhance self-development and broaden personal experiences.

The attitude of the mentor is positive and open. Working effectively with diverse groups as team players is a key ingredient to developing a mentoring attitude. The emphasis is on a spirit of collaboration, not competition. Writing goals, then developing, implementing, and evaluating action plans are all part of the mentoring attitude.

Mentors have a "can do" attitude. They believe in themselves and have respect for their own talents and potentials. This is a confident, not cocky, attitude. This confidence derives from a thorough and honest self-appraisal. Mentors must first believe in themselves before expecting protégés to believe in them.

## *Understanding Personality Styles*

In order to assist others, mentors must first understand themselves. Personality profiling is a means by which to gain this understanding. Tests such as Myers-Briggs assist in identifying strengths and weaknesses and are often used in career counseling. There are other models that take less time to administer but still give individuals helpful information about themselves and how they may be perceived by others.

The secret to getting along with others is to identify others' needs and be willing to meet those needs. Personality profiling can help identify those needs. These measures have been identified as effective tools for promoting team building and managing conflict.

Personality profiling can also be used as part of the curriculum in developing a mentoring program. These profiles give people insight into how they are perceived by others and provide opportunities to improve weaknesses. As a cautionary note, personality profiles should not be used to stereotype; each person is an individual (refer to chapters in this book titled Learning Styles and Teaching Styles, by Sandy Forrest, for further discussion on this topic).

### *Walking and Talking Mentoring*

In the present-day dynamic healthcare environment, walking and talking mentoring is a quick yet effective means to mentor individuals. Walking and talking begins by acting as a servant leader. A servant leader **serves** others and asks what they can do to help or assist. Frequently, it simply involves listening to a particular situation and providing input or feedback to the individual. Walking and talking mentoring uses "impact moments." Impact moments are unplanned situations or occurrences that provide opportunities to teach and influence protégés. Frequently, impact moments occur in the clinical area where a mentor can have a positive impact on a protégé by addressing the situation in the current moment. For example, the student is about to make a medication error. The teacher working with the student uses that impact moment to discuss how to prevent that error in the future. The situation is addressed immediately rather than later. This method of mentoring is less time consuming as situations are addressed at the time of occurrence and protégé receives immediate feedback and learns from the situation. Walking and talking mentoring can be an everyday occurrence and does not need to be formalized.

### *Ask Questions*

Questioning can be an effective means for mentors to gain insight into the thinking of protégés. Mentors should ask open-ended questions such as, "Tell me more about . . ." Questions need to be clear, concise, direct, and easily understood by the protégés. Questions should also be intriguing and thought provoking to encourage protégés to use critical thinking skills and to look at the whole picture. Intriguing questions encourage creativity, innovation, critical thinking, and thinking "outside the box."

## *Become a Storyteller*

Mentors are often storytellers. Stories often have a greater impact than **telling** or lecturing. Stories encourage retention of information because the main points of a story are often remembered. Stories also provide insight and stimulate critical thinking

Stories can be easily incorporated into both the classroom and clinical setting. For example, acting out a scenario in the classroom is an exciting way to highlight the major points protégés or learners need to understand. Several approaches can be used to act out stories in the classroom. Faculty can:

- Collaborate with the drama department to act out a particular story for the class.
- Dress up and act out a particular scenario.
- Create an ongoing audiotape or videotape of a "soap opera" that focuses on a specific healthcare topic.

Regardless of which approach is taken, remember that the protégés tend to recall the major points of a story.

## *Five-Minute Mentoring*

Vance (2000) discussed five-minute mentoring as a means to provide mentoring when time is short. Five-minute mentoring is a quick fix, informal form of mentoring that can be used anywhere. This type of mentoring can be as simple as providing a few words of encouragement or guidance. It can also take the form of just listening to someone. Sometimes just listening or providing encouragement can have a major impact. These seemingly little things tend to accumulate over time and can have a major influence on retention.

## *Mentored Journaling*

Mentored journaling provides the ability to guide the thinking skills and learning of students. The mentored journal forms a synergistic partnership between a novice student and expert faculty. The mentored journal is a mentoring process that can be used as a first exposure to mentoring. From this process, learners are able to appreciate the value of experienced faculty providing assistance in their professional as well as personal lives.

The mentored journal has a clear purpose for both learners and faculty – giving the learners the opportunity to "think out loud" within a mentored environment. The focus of the teachers' feedback is to promote critical thinking and growth of the learners. Journals are a communication tool shared between faculty and learners. The entries can be both personal and professional, using a dialogue format. Learners are encouraged to be creative in their approach to journal writing to promote their uniqueness.

Faculty mentors use mentored journals to support, challenge, and provide vision to learners as they focus on linking theory and research to practice. Learners must consistently take time to write in the journal throughout the term, culminating with an evaluative conclusion at the end of the course.

Bilinski (2002) used the Circles of Meaning Model to promote critical thinking and reflection in mentored journaling. In this model, students are asked to explore and analyze experiences, situations, feelings, and hunches. They seek connections, identify possible solutions, and evaluate those solutions.

Grading the mentored journal is controversial. Biliniski (2002) suggested assigning a portion of the final grade, i.e., 10%, as a compromise to grading versus not grading the journal.

### *Group Mentoring*

With the aging workforce and shortage of nurses, there may soon be a shortage of mentors. To address this shortage of mentors, some members of the business world have developed group mentoring as an alternative to traditional one-to-one mentoring. Group mentoring places an experienced individual or leader with a group of four to six protégés. With the mentor as the facilitator, the group members exchange ideas, analyze issues, and receive feedback and guidance as a group. The group in essence becomes a learning group. This approach provides additional opportunities for the group members to learn from each other as well as from the mentor.

The mentor or group leader continues to offer counsel, guidance, encouragement, support, and feedback. The mentor asks questions and makes suggestions, becoming an ally and advocate for the group in promoting professional growth. With the guidance of the mentor or group leader, the members have the opportunity to explore pertinent issues and increase their ability to engage in innovative thinking. With the increasing use of interdisciplinary teams in health care, group mentoring can also provide experience for protégés in working in a group setting, learning all the dynamics of the group process and team building.

Group mentoring should be considered if more than one new faculty member needs to be oriented and there is a shortage of mentors. Group mentoring may also be effective when faculty serve as mentors for a group of students.

As with all methods of mentoring, guidelines need to be established. One mentor working with a group of protégés can be overwhelming for the mentor. Guidelines can help keep the mentoring experience a pleasant one for the mentor as well as the protégé.

## *Internet Mentoring*

Internet mentoring is a form of mentoring that is becoming increasingly popular in health care. This mentoring is available 24 hours a day, seven days a week, and can be an invaluable tool, considering the present milieu in health care, specifically increased workloads, and decreased staff. Internet mentoring gives students or protégés opportunities to ask questions and receive guidance more expeditiously than in the traditional mentoring models. Two nurses, Linda Anderson and Mark Carroway (1997), together developed the internet mentoring program available through the NursingNet website. For easy launching this website about internet mentoring is located on the CD accompanying this book. Simply launch your internet browser, put the CD-ROM in the in the drive, go to Chapter 49 on the CD, and then click on the website. address. Mentoring opportunities are available at this site through e-mail or chat rooms. Other healthcare-related websites that offer mentoring programs provide students with opportunities to ask questions through a mailing list from which students may receive responses from several mentors. Students may also communicate with specialists to further enhance their knowledge.

Some suggestions for online mentors include:
- Answer questions quickly.
- Set parameters regarding the role of a mentor.
- Give feedback promptly.
- Recognize that learning is a two way process (Federwisch, 1997).

To avoid potential misunderstandings or offenses, both the mentors and the protégés need to apply the principles of **netiquette**. Netiquette provides guidelines for proper communication via e-mail. Refer to the chapter in this book titled *The Cyberstudent*, by Gail Baumlein, for more information on netiquette.

## *Mentoring Programs for Nursing Students*

As the healthcare industry and the nursing profession come to grips with workforce shortages, recruitment, and retention issues, many nursing schools and healthcare systems are developing student nurse mentoring programs. One such collaborative program, which began in 2001, is the Adopt-a-Student-Nurse program developed by Carilion Health System (2002) in Roanoke, Virginia. Students preparing for their senior year are paired with an experienced nurse in a client care setting. The mentors are volunteers who receive formalized training on mentoring and the Adopt-a-Student-Nurse program. The nurse mentors are chosen to be mentors by their managers because they possess qualities that exemplify what excellent nursing is. Each nurse mentors a student one-on-one during an initial six-week assignment, then periodically throughout that student's senior year. If a enroll in two six-week experiences in specialty areas of their choice. During this time, students are considered employees of Carilion and receive salaries. The mentors keep in touch with the students throughout their senior year via e-mail or telephone.

Nursing administration at Carilion considers the Adopt-a-Student-Nurse mentoring program successful based on positive feedback from the students, nursing staff, and nursing faculty involved in the program. Many nurse mentors have stated that they felt rejuvenated because they were contributing to the nursing profession.

Other nursing programs have established similar programs in which students earn college credit for clinical instruction by preceptors or clinical nursing instructors. Additional student mentoring opportunities may be developed through NSNA. Many nursing schools are also developing student mentoring programs with assistance from their nursing alumni.

## *Faculty Mentoring Programs*

Many colleges and universities are developing mentoring programs for new faculty throughout all academic areas. Kent State University, College of Nursing, offers a voluntary mentoring program in which new faculty are coupled with experienced faculty. Several group meetings are held throughout the year for those participants in the program. Additionally, all faculty have the opportunity for peer review of their teaching.

When considering developing faculty mentoring programs, some topics to consider include:
- Adjusting to academic life.
- The appointment process.
- Classroom and clinical instruction.
- Evaluation.
- Problem solving student issues.

## Words of Wisdom to the Protégé

To begin the process, protégés must accept responsibility to:
- Know what they need to master.
- Remember that the relationship is give and take.

Protégés are obligated to apply what they have learned and to appreciate the time their mentor spends with them. After the formal mentoring relationship has ended, protégés may want to keep in touch with their mentors and continue sharing new experiences. When this happens, mentors continue to grow and learn from the relationship. Protégés who have had a positive mentoring experience are likely to serve as mentors themselves, strengthening and reinforcing the use of mentoring in nursing.

## Summary

Mentoring is vital to the future of nursing and nursing education. Nurses must be willing to share their knowledge and expertise. It is an investment in nursing's future. As professionals, nurses accept the responsibility to mentor others – to continue to pass the torch to the next generation. Vance (2000) stated that "we must acknowledge the natural human need to offer and accept mentoring and that it is our priceless gift to each other" (p. 4).

## Learning Activities

Take some time to consider your own mentoring experiences. Answer the following questions:

- Did you seek a mentor as a student nurse or as a newly licensed nurse?
- What qualities do you look for in a mentor?
- If you have had a mentor, was your mentor helpful?
- What was your experience as the protégé?
- What are your skills, strengths, and talents?
- What are your mentoring abilities?
- Have you ever mentored someone? If so, what were the outcomes? Is there anything you might do differently in the future?
- What skills do you need to develop your mentoring abilities?
- What can you do to develop your attitude or skills as a mentor?
- If your institution does not have a mentoring program for students or faculty, what steps can be taken to develop a program? What would the program look like?

### References

Anderson, C. A., & Carroway, M. (1997). *Nursing Student to Nursing Leader: The Critical Path to Leadership Development.* Albany, NY: Delmar Publishers.

Bilinski, H. (January/February 2002). The mentored journal. *Nurse Educator,* 27(1), 37-41.

Bureau of Labor Statistics, Department of Labor, Statistics issued 12/12/01.

Carilion Health System. Interview with Pat Conway-Morana, Sr. Vice President, Nursing Services and Teresa Smith, Nursing New Hire Coordinator, Nursing Services. June 11, 2002.

Huang, C.A., & Lynch, J. (1995). *Mentoring: The Two of Giving and Receiving Wisdom.* New York: Harper.

Murray, Margo. (2001). *Beyond the Myths of Mentoring.* 2nd ed. San Francisco: CA: Jossey- Bass.

Kaye, B., & Jacobson B. (April 1995). Mentoring: A group guide. *Training and Development.* 49(4): 22-27.

Kent State University College of Nursing—Scholarship in Teaching, Faculty Mentoring Program. Available at http://www.dept.kent.edu/nursing/about/PeerRevi.htm Accessed July 4, 2002.

Merriam-Webster Dictionary Web site: http://www.m-w/cgi-bin/dictionary. Accessed July 4, 2002.

National Student Nurses Association. (1996). *Resolution in Support of the Promotion and Awareness, and Development of Mentorship Programs.* New Orleans, LA: National Student Nurses' Association, House of Delegates.

Nurses for a Healthier Tomorrow: Facts about the Nursing Shortage, Sigma Theta Tau International. http://www.nursesource.org/facts_shortage.html.

Vance, C. Mentoring at the Edge of Chaos. *Nursing Spectrum.* http://community.nursingspectrum.com/MagazineArticles/article.cfm?AID=2023. Accessed July 4, 2002.

Vance, C., & Olson, R. (1998). *The Mentor Connection in Nursing.* New York: Springer Publishing Co.


## Bibliography

Carey, S.J., & Campbell, S.T. (1994). Preceptor, mentor, and sponsor roles. *Journal of Nursing Administration,* 24(12), 39-48.

Federwsich, A. The internet gives mentoring programs a boost. *NurseWeek.* Available at http://www.nurseweek.com/features/97-11/mentor2.html. Accessed July 4, 2002.

Ruiz, M. (Third Quarter 2001). How to get the most out of your mentor. *Sigma Theta Tau International Honor Society of Nursing Excellence in Clinical Practice,* 2(3).

Restifo, V. Partnership: Making the most of mentoring. *Nursing Spectrum.* http://nsweb.nursingspectrum.com/ce/ce190.htm Accessed July 4, 2002. www.mentorsforum.co.uk/cOL1/tools/facts/Sheet1.htm Accessed July 4, 2002.

Vance, C. (1982). The mentor connection. *Journal of Nursing Administration,* 12, (4) 7-13.

# Chapter 50: EXPANDING YOUR ROLE: BECOMING A NURSE ENTREPRENEUR

### Linda Caputi, MSN, EdD, RN and Dave Johnson, MA, DNS, RN, CS, LCSW, LMFT

*Picture this: It is faculty in-service day, and you just sat through eight hours listening to a consultant talk about a very important topic for your faculty. As you are driving home, you think, "I could do that! Sure, that consultant was good and knew a lot about that topic, but I know about _____ topic. I could be a consultant!" I say, "Yes! You can!" Especially if you have just finished writing a master's thesis or a doctoral dissertation, you can bet you know more about that topic than almost anyone, even your thesis/dissertation committee. And that's the truth! – Linda Caputi*

## Introduction

This chapter provides an overview of entrepreneurship. Dr. Caputi describes the general steps in putting together a small business then Dr. Johnson shares his experiences as a successful nurse consultant. The goal of this chapter is to provide insights of the lived experiences of the authors for the purpose of providing support and mentoring for all those who have creative ideas waiting to unfold.

### Educational Philosophy

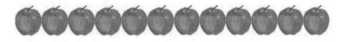

My educational philosophy is succinct: Give the best educational experience possible. I feel faculty should continuously challenge themselves to provide creative, interesting, and sound education – students soon learn that education doesn't have to be boring; they become self-motivated, enthusiastic, and interested…..learning then follows. – Linda Caputi

Life is a journey of many lessons to be learned. As a teacher, my role is to be a facilitator of learning whether in the classroom, corporate, or individual setting. I appreciate having mentors and being a mentor for others in this process. Often, the lessons to be learned are difficult or challenging and being a teacher is both a responsibility and an honor. – Dave Johnson

## Reasons for Starting a Business

Starting a business as a nurse entrepreneur can be exciting and, at the same time, a lot of work. Why would a nurse leave a secure, safe, steady, full-time paycheck to start a business with an unknown future? Many nurse entrepreneurs do not leave their full-time positions. They are full-time employees and part-time small business owners. However, many eventually turn their part-time small business into a full-time job.

But what drives nurses to go into business? Some of the reasons nurses have started small businesses include:

- They have a talent, art, or expertise they want to share with others.
- They want/need to supplement their income.
- They aim to establish a business they can continue after retirement from their full-time position.
- They desire the chance to control their destiny.
- They want to travel.
- They want to enhance networking with other professionals.
- They are ready for a change.

There are probably many more reasons for starting a small business. Consider what your reasons might be. The reason for starting your business is what will sustain your motivation and drive to succeed over the long term.


## The Three Dimensions of the Entrepreneur

Every successful entrepreneur has three dimensions (Gerber, 1995). Consider these dimensions and your capacity for each as you begin your adventure. Figure 50.1 shows the main responsibilities of each of these three dimensions.

Figure 50.1 - The Three Dimensions of the Entrepreneur

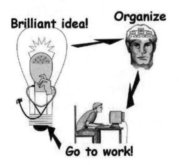

**Idea generator.** The first dimension is the creative, idea-generating person who has a wonderful idea just waiting to come to life. In fact, there may be many new ideas scampering around in the entrepreneur's mind. This is the start, where it begins. These ideas are often vague, not well-defined, but very exciting.

**Organizer.** The second dimension is the organizer. The organizer takes the idea and converts it into a working idea – something that can be realized, something that can produce a deliverable. Just what is the deliverable? The deliverable may be a product – a book or series of books, software programs, or educational videos. Or the deliverable may be a service – a public speaking business, legal nurse consulting, or a nurse staffing agency.

**Worker.** Thomas Edison once said that genius is 1% inspiration and 99% perspiration. This applies to the worker dimension. The worker makes the idea happen and, in the process, dreams of new ideas that are passed back to the idea-generating dimension, and the whole cycle repeats. In fact, success is most assured when ideas are churning for the next project at the same time the current project is just beginning. Many entrepreneurs are successful because they are able to concurrently handle many projects, all in different stages of development.

Many ideas that pass through the organizer dimension fade and die in the worker dimension. This is not to say that the worker is lazy. Many factors can prevent the creative soul from completing the work required to see the idea to fruition.

These three dimensions have been described in extremely general terms. Consider each of these and their related roles as you read through the rest of this chapter.


### Types of Nurse Entrepreneurial Businesses

Now that you have decided that you have good reason to start a small business and that you have what it takes–ideas, organization, and hard work–think about the type of business that interests you. Many types of businesses can be considered by a nurse entrepreneur. But which is best for you? Take a look at:

- http://www.nursefriendly.com/nursing/directory/nursingentrepreneurs/nurse.owned. businesses.nursing.entrepreneurs.by.state.htm  This site lists businesses owned-and-operated by nurses in the United States.
- http://www.nursefriendly.com/nursing/directory/nursingentrepreneurs/canadian. owned.businesses.nursing.entrepreneurs.htm This site lists nurse-owned-and-operated businesses in Canada.

These lists can overwhelm you or they can spark ideas and ignite the entrepreneur inside.

# Learning about the Business

One of the best ways to learn about what others have done to start and succeed in an entrepreneurial adventure is to network. There is much encouragement and psychological benefit to talking with other entrepreneurs. Networking can be done face-to-face or via the internet.

Face-to-face encounters can be local. Find other nurses near you who are owners of small businesses. Talk with people who are currently or were formerly employed with the institution in which you work. You may be surprised to find others who are involved in such activities.

Local networking also involves nonnurse entities. For example, a local group may offer assistance with starting a small business. Also, if your plans involve public speaking, attending meetings of your local speakers' bureaus may be helpful.

To expand your face-to-face networking, attend professional conferences. Many of the speakers at these conferences are also independent consultants or small-business owners. Most of these people would love to talk with you and share their experiences.

Most professional conferences also have areas where vendors exhibit. These exhibit spaces are often reasonably priced so provide an attractive venue for small-business owners. Visit this area and talk with these creative nurses about their businesses and how they got started. Personally, I remember a conference a number of years back. I was tending to my exhibit table when a budding entrepreneur stopped by and asked me lots of questions about my business. I enjoyed several hours discussing my venture. He was extremely honest and shared with me that he was planning to start a similar business. At this same conference the following year, there he was with his new company, exhibiting his products. Presently, five years after our first meeting, his entrepreneurial dream is an award-winning educational software company. I quietly smile to myself when I hear other nurses speak positively about the software from that company.

The internet can also be used for networking. To start, visit the National Nurses in Business site at http://nnba.net/

# Getting Down to Business

Now that it is apparent that nurses are very creative and capable of starting their own businesses, how does one actually get started? Let's take a look.

### *Start as a Consultant*

As discussed earlier, there are many types of nurse-owned businesses. If the company produces a product and requires a financial investment, a detailed business plan is needed before eliciting financial backing. This type of business can be very complex but very doable.

Many nurses start by establishing themselves as consultants. This requires less up-front money and can be run from a home office. Because a consulting business is less complex but nonetheless exciting, we will use consulting as the example throughout the remainder of this chapter.

Just as the nursing process starts with assessment, so does the establishment of a consulting business. Here is where the idea dimension goes to work. Assess what you know, your strengths, and what you have to offer others. You may wonder what kinds of topics you would be qualified to offer as a consultant. Take an honest look and think about the following:

- Positions you have held in your career.
- Your interests as you pursued your educational goals.
- Your main interests in your current position.

For example, during your nursing career, you functioned as a manager, perhaps a unit manager in a hospital, and as nursing faculty, you now teach leadership courses. Your consulting business might offer solutions to management problems in healthcare organizations.

Another example involves test construction. As a nursing faculty, you have worked hard on learning to write valid, reliable, critical-thinking test items. You develop a test blueprint that is the envy of all your colleagues. Your test statistics are admirable. You attend workshops on item writing and read all the latest information. In fact, you have published a journal article or a chapter in a book. Your new consulting business offers a service that analyzes a nursing program's tests and provides assistance to faculty with writing test items.

You do not need to be an expert, but you do need experience and an interest in staying current in the topic of your consulting business. You also need confidence in yourself and your ability to offer this advice and service. Think of it as mentoring new faculty or employees. You share tips, advice, and techniques that work. In so doing, you will also learn.

It is important to know and feel comfortable with the idea that at times your clients may offer you information. I have had the personal experience of consulting and learning from my clients. In one instance, I was delivering a presentation on instructional strategies. The faculty were highly positive, receptive, and enthusiastic. Throughout the day they continuously offered wonderful ideas of their own. At one point, I stopped my presentation and stated that I was very impressed with this group of creative teachers. I shared with them that I believed they were doing a wonderful job and probably did not really need me!

They all smiled and said, "Oh, no. We need you. You're our catalyst for generating our own ideas!" I have since used many of their ideas in my own teaching.

## *Organize Your Ideas*

Now the organizer dimension takes over. Recognize your talents. Be very specific about what it is you know, what you will offer in your consulting business, and to whom you will offer your services. Define yourself and your business.

## *The Worker Dimension Takes Charge*

Once you know who you are and the scope of your consulting business, you can now get to work. There are many aspects of running a business. Many excellent books can help you with these specifics. The following is offered as a minimal list of important issues to consider.

- Construct a business plan. A business plan can be very simple or very complex. A simple business plan includes:
  - A thorough description of your consulting business.
  - Goals for a specified period of time, such as two to five years.
  - Strategies for marketing your business, marketing goals, and how to achieve those goals.
  - A list of potential clients.
  - Projected start-up costs for equipment, marketing, etc.
  - A list of capital equipment, including computers and other office equipment.
  - A description of any loans or financing (Colorado Business Resource Guide, 2003).
- Establish your business address. Many nurse consultants quite capably run their business from their homes. A home business can have both advantages and disadvantages. The advantages include saving time by eliminating the commute to work and saving money for rent. The disadvantages include giving up some living space for the office and always being at work. One very successful nurse with a small business shared with me that she never works on weekends. She closes the door to her home office on Friday evening and does not open it until Monday morning. This helps her cope with the "always being at work" feeling.
- Market your business. It does not matter how wonderful your idea is if no one knows about it. Two factors to consider when developing a marketing plan are exposure and cost. Your marketing should yield the most exposure for the dollars you invest. Some ways to market include the following:
  - Conference exhibits. This is perhaps a great way to start your marketing campaign. The cost of renting an exhibit space can range from a few hundred to a few thousand

dollars. Starting small may be your preference. The least expensive exhibits involve a draped table to display information about your product or service. You are present during exhibit hours talking with conference participants about your business. This is a nice way to start and provides direct feedback from potential clients about what you have to offer. It is important to have print materials and your business card to distribute to potential clients.

- Referrals. Most small businesses are limited in scope and their client base is drawn from a small segment of the profession. This small segment may have a highly extensive network that shares information about products and services. Once you have a few satisfied customers, referrals from within this client-based network becomes a very powerful marketing force for your business.

- Direct mail. To market without leaving home, try direct mail. You will need to design marketing materials that very clearly define who you are and what you have to offer. These materials should command attention, interest, desire, and action from your potential clients.

- Advertisement in publications. Become familiar with the publications your clients are reading. Although advertising in some publications may be expensive, you must weigh the cost with the number of clients who will be reached with your advertisement.

- Articles, chapters, and books. Being published helps establish a reputation in your area. Writing articles, chapters in books, or even an entire book itself can be well worth the time and effort. Talk with editors of both print and online publications about your ideas for articles. Some nurse entrepreneurs contribute a monthly column to professional journals.

• Develop a contract. When a client hires you to consult or perform a service, it is extremely important to have a signed contract. The contract is a clearly constructed, formal agreement. This contract prevents misunderstandings and disappointments. Figure 50.2 shows a simple contract with sample information to include in a contract. Use this only as a sample. The details of your contract will be specific to your business.

### *Making Your Business a Legal Entity*

Once you begin to experience success in your business, you may want to consider establishing a legal entity. Setting up a legal business entity is not difficult. You may hire a lawyer or an accountant to give you advice. But you may also complete and file all the papers yourself. Contact your state agency for information on the requirements in your state.

There are six legal structures to consider:

Figure 50.2 - Sample Contract

---

**ABC Consulting**
{Date}

Name of Event:   **State University Workshop on Test Item Writing**

Workshop Date(s):

Contact Person:   {State University representative.}

Thank you for inviting me to conduct this workshop.  The workshop will run from 8 am until 5 pm on the above date.  The workshop fee is \$ _____.  The workshop fee covers all materials for 15 participants.  Please add \$50.00 for each additional participant.

**State University** will pay {your name or company name} the agreed-upon fee as well as travel/accommodation expenses.  These include the following:

1.   Round trip air fare from _____ to _____.
2.   Transportation to and from each airport.
3.   One night lodging.
4.   Meals, including dinner on _____ and lunch, breakfast, and dinner on _____.

Air fare and hotel to be arranged and paid directly by **State University**.  Other expenses will be paid after incurred and submission of an expense report to **State University**.
Cancellation clause: Both {your company} and **State University** have the option to cancel this agreement within 72 hours of the scheduled date of service.

*By my signature below, I accept these conditions on behalf of the above-named organization.*

_____        _____
Signature                    Date            Signature                        Date
{Your name or company name}          **State University**
{address}                    {Representative's name}
{phone and e-mail}

---

- Sole proprietorship.
- Partnership.
- Regular corporation (C-Corp).
- S-corporation.
- Limited liability company (LLC).
- Registered limited liability partnership.

These business structures vary in terms of liability, taxation, number of shareholders, and other concerns. To determine which structure best fits your needs, start with your state website. Here you will find helpful information. For example, the Illinois website at http: //illinoisbiz.biz/bus/step_by_step.html#3d describes these six types of business structures.

## *Staying Positive*

As with all ventures, running your small business may be discouraging at times. You may feel overwhelmed or self-conscious, especially if evaluations from your last client were not as positive as you expected. Know that everyone has had these experiences. The true professional takes it on the chin, learns from the experience, and changes the plan for future clients.

Sustaining motivation in your work, especially during down times, can be very challenging. This is why a compelling reason for starting the business is so important. Hang on to that reason and work through the down times.

Running a small business can also be a very lonely experience, especially if you are the only employee. There are times when you will spend months working by yourself in your home office, preparing for future clients. Remember the joys and rewards from experiences with past clients. In a conspicuous place, keep positive evaluations from previous experiences and read them often. These will help keep you enthusiastic and motivated. With hard work and dedication, those positive experiences will happen again and again.

## The Story of a Successful Nurse Consultant

This chapter has presented many ideas, guidelines, and hopefully inspiration to all aspiring entrepreneurs. A conversation with a successful nurse consultant can crystallize these thoughts and demonstrate their application.

Let's meet Dave Johnson. Dr. Johnson is a professor of nursing at the University of Saint Francis in Fort Wayne, Indiana. He is also a clinical nurse specialist in adult mental health nursing, a licensed clinical social worker, and a licensed marriage and family therapist. Last, he is a nurse consultant. Following is an account in his own words of how he established himself as a nurse consultant.

### *Introduction*

Although I had been teaching nursing for several years as an adjunct faculty member, in 1990, I decided to pursue my passion of teaching full time at the University of Saint Francis in Fort Wayne, Indiana. Having worked as a nursing administrator for a 10-year period, my role transition to full-time academia resulted in approximately a 50% salary cut. Married and with five children, I recognized the need to supplement my university salary.

Consulting became the tool that allowed me to pursue my academic career yet support my family with a salary comparable to what I was earning as an administrator.

The challenge before me was how to develop a consulting practice deemed worthy by clients. In my previous position as an administrator, I had helped establish an employee assistance program (EAP) with Parkview Behavior Health in Fort Wayne, Indiana. As a clinical nurse specialist in psychiatric mental health nursing, I identified systems thinking and processes for helping individuals, families, and corporations cope with change, conflict, and stress.

My consulting practice was taking shape. I conceptualized my new consulting practice around the notion that therapy, administration, and teaching skills were transferable to both healthcare and non-healthcare corporations. I negotiated a fee-splitting arrangement with Parkview Behavioral to maximize profits for my time and experience.

### A Multifaceted Consulting Business

My beginning idea was taking shape, and it grew as I incorporated additional dimensions. In addition to providing clinical counseling services as part of the EAP, my consulting practice now includes:
- Employee assistance programming consulting.
- Public-speaking and management training.
- Corporate teambuilding and management coaching.

### Employee Assistance Programs (EAPs)

EAPs assist individuals and companies with stress and change. This counseling program addresses individual issues of marital and family discord; conflict; drug and alcohol abuse; financial stress and bankruptcy; domestic violence; and workplace issues. Most EAPs operate on a capitated fee structure whereby the company pays a fixed amount of dollars per employee per year regardless of utilization. Employees and their immediate family members then have access to services with a specified number of sessions allotted per calendar year. Various rate plans are available from a one- to two-session assessment and referral model through a six- to eight-session brief treatment model. Individuals who have needs beyond the scope of the EAP are referred to community mental-health providers and their mental-health insurance benefits accessed. Although most individuals who access the EAP do so on their own volition, a management referral structure is established for mandatory referrals of individuals whose work performance has declined or who are in violation of company policy. Violations may include such issues of absenteeism, harassment, performance decline, or positive drug screens.

The EAP client extends beyond the individual employee and includes management and human resources. A key contact relationship is established within each company for orienting employees to the program, review of utilization reports, and ongoing identification and management of company needs. Having established trusting relationships with key contacts, additional corporate needs can be identified, such as management coaching, teambuilding, strategic planning, and motivational workshops. These consultation services are provided at a discounted rate for companies that have a current contract for EAP services and are perceived as value-added programming. I liken the model to the cell phone or cable television industry. Customers buy a base-priced service, but additional options and add-ons are available. The EAP became a launching pad for development of other corporate consulting services. For additional resources on employee assistance, see the employee assistance professional's association web page at www.eapassn.org

### Public Speaking and Management Training

Going "corporate" is often a minor adaptation to an existing role with a creative twist, a marketing strategy, and an edge of confidence. Public speaking and management training are two areas that are closely connected and were easily transformed from my university teaching skill set. Conceptualizing the classroom as a learning laboratory, mastering the art of storytelling, and using props and process groups launched my teaching to a presentation level, commanding $125 to $1,000 per presentation hour.

***The learning laboratory and repackaging of skills.*** I love to teach, as I am certain that most faculty and staff development instructors do as well. Engaging students in the process of learning and viewing each class as a learning laboratory has helped launch this side of my consulting practice. The classroom becomes a laboratory, not only in the sense that learners entertain new ideas and experiment with new knowledge but in the sense that I am a facilitator of learning. What can I do to make the learning lab more fun? Efficient? Effective? How can each contact with students in the lab stand alone as an event yet build upon other experiences to facilitate comprehensive learning outcomes? My goal is to have enough energy and passion for the topic generated in the classroom for students to experience a "WOW" . . . I want to WOW them! WOW with new insights, applications, and passion to move forward in their careers as nurses with the additional information gained in the course.

Transforming the classroom into a learning laboratory requires the expertise of the teacher to "repackage" the content for use with other audiences. For example, a stress and mental-health lecture for nursing students can be transformed into a module of self-care for staff nurses experiencing job burnout and overload. Or a leadership and management course taught at the university can be transformed into a four-module lunch-and-learn series offered to corporations for new managers. The contemporary movie snippets that are used at the start of many mental health nursing classes to amplify course themes get reused for a continuing education course for advance practice nurses and therapists interested in "cinematherapy" as a methodology for creative therapy.

*Mastering the art of storytelling.* Along with using the classroom as a learning laboratory is practicing the art of story-telling. Students love to hear stories, and nurse educators have many to tell. The anecdotes and case scenarios can be woven and adapted to the classroom content. Becoming a masterful storyteller not only makes classes more interesting and invigorating to the techno-frenzied, dependent, and easily bored student, but becoming masterful with this art transforms a good teacher in the classroom to a polished presenter in the corporate world. Stories and anecdotes are more likely to be remembered than abstract or sophisticated information. Telling a story is one method of impressing an audience with the brilliance and creativity of the speaker. Professional presenters become adept at weaving a number of stories into each presentation. Once memorized, the story can be reformatted and adapted to meet the needs of various audiences both in the classroom and in the corporate training arena. The storyteller's delivery, passion, and emotion for these stories are as important, or even more important than the actual content when making the transition from the college classroom to the corporate classroom. Success in the college classroom is measured with learning outcomes; success in the corporate setting is measured by WOW, which includes being "invited" to present this and other topics to other corporations and at conventions or seminars.

*Using props and experiential processes.* Students and audiences love to make sense of experiential processes and games. The tools that transform classrooms into creative learning environments are readily adapted to corporate settings. Believing in and experimenting with these tools and experiential processes is part of this transformation. One should also recognize that creating meaning and projecting insights onto a prop is psychologically rewarding to both the teacher and students. For me, this is analogous to the Rorschach test. The inkblots become the creative tools and props identified by the presenter. The projections, connections, and insights made by students and workshop attendees are the psychological rewards!

For example, in teaching team dynamics in a nursing leadership class, I use a coin tapping game. Each student is given a penny and is asked to replicate a pattern of tapping that I lead them in doing. I use a fairly simple pattern. Once the whole group is tapping in unison, I begin varying the tapping sequence, slightly at first, then more rapidly. Students become a little stressed or annoyed with my pattern changing but quickly adapt. I continue the process for about 90 seconds. I then give instructions to the participants to start a second set of taps but, this time, to create their own tapping sequence. I invite two students to be observers and just listen and not tap.

Following the second exercise of individual taps, I begin to process with the class how this exercise is similar to the work team. Students create meaning and often suggest content covered in the readings, classroom discussion, or personal experiences from the work setting. They construct that tapping in unison was easy and that as humans, we are readily adaptable to change. Some may note that rapid change and frequent change is stressful or anxiety provoking. Usually someone will add that going over the same pattern a number of times was initially fun but became boring, redundant, or irritating. Someone from the class identifies that watching movements and nonverbal behavior was just as important as the verbal cues preparing for change.

In asking how the second set of taps – the ones for which the students created their own rhythms or patterns – is like the workplace, students again project meaning. They highlight examples such as, "When team members do their own thing without regard to the group, noise and chaos ensue." Some report that they have difficulty expressing their own creative pattern and inadvertently acquiesce to another's louder or more dominant patterns. They readily identify that this is similar to dominance and groupthink in the workplace.

The two students who were observers note other details not readily identified by the group involved in the tapping process. They reveal that although noise is evident early in the pattern with everyone doing their own thing, over time, a pattern begins to emerge, not unison but harmony. The group gains insight on how an outsider-observer role has utility and is helpful for teams that are conflicted or lack synchrony. The class reflects on forces in the workplace that encourage creativity, teambuilding, and harmony. They acknowledge the challenges that exist with conflict, discord, and lack of synchrony. Adaptability to change and the acknowledgment of paradigms or rigid patterns are more easily understood as a result of this lesson.

***Engaging participants in the learning process.*** Recently, I created a format for an on-line nursing leadership and management course, asking students to post at the onset of each module their "insights, resources, and applications" (IRA). Students reveal three insights about the assigned readings for class each module; share a resource (book, website, contemporary film) that amplifies the themes from the readings; and share a personal application or example from their practice or clinical situation that reinforces concepts from the class. The purpose of this activity is to engage students in their learning investments before entering into an electronic discussion-board case scenario. Although I was new to the electronic classroom, the IRA format rapidly became a wonderful tool that students and teacher both enjoyed.

Repackaging the IRA for an on-ground group of healthcare managers desiring to build their networking and supervisory management skills was easy. I constructed a four-module series using a contemporary leadership and management textbook. Structuring the corporate syllabus using the IRA as a teaching strategy assists participants in engaging in the learning process. At the start of each module, participants bullet-point their insights and resources on flip charts at the front of the classroom. We review this homework and their specific ideas on application at the onset of the class. Resources are added each week. At the end of the course, this list is distributed in hard copy to all participants. More information on this exercise can be found in the book, *Engaging the Online Learner: Activities for Creative Instruction* (Conrad & Donaldson, 2003).

***Other tips on expanding the walls of the classroom into the corporate setting.*** Adapting experiential processes, props, and stories is easy with most corporate groups. Although individuals within corporations believe their team needs are unique – and to some degree, perhaps they are – as a facilitator of learning, one can use the spontaneity, energy, and unique differences of any audience and construct an engaging learning process. The following are some guidelines and questions to assist with this adaptation.

***Seek additional resources.*** Seeking additional resources is about building your bag of tricks and experiential processes. I carry a bag of toys in my car. In addition to coins for the tapping exercise, my tool chest includes plastic children farm animals, multiple balls of all sizes and shapes, paper clips, colored paper and note cards, a parachute (great for outdoor activities), and even a roll of toilet paper! These objects are readily adaptable to facilitate learning. For additional ideas, consult *The Big Book of Humorous Training Games* (Tamblyn & Weiss, 2000) or join a professional organization, such as the American Society for Training and Development (www.astd.org).

***Identify common themes.*** Identifying common themes that transcend audiences inside and outside healthcare environments expands your marketing niche. For example, stress, teambuilding, leadership, management, conflict, change management, creativity, critical thinking, problem solving, marketing, and strategic planning are important to all organizations. Becoming masterful in assisting corporations to become ongoing learning environments is a needed and highly marketable consulting skill set.

***Remember who you are working for.*** Keep in mind who is paying your speaking or consulting fee and what a successful program means for them. Are they interested in entertainment and learning, or is this a beginning launching pad for gaining insights and change within the organization? Do not lose sight of who your primary customer is. It is easy to become triangulated between the audience and the individual who hired you.

***Assess, assess, assess.*** Remember to assess. A well-intentioned but novice administrator may desire teambuilding and conceptualize the consultant as:
• Someone who will provide a quick fix of a long-term conflicted group.

- A way to address one or two individuals who are nonproductive members.

Assessing the organization's needs through the eyes of the hiring person assists you in more closely meeting the institution's needs. You also become a conduit for offering additional consultative or management coaching services.

***Entertainment?*** Entertainment is marketable. Managers and administrators often simply desire entertainment with a hint of content for presentations. These speaking engagements are common during retreats, graduations, employee appreciation dinners, or recognition days for specific groups such as nurses, secretaries, social workers, caregivers, managers, etc. Recognize that your knowledge of facilitating learning and working with groups transcends traditional nursing-care populations. As holistic professionals, we are capable of assessing the needs of specific target audiences and amplifying and appreciating the commonalties that all humans possess, such as the need for attention, appreciation, and recognition. Assess the strengths, challenges, and needs of the particular group or organization. Use your stories, props, and experimental processes to engage the group.

***Touch.*** Touch the audience with your words, your hands, and your spirit. Arriving early on the day of the presentation is important. Shaking hands, learning names, and asking questions of the group immediately reduces the barriers of speaking to a cold audience. Ask individuals to share the most challenging or most rewarding aspects of their job. Take notes and use content derived during this informal, prespeaking assessment. Feeling you are a part of the group lessens pubic-speaking anxiety and facilitates your connection with the spirit of the audience.

***Stage your performance!*** Recognize the platform for speaking is a stage and you are an actor or actress. If your personality is more reserved, ask yourself if you can choose to act a different role to set the stage for a particular group. I once had difficulty masking anxiety when presenting to corporate groups. Public speaking is widely recognized as one of the most anxiety-producing phenomena. Faking confidence and acting the role of "presenter" helped me to mask my underlying anxiety. This is especially important during that first three to five minutes of any talk. It also facilitates reduction of negative autogenic – self-doubting – messages.

Becoming masterful in the art of public speaking requires listening, studying, and acting the role learned from other master presenters. The public library is full of tapes and films of the masters. I especially love the films of my all-time favorite orator, Winston Churchill. Another great resource for "staging" your consultation and public speaking skills is Pine and Gilmore's (1998), *The Experience Economy: Work is Theatre and Every Business is a Stage*.

## Corporate Teambuilding and Management Coaching

Conceptual work with teams began in the early 1950s and 1960s. Team building as strategy became popular in the 1960s, with the primary emphasis on removing barriers that prevent effective work-group functioning as well as building the group's ability to more effectively solve future problems. The request to conduct an in-service or educational program on teambuilding is most likely symptomatic of needs beyond the scope of a one- or two-hour program. Models on team assessments and interventions are available and helpful for diagnosing root disturbances and providing strategies for moving teams forward. Action research (AR), appreciative inquiry (AI), and learning organization (LO) frameworks are the models I have found most helpful in this endeavor. Refer to the bibliography for multiple citations on team building, action research, and workplace assessments.

Segueing from workshops to teambuilding and management coaching is a natural transition. Management coaching is a partnership between a manager and coach to promote exploration of issues, decision making, and problem solving. The top reasons given by organizations that implement coaching programs for managers include sharpening leadership skills, promoting success of newly appointed managers, and improving employee relations. Coaching is now part of many standard leadership training programs for executives and up-and-comers in larger organizations. For additional information on executive coaching visit www.executivecoachcollege.com

### Lessons Learned

Throughout my experiences as a nurse consultant I have learned many lessons. Following is a list of some of those lessons.

### Market Your Skills

Consulting can be as close as your own backyard. Some individuals have the idea that consulting is always done in far-away lands and that you cannot be a prophet in your hometown. Although it sometimes is easier to be recognized as an expert when outside your local area, I have found multiple opportunities very close to home. For example, it is not unusual to hear about or have requests from colleagues to network an open position or job opportunity. This is an ideal situation to inquire about the business, their needs, and future direction and strategic planning. I also begin to think about what intellectual property I possess that might be of value to their company. As I decline the full-time position, I offer to network their request to friends and colleagues. I also take the opportunity to inform them of services that I can provide as an external consultant. Aware of their current needs,

I am in a unique position for marketing, or at least soft-selling, my capacity as an educator, corporate teambuilder, or management coach.

## *Talk Money*

Do not be embarrassed to ask for payment. Have a fee schedule that is reasonable for your services. Consult with others in your area who charge a fee for service and adapt your structure to be consistent with similar practices. I recall the first time I asked to be paid for pubic speaking. A mentor colleague and gifted speaker told me her fee structure was $200 per hour and $1,000 per day for workshops and presentations. She offered the same programs to nonprofit agencies at a 50% discount. She coached me in the art of feeling comfortable saying the words, "these are rates for organizations . . ." but then quickly adding the concept of the price break for nonprofit organizations. This approach seemed to ease my discomfort in that many organizations using my services are nonprofit and seem to appreciate the cost break. My colleague convinced me that my sense of worth and value started with me and that to project less than what I deserved undermined my own self-esteem as well as reduced credibility in the eyes of my customers. The old adage that people value to the tune of what things cost is true in consulting as well! I quickly learned that although budgets are tight in most organizations, almost all budgets have a built-in miscellaneous section for consulting or education.

## *Partner, Partner, Partner!*

Although working with other professionals is fun and rewarding in and of itself, the synergy that occurs with partnering a project optimizes one's individual energy and transforms collective energy into completed projects – book chapters, journal articles, workplace presentations, and consultations. Partnering enhances commitment to action and task completion as well as captures individual and collective strengths. Over the last two years, I have partnered with a freelance writer, Shirley Kawa-Jump. Shirley is an excellent writer who is well respected in her writing circles. Using her writing talents and contacts, Shirley has partnered with me to write a monthly column on parenting and stress. Shirley is a great mentor. Specifically, she has facilitated my learning of the electronic interview with other professionals. This skill set alone has aided my ability to obtain efficient, practice-based information that is readily transformed into articles suitable for contemporary publications, newsletters, and public journals. Shirley interviews parents and weaves their stories with the clinical information that I provide. Shirley also enhances the marketing of our joint efforts by reselling our articles to several home journals and community newsletters as we retain rights for republishing. For additional information, check Shirley's website at www.shirleyjump.net

## Who Said Marketing Has to Be Expensive?

Consider offering continuing education programs at a university regional provider location. Several years ago, I offered a workshop on professionalism and burnout-prevention strategies for nursing assistants and unit secretaries of healthcare facilities. I partnered with another nurse and offered the same program throughout Indiana through the continuing education departments of the regional providers of Indiana and Purdue Universities. We negotiated a 50% fee split arrangement, and they provided the room, lunch, registration personnel, and marketing. At $75 per participant, we felt successful when we were able to present to groups of 50 to100 individuals.

What we had not anticipated was that individuals who attended the workshops returned to their individual institutions and requested we provide the same program on-site to their employees. The benefit of the marketing in each region was rapidly realized beyond the initial program. As individual free agents of the program, success was measured in being invited to present for two or three other provider locations. We launched a regional public speaking enterprise without incurring any further marketing expenses. This is an example of how word-of-mouth marketing – cost-free marketing – may be your best marketing strategy!

## Get Unstuck!

Fear, self-sabotage, jealousy, guilt, apathy, or feelings of being overwhelmed often zaps creative energy that moves us toward our goals of consulting, speaking, writing, acting, or any other entrepreneurial endeavor. Getting unstuck is central to moving through mind over mattress – procrastination, stagnation, or rolling over in bed and not taking action. It is important to discover what gets you "unstuck." The following list presents suggestions that others have used to sort out priorities and remove underlying blocks to achievement:
- Keep a journal.
- Find a mentor.
- Get counseling.
- Meditate.
- Pray.
- Exercise.
- Attend workshops.
- Read.
- Listen to audiotapes.

One resource particularly helpful in my own stagnation was Julia Cameron's (1992) *The Artist's Way*. Cameron provided recommendations and a process for connecting human creativity with the creative energies of the universe through exercises and activities.

### *Create a Follow-up Letter and Build Leads*

If the client is satisfied with your performance, ask for feedback in writing and permission to use this feedback in your marketing materials. Ask also for names of other corporate clients who may need your services.

### *Contracts and Billing*

My method of writing contracts and billing is highly informal. My contract consists of an e-mail. After initial discussions with the client, I e-mail specifics relative to what I will need during the presentation, along with my fees and anticipated expenses. I keep it simple. I note what materials I am bringing and what accommodations I will need. For example, I always request a cordless microphone for large groups and a projector. Airfare, accommodations, mileage, food, etc., are all negotiable. Plan ahead what your costs will be and simply request payment for those expenditures. Some presenters have fairly elaborate contracts with cancellation clauses and minimal attendance requirements.

For ongoing management consulting and coaching services, the client and I discuss frequency of billing, such as monthly or quarterly. A simple letter listing services provided, dates of services, and total fee is sent to the client. Most organizations are quite comfortable with e-mail submission, which makes this part of the practice painless and readily accomplished.

### *Believe in Yourself*

Last is the notion of believing in yourself and your competence to be effective. You are the expert in facilitating learning environments. Recognize the transferability of the tools of your trade to other settings. I agree with Linda Caputi 100%: you can be a consultant, and that's the truth!

## Any Way to Fail?

Dave Johnson is a very successful nurse consultant. Sounds easy, and many times it is. However, no matter how easy it may seem, being an entrepreneur is a lot of work. Consulting businesses can and do fail. Some of the reasons they fail include:
- Not articulating a clear goal and working to accomplish that goal.
- Making promises to client you can not keep.

- Ineffective advertising.
- Failing to individualize your work to meet your client's unique needs.
- Failing to conduct background research on the special characteristics of your client.

It is so very important to treat all consulting clients as individuals. For example, when conducting a workshop that you may have given numerous times, it is very disheartening for the client to perceive the presentation as off-the-shelf or canned. Research the school or organization. Find out what is happening in that entity that is new or different. Web pages make this very easy. For example, if hired by a school of nursing, read about that school. Many web pages have the nursing school's philosophy, goals, and even their school handbook. Weaving that information into the content individualizes the presentation. This takes very little time, perhaps only a few hours, but goes a long way in showing clients they are important.

## Conclusion

Being a nurse entrepreneurial can be very rewarding. However, before you start any business, do your homework. Visit the websites listed throughout this chapter. They are listed on the CD-ROM accompanying this book for your convenience. Write your business plan, do your homework, work hard, then enjoy!

## Websites

For easy launching, all of the websites referenced in this chapter are located on the CD accompanying this book. Simply launch your internet browser, put the CD-ROM in the drive, go to Chapter 50 on the CD, and then click on the website address.

## Learning Activities

1. Interview a nurse entrepreneur. Discuss the nature of the business, what works, and what does not work. Review with the entrepreneur the business plan, individual goals, and how those goals are being met.
2. Conceive an idea for a consulting business. Develop a business plan. Address what activities would take place during each of the three dimensions of the entrepreneur: idea generator, organizer, and worker.

# References

American Society for Training and Development. (2003). *Homepage*. Retrieved March 29, 2003, from http://www.astd.org/index_IE.html

Cameron, J. (1992). *The artist's way: A spiritual path to higher creativity*. New York: Penguin Putnam.

Colorado Business Resource Guide. (2003). *Business plan*. Retrieved February 6, 2003, from http://www.state.co.us/oed/guide/11-1print.html

Conrad, R., & Donaldson, J. (2003). *Engaging the online learner: Activities for creative instruction*. San Francisco: Jossey-Bass.

Gerber, M. E. (1995). *The e-myth revised*. New York: Harper Collins.

Pine, B., & Gilmore, J. (1998). *The experience economy: Work is theatre and every business is a stage*. Boston, MA: Harvard Business School Press.

Tamblyn, D., & Weiss, S. (2000). *The big book of humorous training games*. New York: McGraw-Hill.

# Bibliography

Argyris, C. (1998, May-June). Empowerment: The emperor's new clothes. *Harvard Business Review, 98-*105.

Bellman, L. (1996). Changing nursing practice through reflection on the Roper, Logan, and Tierney model: The enhancement approach to action research. *Journal of Advanced Nursing, 24*, 129-138.

Bennett, B. (1998). Increasing collaboration within a multidisciplinary neurorehabilitation team: The early stages of a small action research project. *Journal of Clinical Nursing, 7*(3), 227-231.

Blount, K., & Hahigian, E. (1998, August). How to build teams in the midst of change. *Nursing Management*, 27-29.

Breda, K. L., Anderson, M. A., Hansen, L., Hayes, D., Pillion, C., & Lyon, P. (1997). Enhanced nursing autonomy through participatory action research. *Nursing Outlook, 45*(2), 76-81.

Bruffey, N. G. (1997). Job satisfaction and work excitement: Organizational considerations. *Seminars for Nurse Managers, 5*(4), 202-208.

College of Executive Coaching (2003). *Homepage*. Retrieved March 29, 2003, from http://www.executivecoachcollege.com/

Crowell, D. M. (1998). Organizations are relationships: A new view of management. *Nursing Management, 29*(5), 28-29.

Drucker, P. F., Dyson, E., Handy, C., Saffo, P., & Senge, P. M. (1997, September/October). Looking ahead: Implications of the present. *Harvard Business Review*, 18-32.

Dyer, W. G. (1995). *Team building: Current issues and new alternatives*. New York: Addison-Wesley.

Eden, C., & Huxham, C. (1996). Action research for the study of organizations. In C. R. Stewart, C. Hardy, & W. R. Nord (Eds.), *Handbook of organization studies* (pp. 526-542). Thousand Oaks, CA: Sage.

Employee Assistance Professional Association. (2003). *Homepage*. Retrieved March 29, 2003, from http://www.eapassn.org/public/pages/index.cfm?pageid=1

Forte, P. S. (1997). The high cost of conflict. *Nursing Economic$, 15*(3), 119-123.

Furnham, A., & Gunter, B. (1993). *Corporate assessment: Auditing a company's personality*. New York: Routledge.

Glanton, E. (1997, September 13). Companies play at boosting morale, teamwork. *The Indianapolis Star,* C2.

Glasscock, F. E., & Hales, A. (1998). Bowen's family systems theory: A useful approach for a nurse administrator's practice. *Journal of Nursing Administration, 28*(6), 37-42.

Hannigan, G. G. (1997). Action research: Methods that make sense. *Medical Reference Services Quarterly, 16*(1), 53-58.

Harrison, M. I. (1987). *Diagnosing organizations: Methods, models, and processes.* Newbury Park, CA: Sage.

Hart, E. (1996). Action research as a professionalizing strategy: Issues and dilemmas. *Journal of Advanced Nursing, 23*, 454-461.

Hinton, J. E. (1997). Diagnosis: Poor morale. *Nursing Management, 28*(6), 40G.

Horgen, T., Joroff, M., Porter, W., & Schon, D. (1998). Process architecture: Transforming the workplace for effective work. *Employment Relations Today, 25*(3), 77-93.

Huffington, C., Cole, C., & Brunning, H. (1997). *A manual of organizational development: The psychology of change.* London: Karnac.

Hugentobler, M. K., Israel, B. A., & Schurman, S. J. (1992). An action research approach to workplace health: Integrating methods. *Health Education Quarterly, 19*(1), 55-76.

Johnson, D. R. (1999). *Team building through action research and genograms: The case of a nursing care delivery work team.* (Doctoral dissertation, Indiana University). Dissertation Abstracts International, 60, No. 07B (1999), p. 3202.

Jump, S. (2003). *Webpage.* Retrieved March 29, 2003, from http://www.shirleyjump.com/

Kreitzer, M. J., Wright, D., Hamlin, C., Towey, S., Marko, M., & Disch, J. (1997). Creating a healthy work environment in the midst of organizational change and transition. *Journal of Nursing Administration, 27*(6), 35-41.

Lengacher, C. A., Mabe, P. R., VanCott, M. L., Heinemann, D., & Kent, K. (1995, Summer). Team-building process in launching a practice model. *Nursing Connections, 8*(2), 51-59.

Lynch, D. (1997, May). Unresolved conflicts affect the bottom line. *HR Magazine*, 49-50.

Maxwell, L. (1993). Action research: A useful strategy for combining action and research in nursing? *Canadian Journal of Cardiovascular Nurses, 4*(1), 19-20.

Moch, S. D., Roth, D., Pederson, A., Groh-Demers, L., & Siler, J. (1994). Healthier work environments through action research. *Nursing Management, 25*(9), 38-40.

Morgan, G. (1997). *Images of organization* (2nd ed.). Thousand Oaks, CA: Sage.

Nelson-Gardell, D. (1995). Feminism and family social work. *Journal of Family Social Work, 1*(1), 77-95.

Norwood, S. L. (2003). *Nursing consultation: A framework for working with communities.* Englewood Cliffs: New Jersey: Prentice Hall.

Paradise, C. A. (1991). Team building: The role of teams in organizations. In J. W. Jones, R. D. Steffy, & D. W. Bray (Eds.), *Applying psychology in business* (pp. 587-594). Lexington, MA: Lexington Books.

Senge, P. (1998). Sharing knowledge. *Executive Excellence, 15*(6), 11-12.

Senge, P. (1990). The leader's new work: Building learning organizations. *Sloan Management Review, 32*(1), 7-23.

Senge, P. (1990). *The fifth discipline: The art and practice of the learning organization.* New York: Doubleday.

Senge, P., Kleiner, A., Roberts, C., Ross, R., & Smith, B. (1994). *The fifth discipline fieldbook: Strategies and tools for building a learning organization.* New York: Doubleday.

Sessa, V. I., Bennett, J. A., & Birdsall, C. (1993). Conflict with less distress: promoting team effectiveness. *Nursing Administration Quarterly, 18*(1), 57-65.

Schon, D. A. (1998). *The reflecive practitioner: How professionals think in action.* Aldershot, England: Ashgate Publishing Limited.

*Starting a small business in Illinois: Cutting through the red tape.* (2003). Retrieved February 8, 2003, from http://illinoisbiz.biz/bus/step_by_step.html#3d

Stringer, E. T. (1996). *Action research: A handbook for practitioners.* Thousand Oaks, CA: Sage.

Tolley, N. S. (1994). Oncology social work, family systems theory, and workplace consultations. *Health and Social Work, 19,* 227-230.

Tonges, M. C. (1997). Using systems thinking for health care reform. *The New Definition, 12*(1), 1-2.

Tumulty, G., Jernigan, I. E., & Kohut, G. F. (1994). The impact of perceived work environment on job satisfaction of hospital staff nurses. *Applied Nursing Research, 7*(2), 84-90.

Waterman, H. (1998). Embracing ambiguities and valuing ourselves: Issues of validity in action research. *Journal of Advanced Nursing, 28*(1), 101-105.

# Chapter 51: KEEPING YOUR PASSION FOR TEACHING NURSING ALIVE

Laura Brown, BS, MA, RN

*I have had the pleasure of knowing Laura Brown for several years. She is a delightful person, with a realistic view of life and a relentless passion for nursing. I asked Laura to write this chapter for the book after hearing her speak on the topic of keeping one's passion for teaching nursing alive. She graciously agreed, and I am delighted that all readers of this book will have the extreme pleasure of hearing Laura's message. – Linda Caputi*

## Introduction

So, now you've read the book on how to successfully teach nurses. My expert colleagues have shared some wonderful ideas from their many years of experience. I hope you are excited about getting started; eager to try some things you've learned. And I also hope that your enthusiasm for teaching and your passion for this career never wanes. But let's be realistic. You know and I know that you will experience emotional peaks and valleys in your work. There will be days when you go home fulfilled, knowing that you've made a difference; and then there will be those **other** days. You know the kind of days I'm talking about. The days when you get in your car to drive home and you have to adjust the rearview mirror down a bit. It was fine on the way to work, but somehow, you're shorter now, beaten down by frustration, overwhelmed, and not sure this is what you bargained for when you became a nurse educator.

### Educational Philosophy

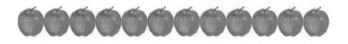

I see a teacher as a guide, a facilitator, and a coach, not as an imparter of all wisdom and knowledge. Because learning is a lifelong process, teaching and learning should be fun. I see teaching as a little theory and a lot of real-world, practical application. – Laura Brown

So, how do we keep our passion for teaching alive? What coping techniques can we develop to deal with some of the passion killers that we encounter? Nursing is a special career. Some might even say it's a calling. Students deserve teachers who are caring and enthusiastic and full of passion for nursing and for teaching nurses.

In my many years in nursing and health care, I've learned – sometimes the hard way – some strategies that have helped me to renew my passion for my work. In this chapter, I'd like to share some of those ideas with you.

## Recognizing Passion

Over the past two years, I have presented at several nurse educator conferences on the topic of keeping one's passion for one's job alive. I generally start with a warm-up activity in which participants are asked to find a series of partners and discuss a different question with each partner.

The first question, "Why did you become a nurse educator?" produces a variety of different responses. Common ones include:
- "To make a difference."
- "Because I had a great instructor once, and I wanted to be just like her."
- "So there would be good nurses to take care of me when I get older."
- "To get out of working nights and holidays."
- "I love to teach; it's in my blood."
- "Summers off!"

My second question is "What are your passion killers in nursing education?" They respond with remarks such as:
- "Bureaucracy, having to jump through too many hoops to get things done."
- "The politics of the organization."
- "Students who don't really care."
- "Faculty who don't really care."
- "Negative attitudes."
- "People who are unwilling to change."
- "Lack of teamwork."
- "Budget cuts."

When I ask the third question, "What rekindles your passion for nursing education?", faces brighten, eyes light up, and I get these rapid-fire responses:
- "When I see the light-bulb go on for a student."
- "When I can tell I've made a difference with a student."

- "When a student thanks me."
- "When I work with a student to ease a client's pain."
- "When faculty work together as a team."
- "When my ideas are listened to."
- "When I watch my students graduate."
- "When my students pass NCLEX®."

The final question – and always a fun one – is, "When you retire, what do you want your students and your colleagues to say about you?" I have heard the gamut of interesting remarks, such as:

- "She really cared."
- "He made a difference."
- "She's why I stayed in school."
- "He's a great team player."
- "We'll miss him."
- "Don't leave."
- "Who will bring in the treats now?"
- "What a great teacher!"
- "She looks pretty good for 95!"
- "He had some fantastic ideas."
- "Ding dong, the witch is dead!" (which came from a faculty member who was considered to be tough and demanding with her students).

These questions are a wonderful way to get people thinking about why they do what they do and, even though there are day-to-day passion killers, why they keep teaching nursing students, sometimes for as long as 30 years or more.

Maybe we all need to stop now and then to take stock of all the positives in our work. It is so easy to get caught up in whining about little negative distractions.

One of the ways in which we are reminded of why we went into nursing and nursing education is through telling the stories of our memorable moments in nursing. We all have experienced situations that made it all worthwhile or helped us to deal with some of the times when we have wondered if this is really the career for us or if anyone really appreciates what we do. When working as a director of education in an acute care hospital setting, I had an especially memorable experience that rekindled my passion for teaching cardiopulmonary resuscitation (CPR).

Having been a CPR instructor trainer for over 20 years, I was sick to death of teaching CPR. It seemed boring and not very challenging, to the extent that I felt I could hardly look another Rususci Annie in the eye. It was our annual CPR refresher time for all employees having direct client contact, and I was not a happy CPR instructor.

One particular class was composed primarily of laboratory staff, and one of the medical technologists, Sherry, had called our department to request the class, even though she did not have direct client contact. We welcomed Sherry, and as the class was nearly completed and most of the other students had gone, Sherry was still working with Ann, an instructor in my department.

I remember hearing Sherry say to Ann, "Why don't we just quit, Ann? Most of the students have finished, and I know you have lots of work to do. It's taking me a long time to learn this; let's just stop now. I don't have to get a course completion card." Ann patiently responded, "No, it's okay, Sherry. I have time. You're doing very well. Remember, the others in the class are refresher students. This is your first CPR class. You're almost there; let's not quit now." Thinking I was pleased with Ann's response, I finished tidying up and left without another thought about the interaction I had witnessed.

Several months later, Sherry and her husband were driving home, and as they passed a popular fishing spot in their hometown, a young man was standing at the side of the road, waving his arms and screaming for help. Sherry and her husband stopped the car and ran with him to the edge of the lake, where his uncle and little brother, Chad, had fallen into the lake while they were fishing. The uncle had been able to pull Chad out of the water, and the little guy was lying unconscious on the ground.

Sherry said she prayed she would remember what to do, that what she had learned in class would come back to her. As she knelt beside Chad, Sherry said she heard Ann's calm, patient words in her head, saying, "Open the airway; look, listen, and feel for breath; give two breaths – " Sherry followed the instructions perfectly and proceeded to do CPR on Chad until an off-duty firefighter arrived on the scene and assisted her. By the time the paramedics arrived, Chad was breathing on his own and conscious. He was discharged two days later from the hospital. His prognosis indicated he would have no ill effects from the incident.

As director of education, one of my "other duties as assigned" functions was to chair the hospital's employee-of-the-month committee. One of Sherry's colleagues in the laboratory nominated her for saving a life and for the recognition she brought to the hospital. The committee selected Sherry as the employee of the month, and the laboratory staff planned a wonderful surprise ceremony with food and decorations to honor her. The CEO of the hospital always accompanied me to present the award. He did a wonderful job of describing what Sherry had done and praised her for her skill and quick action. She was surprised and pleased and even a little teary-eyed.

Just then, there was a knock on the lab lounge door. Unbeknown to Sherry, her colleagues had invited Chad, his big brother, and his mom and dad to the award ceremony. As the door opened, Chad was the first to enter the room. His eyes scanned the room, searching. When he spotted Sherry, he screamed her name joyfully and ran to her, his arms outstretched. Sherry knelt down and enfolded Chad in the biggest, warmest hug I think I had ever witnessed. When Chad said, "Oh, Sherry, I love you so," there was not a dry eye in the room.

As I watched this glorious human interaction, I remember thinking to myself, "Of all the things you teach, what could be more important than CPR? What could be more important than saving lives?" It was one of those moments one never forgets. And it was a moment that rekindled my passion for teaching CPR.

## Symptoms of Declining Passion

As nurses, we feel it is important to learn the symptoms of diseases and conditions. We have to recognize the problem before we can treat it. So how do we recognize reduced morale, burnout, or a loss of passion for our work? The symptoms may vary from person to person, but there are some common threads.

Individuals who have lost passion for their work report fatigue, depression, lack of enthusiasm, negative attitudes, and stress-related physical symptoms. They talk about not wanting to go to work, unwillingness to take on new challenges, resistance to change, and impatience with others. Recently, a young woman told me that she recognizes a loss of passion in herself when she just can not tolerate interacting with people any longer, so she shuts the office door and works on that project for a long time.

When several people in a work group are all struggling with a loss of passion, we see organizational symptoms develop. Absenteeism and tardiness increase, as does the staff turnover rate. When people are not passionate about their work, they may do one of two things – resign and leave or, worse yet, resign and stay. Everyone knows someone who has resigned and stayed in an organization. Their body shows up to work, but their heart is just not in it anymore.

A common organizational symptom is "turfism," sometimes called "silo thinking." Individuals or groups become very self-protective, guarding their resources and refusing to collaborate with others. One can often recognize this turfism from statements such as, "Whose budget is that coming out of?" or "Don't look at me; I'm not paying for that!"

There is an interesting story that illustrates this turfism and concern only for self. Two men were hiking through the woods. Through a grove of trees, they spotted a grizzly bear that seemed to be stalking them. One hiker immediately threw off his backpack and began to run as fast as he could in the opposite direction from the bear. His buddy yelled after him, "What are you doing? You know you can't outrun a grizzly bear." His friend, still running, shouted back over his shoulder, "I don't have to outrun the grizzly bear; I just have to outrun you!"

When a nurse educator loses passion for teaching, the impact is wide-reaching, effecting not only the educator and his/her family and friends but also the educator's colleagues, students, and even their clients. In the past few years, I have witnessed many people in health care trying to outrun each other, competing instead of cooperating.

## Qualities of Those Who Have Passion for their Work

It is easy to recognize those who are passionate about their work. I have two adult sons whose careers are very diverse. One is an attorney who specializes in appellate law; the other is a NASCAR Winston Cup pit crewmember. Both are passionate about their work. How do I know that? I can tell when I hear them talk about their jobs. There is a light in their eyes, an enthusiasm in their voices, and a fire in their hearts that is unmistakable. They work extended hours without complaining or feeling used by their organizations. They're willing to take on new responsibilities, make changes, or take risks. Their jobs are very different, but what creates passion for them in their work is the same. Whether the older son just won a unanimous decision in the Ohio Supreme Court or the younger son and his team just performed a 14-second pit stop, the fulfilling sense of accomplishment is the same. Those who are passionate about their work are enthusiastic about change, volunteer to take on new challenges, have a positive attitude, and focus on the future rather than dwelling on the past.

## Strategies for Keeping Your Passion Alive

### *Organizational Strategies*

### *Focus on the Future and on Growth*

Having worked with many healthcare organizations, I have observed how they respond to difficult challenges and financial crunches. Those organizations that seem to have higher employee morale and people who are passionate about their work focus on the future. They look for ways to grow and to bring in more revenue. Their employees see this visionary focus and have a sense of hope. They can concentrate on doing their work well rather than on whether or not they'll have a job next week or next month.

In one Midwest city, the two hospitals have always been very competitive. Both have felt the pinch of tough economic times in health care. One hospital began cutting back on staff and expenses in the mid-1990s and continued to focus its energies on downsizing and reducing expenses through 2002. Many talented staff members left for greener pastures. Remaining staff were demoralized and cynical. There was an atmosphere of lack of trust for senior leadership and a serious loss of hope.

In the organization across town, proactive planning led to recruiting more physicians, constructing office buildings, and adding new services. Staff felt a sense of pride in their visionary leadership. They saw the forward progress and growth as a sign that their leaders were making proactive decisions to position the hospital well for the future. They did not spend so much time talking in the parking lot with colleagues about whether or not they had a future in the organization. And they had more time and energy to devote to doing a good job, whatever their job was.

## *Hire Appropriately*

Whenever I read the latest Human Resource (HR) study on how much it costs to hire or replace an employee, I am always amazed at the lack of time and energy that some leaders and managers put into the hiring process. Selection of new employees is often done using the warm-body approach. If the person is able to walk in and has the appropriate license or education for the job, he or she is put on the payroll. Later, we sometimes pay a heavy price for creating a job-employee match that was definitely not made in heaven.

One Midwestern hospital has created a video that features employees from a variety of departments sharing their perspectives on the organization's culture. They show the tape to prospective employees early in the interviewing process and report that it has been very effective in helping job candidates to get a feel for what it is like to work in that organization and if there is a fit between the employee and the organizational culture.

## *Help People See How Their Work*
## *Contributes to a Higher Purpose*

How sad it is to hear an employee say "I'm just a housekeeper" or "I'm only a food service worker." How would our organizations operate without housekeepers and food service workers? Everyone in your school, including your students, must be helped to realize that what they do is critical to the school's success. I have noticed the same interesting phenomenon in both health care and academia. There is a well-established hierarchy in which people who are at the top are sometimes seen as having more personal worth than those at lower levels. Sometimes, the position one has on the hierarchy has a lot to do with how much education one has or how much money one makes. The reality is, everyone in the hierarchy is critical to the success of the organization. People who feel valued and appreciated and who know how they contribute to the overall mission of the organization have more passion for their work than those who see what they do from a very narrow point of view.

I read a story once about a nursing professor whose first question on a major exam for nursing students was "What is the name of the housekeeper in the School of Nursing?" The students were incredulous and asked if the instructor was serious. The instructor responded that he was very serious and that it was important that they recognize the importance of the work of everyone who worked there. My guess is that the students learned the housekeeper's name very quickly and probably have never forgotten it.

### Recognize Contributions

Mary Kay Ash, the Mary Kay Cosmetics founder, once said, "There are two things people want more than sex or money, that's praise and recognition." Nurses become nurses because they care about people and want to help them. Nurses also thrive on praise and recognition. Sure, it would be wonderful if organizations could reward superior performance with cash bonuses and substantial raises. But the reality is, most organizations do not have that kind of money. There are many ways to recognize people that do not cost a lot of money. I have heard nurses say that a thank you or a pat on the back has sustained them for a week.

In asking that first question in my workshops – "Why did you become a nurse educator?" – I never recall anyone ever saying it was for the money.

Get all staff involved in creating a recognition system and use it generously to recognize people for a job well done. Praise colleagues publicly for their accomplishments. When someone finishes an advanced degree, becomes certified in a specialty, is published, or wins an award, plan a celebration, put it in the newspaper, and announce it to the organization. Success begets success, both in that individual and in others.

### Listen To and Implement Employee Ideas

We all want to feel listened to and we all have ideas for how to make our workplace better. Who is in a better position to recommend changes and improvements than those who are on the "front lines"? But rarely do most organizations openly solicit employee feedback, and even fewer actually try employee ideas.

There are many ways to be open to employee ideas. Suggestion boxes or hot lines can work. One organization put up a 'Spose Board in an employee area. Next to the board were pens and Post-It® notes for employees to suggest ideas to improve the workplace and their customer service. Employees could write their suggestions on the Post-It® notes and stick them on the 'Spose Board. All 'Spose ideas were considered and responded to in the employee newsletter. If a suggestion was implemented, the employee who recommended it received a monetary award. The 'Spose Board was usually full of good ideas.

What an arrogant, passionless workplace it is that has no interest in listening to its employees.

## Support Each Other

There is a saying about nurses that I hope I never hear again. Nurses are sometimes accused of "eating our young," of not supporting less experienced nurses coming into our organizations. It is sad that those who give of themselves in so many ways to help others do not always welcome and willingly mentor the new blood that we need so much in nursing.

There is a myriad of ways in which we can support other nurses. We can collaborate to get the work done when resources are scarce. We can teach and mentor fledgling nurses so that they gain confidence more quickly. We can share our expertise in areas of nursing not familiar to some nurses. We can recognize and celebrate the successes of nurses. We can share memorable moments in nursing to remind ourselves of why we became nurses. People who feel supported and valued are more passionate about their work than those who feel isolated and unappreciated.

### Personal Strategies

## Focusing on the Positive

Research has shown that people who are optimistic are happier, healthier, live longer, and have more friends than those who are pessimistic. Yet when nurse educators experience a loss of passion for their work, they tend to see the glass as half empty, often seeing only the negative side and becoming somewhat paranoid about things happening around them.

My friend, Faith Roberts, (see *Socialization into Nursing: Forming a Professional Attitude*, a chapter in this book by Roberts) tells a story about crab fishermen that illustrates what happens in a negative workplace:

When the New England crab fishermen come in from their day of fishing, one can walk along the dock and see all their crab buckets lined up. Some of the buckets have lids on them, and others are uncovered. The crab fishermen have learned that if they only caught one crab, they have to cover the bucket because the lone crab is able to crawl out of the bucket and escape. However, if they caught more than one crab, there is no need for a lid. As one crab tries to crawl out, the others pull him back down into the bucket. This is just like some work groups. They have all become negative and cynical, and when one person tries to be positive, the others work really hard to pull that person back into the negativity, back into the crab bucket.

Some educators may have even witnessed this phenomenon when they have taken their eager students to a new clinical area and watched the reaction of the seasoned nurses in that setting. No one can miss the eye rolling, the sighs, and the remarks such as, "Here we go again. Just wait until they see what the real world of nursing is like."

In my presentations, I sometimes show several pictures to the audience. I ask them to first put on their negative, pessimistic hat and spontaneously call out their reactions to each picture. Then I ask them to put on their perky, positive hat, and respond again. For example, when I show them a piece of chocolate pie, their negative responses include "too much fat," "too many calories," "weight gain," "probably not homemade," "soggy crust," or "the piece is too small." When asked to switch hats, they respond with things such as, "ummm-looks good, chocolate!", "I love chocolate," "bet that's real whipped cream on top," or "I deserve that piece of pie." I have tried this with a variety of different pictures, and my audiences do a great job of responding from both perspectives.

The point of this activity is that we all choose which hat we wear when we respond to situations in our lives. We can choose to be optimistic and see the possible positive outcomes in a situation, or we can choose to view it negatively. Granted, there are some things that happen in our lives that are a bit difficult to see positively at first. Things such as divorce, the death of a loved one, chronic illness, or the loss of a job can be extremely devastating. But we often hear someone who has survived one of life's challenges say that it was the best thing that ever happened to them or how much they learned from the experience, or even how much more they appreciate life and loved ones after the dust from the situation settles.

### Focusing on What We Can Control

In my many years of teaching in the acute-care healthcare setting, I remember that the times when I felt the most frustrated and helpless were the times when I disagreed with the decisions of the senior leadership team and thought they were not listening to managers or staff in the organization. I was especially irritated when top management hired consultants who came in, interviewed some of us who were considered opinion leaders in the organization, then regurgitated what we told them in a fancy looking, glossy report. The consultants were praised for their insightful work and their ability to diagnose problem areas in a brief time. They went away smiling, wallets bulging, and we were left shaking our heads in disbelief once more. Lots of paper was wasted making copies of this report, and all the managers who read it said, "Duh," and tucked it away in a file drawer never to be discussed again. Been there? Done that?

Somewhere along the way, as this process repeated itself many times in my career, I learned to focus on what I could control and let go of the rest. When we think about it, there is a lot we can control. We have total control over our attitude when we come to work, the way we interact with students and coworkers, and how we teach our students. We can decide that, despite the frustrations, we can be the best nursing faculty our students have ever had. Focusing on what we can control, not what is outside our control, can truly help us to keep our passion for teaching alive.

## Ending Perfectionistic Thinking

In my workshops, I frequently ask for the perfectionists in the group to raise their hands. I am amazed by the number of nursing educators who say they are perfectionists. My next question is, "So how many of you are perfect?" No hands go up. Then I ask, "How many of you know someone living today who is perfect?" Other than one delightful woman who raised her hand and responded, "My grandson is!", I have never had anyone else answer affirmatively to the last question.

So what is the lesson learned here? Obviously, if none of the proclaimed perfectionists are perfect, and no one actually knows anyone who is perfect, what does this tell us about perfectionism? Give it up! It is never going to happen! It is great to strive to do your best or to work toward continuous improvement, but if perfection is the goal, then who among us ever achieves it? Perfectionists are always frustrated because they never measure up to the impossible standards they set for themselves.

## Being Our Own Cheerleaders

I have made a career out of cheerleading. My training started in eighth grade when I was selected for my school's cheerleading squad, continued through high school, and has never stopped. I often give "motivational" presentations, which basically consist of a series of cheers, albeit more sophisticated cheers than we used in high school, but have the same basic purpose – to energize people and to convince them that they can achieve their goals.

Think about cheerleaders and what they do for the sports team and the fans. When the team does something really well – scores a touchdown or a goal, takes possession of the ball, or makes a great play in some way – the cheerleaders jump up and down, wave their pompoms wildly, and chant things such as, "Let's have another one, just like the other one. Go team, go!" But what about those times when the team plays poorly and really messes up? They are on the one-yard line and do not score the touchdown; they allow the other team to steal the ball and go in for a lay-up; or they just do not seem to be working as a team? What do the cheerleaders do? Yes – they jump up and down, wave their pompoms wildly, and chant things such as, "That's all right, that's okay; we're gonna beat them any way!" (I really dated myself with that one, didn't I?) Think about this. The cheerleaders do not stop cheering. They do not say things such as, "That was really stupid! Can't you guys do anything right? How embarrassing. I think I'll just go sit on the fan bus, and if you guys don't play any better, don't expect me to be here cheering for you next game!"

So what do we say to ourselves when we make mistakes? "That was really stupid. Can't you do anything right?" Or are we our own cheerleaders? Do we say things such as, "That's all right. You made a mistake. You're only human. Just learn from it and move on." We can be our own cheerleaders!

## *Recognizing That We Do Have Options*

Having worked in the same organization for 27 years, I became a slave to a mentality that said things such as, "I can't leave here. All my friends are here. This is the only job I really know well. What about my pension? I need the benefits. Who would hire me now? What would I do?" Many long-term employees there had the same mentality. When we felt we had no options, it was very difficult to remain passionate about our work during difficult times.

When I finally decided to investigate some other alternatives, I was amazed to find that I did have options, as do we all. This is not to say that every time we get a little frustrated with teaching nursing students, we can quit our jobs. The key here is that if we feel we do not have options or we're stuck in a bad situation, it is more difficult to be passionate about our work. The mere recognition that we **do** have other options makes it easier to stay and to deal with the passion killers.

## *Achieving Balance in Our Lives*

Sometimes when we're feeling overwhelmed by our work, we work longer and harder to try to get on top of the load in some way. Yet it never seems that our work is done, and we find ourselves getting more tired and discouraged. A skill that is critical if we wish to remain passionate about nursing education is to be able to find a balance between work and play, between our jobs and family or home life.

When we feel ourselves losing our passion for work, we need to spend time with people who re-energize us, people we love and who make us laugh. We must balance our lives with hobbies that relax us or with activities that refresh our bodies and our minds.

When I ask workshop participants what activities recharge them, they respond with everything from warm bubble baths to listening to music to fishing to vigorous exercise. Anyone who does not have a battery-charging hobby ought to find one and practice it often. It is amazing how much better we can feel about dealing with frustrations at work.

## *Developing Our Sense of Humor*

Research shows that the average toddler laughs about 350-400 times a day, and the average 8-10-year-old laughs 150-200 times a day. The average adult laughs about 10 times a day. Laughter is a natural mechanism that helps us deal with the stressors in our lives. So what happens between toddler age and adulthood to diminish that powerful stress reliever? I think it is things like our third-grade teachers, with hands on hips, saying, "What's so funny? Wipe that silly smile off your face," or our nursing school clinical instructors, who catch us with several other nursing students giggling hysterically in the nurse's lounge, and say, "This is a serious place. People are dying here. Act like professionals." We often get the message that laughter is not mature or professional. Is that not sad?

Study after study has proven the physical and emotional benefits of laughter. People have written entire books on how laughter helps us to cope and to heal. King Solomon said in Proverbs, "A merry heart doeth good like medicine, but a broken spirit drieth the bones." And Bill Cosby once said, "If you can find humor in anything, you can survive it." Seasoned healthcare professionals, especially those who work in extremely stressful, fast-paced, acute-care settings such as critical-care units and emergency departments, know the value of survivor humor. They sometimes call it "medical humor" or even "sick humor." They often laugh to keep from crying, and the laughter serves as a wonderful outlet for their stress and helps them continue to function effectively in day after day of dealing with human trauma and tragedy.

One of my favorite quotes about laughter's positive effects is from Alan Klein, a humorist and speaker, who said, "Laughter is a powerful tool in a powerless situation." That quote reminds me of a memorable personal experience. A year ago, my husband Ron, who is also a nurse, was diagnosed with colon cancer. He had been having some of the symptoms that all nurses know are warning signs of cancer, but like many nurses, he denied them and was too busy with his work to go to the doctor. When I finally insisted he see his physician, a video rectal exam in the office led to an immediate visit to a surgeon, and a hospital admission for a colonoscopy under general anesthetic. The surgeon found me pacing in the surgery waiting room; showed me the ugly, frightening photos from the colonoscopy; and said, "He has a big colon tumor that needs to come out now. I'd like to keep him overnight and do the colon resection in the morning. Is that okay with you?"

Trying to stay calm and in control but unable to stop crying, I suggested that we talk to Ron because he was the one who needed the surgery. The surgeon invited me into the post-anesthesia room (PAR), so we could discuss it with Ron, who was just starting to wake up from his Versed-induced sleep. It was late in the day, and Ron was the only client still in the PAR. Several physicians and nurses were there, finishing up for the day.

As the surgeon and I approached Ron, I was trying so hard to be strong and not let him see how upset I was. Ron squinted at me, smiled, and said, "Hi, honey; just let me wake up a little, and you can take me home." I responded, "Well, Ron, I don't think we're going home tonight. Doctor found a tumor in your colon, and he'd like to keep you overnight and take it out tomorrow morning." By now, all eyes in the room were on us, and it was quiet as everyone waited for Ron's response. I knew he could tell how upset I was. He had to know that this was a very serious medical problem we were facing. He said nothing for quite awhile – it seemed like forever – then in the loudest voice he could muster, Ron quipped, "Well, I guess that means no wild sex tonight, huh, honey?" I gasped. No one said anything. Then one of the surgeons started to laugh, then another and another. The nurses were giggling, I was blushing, and Ron, who was so proud of himself, was grinning from ear to ear. He had taken control in a powerless situation. Making us laugh gave him some sense of power. The really interesting part of the situation is that, to this day, he has no recollection of the incident. That Versed is a wonderful drug!

There are a number of strategies for bringing more laughter into both our personal and professional lives. Everyone has a different sense of humor and finds different things funny. The key is for all of us to determine what we and the people around us find funny, then surround ourselves with that type of humor.

Put up a humor bulletin board and have co-workers bring in cartoons and fun pictures. Assign one person each month to be the Ambassador of Fun. That person's job is to change the items on the humor bulletin board and to coordinate one fun activity for the group during the month. Ideas for fun activities could range from photo captioning contests to challenging another work group to a bowling or volleyball game to everyone bringing in food for a theme party, such as a luau, a Mexican feast, or a dessert festival. Give fun prizes for the most creative photo captions and recognize the winners in your in-house newsletter. Another morale-boosting contest is asking people to finish these sentences:

- You might be a nurse educator if . . .
- You might work at the College of Lake County if . . .
- You know it's going to be a stressful day when . . .

Responses will be both amazing and amusing. These activities are supposed to be fun.

The remarks of a very small group of negativists or cynics should never halt efforts to bring more humor and laughter into the workplace.

Start a humor collection. Find an empty cabinet or file drawer and have people start bringing in fun things like rubber chickens, bubbles, cartoons, and joke books. One of my favorite items in my humor collection is a pair of wide, gold bracelets that my friend Lucy gave me. She knew that Wonder Woman was my "she-ro" because she could stay so cool and calm in all circumstances. She always wears these wide metal bracelets, and when bullets or arrows come her way, she just raises an arm and deflects them with her bracelet. I sometimes get out my Wonder Woman bracelets and put them on. This very act helps me to mentally deflect negativity that seems to be coming at me from all directions.

Look for humor everywhere. It is all around us, but we often miss incredibly funny things. Dr. Seuss says, "From there to here, and here to there, funny things are everywhere." Signs can be great fun. I once saw a sign in a laundromat window that said, "Ladies, leave your clothes here and go have fun." When we can't find humor readily, we can create our own. We can make our classes creative and fun. Our students will love us for it, and the best part is, when they have laughed about something, they will remember it better.

My favorite author, Anonymous, once said, "Blessed are we who can laugh at ourselves, for we will never cease to be amused," and "He who laughs, lasts." If we are not laughing, we need to start. If we are, we need to spread it around to our colleagues. Laughter is such a good way to deal with life's insults and challenges, and it is a wonderful tool for keeping our passion for both work and life alive. For ways to incorporate humor into your teaching, see *Humor in the Classroom*, a chapter in this book by Fran London.

## Conclusion

No career or job is perfect, but think about the job of teaching nursing students. What job could be more important? We teach people to help others at the most vulnerable times in their lives. We help nurses learn to share in times of joy and times of sorrow with others as they ease pain and help people die with dignity. What could possibly be more important than the work we are doing? Nursing education needs people who are passionate about what they do. I wish all nursing educators well as they embark upon this very important mission of teaching others to nurse.

## Learning Activities

1. Make a list of the positives and the negatives in your current work situation. Describe how you can deflect the negativity.
2. Discuss a nursing experience that helped you to recall the passion that you have for nursing.
3. Ask colleagues why they went into nursing, what their passion killers are, and what rekindles their passion.
4. Get a group of colleagues together and list ways you can support each other.
5. List the activities you do to achieve a balance in your life. What are your hobbies? Who are the people you spend time with? What are your stress relievers?
6. Create a humor tool kit for your work group or classmates.
7. Put up a humor bulletin board and ask everyone in the class to contribute something to it.
8. Take turns starting class with either a memorable nursing moment or a humorous story or joke.
9. Bring in silly pictures and have a photo-captioning contest.
10. Interview a nursing faculty member or a nurse educator that you believe is passionate about his/her work. Find out what he/she does to keep the passion alive.

# From Student to Practitioner: Supporting Role Transition

# Chapter 52: SOCIALIZATION INTO NURSING: FORMING A PROFESSIONAL ATTITUDE

Faith Bresnan Roberts, BSN, RN, CRRN

*Several months ago, a strange thing happened when I was supervising students in the clinical setting. A surgeon entered the nurses' station accompanied by a medical student. Two nursing students were sitting across from me at the desk. They saw the surgeon and rose from their seats. The surgeon looked at them and said, "I see you are still in nursing school. One thing I want to teach you is this: when you become a nurse, never give your chair to a doctor. Nurses work too hard to be getting up when they can be sitting down." He walked to the other side of the station and took a seat. The world of nursing is changing in so many ways, including the traditional unspoken rules that have often dominated our profession. This chapter offers stimulating insight into how faculty can socialize present-day students into the professional role. – Linda Caputi*

## Introduction

How nurses incorporate or socialize their newer members into the profession is tantamount to that newcomer's success. Transitioning a graduate nurse into the world of clinical practice is difficult, at best. For most graduates, the disparity – both real and perceived – between theoretical frameworks and clinical practice often leave them frustrated and overwhelmed. This dilemma in practice – "how do we make a nurse out of a new grad?" – mirrors the dilemma faced in nursing education. How does one take a person

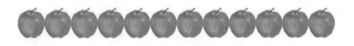

## Educational Philosophy

Teaching nursing is best accomplished by creating a partnership between instructor and student. This partnership should be built on trust and a desire to attain the highest level of understanding of the information provided. Clarity of purpose and joint responsibility for seeking out the best opportunities available for learning are two components necessary for the partnership to be effective. Implicit in such a partnership is an environment that nurtures self-discovery and fosters critical thinking as it encourages the qualities of caring and compassion. – Faith Brensan Roberts off the street and at the end of a two- to five-year curriculum produce a nurse able to begin professional practice?

Just what is this socialization process that is deemed so necessary for professional nurse orientation, nurturance, and survival in the workplace? Socialization has been defined as a process by which "individuals incorporate the roles, values, and beliefs held by the profession into their own value/belief system" (Muff, 1982, p. 96). Another definition is that professional socialization is a process by which "professional attitudes, values, and beliefs become internalized during which the individual develops a sense of occupational identity" (Clayton, Broome, & Ellis, 1989, p. 72). Socialization has to do with "helping the students move into the culture of nursing" (Tanner, 2000, p. 8). The process of socialization in nursing has been the subject of a great deal of research and writing. The groundbreaking work of Kramer (1974) and Benner (1984) still set the standard on this topic. Figure 52.1 lists the stages of reality-shock as first reported by Kramer (1974). A look at Figure 52.2 allows the reader to compare these stages with the work of Benner (1984). Nursing faculty continue to find this information rich with applications to their work with students.

Nursing professionals are divided on the subject of when socialization occurs for nursing students (Nesler, Hanner, Melburg, & McGowan, 2001). There does exist in the literature a debate as to whether this process happens during the student years or in the world of practice. This chapter focuses on the premise that professional socialization begins at the undergraduate level (Scheer, 1994) and continues as a lifelong process.

## Measurement

A socialized nurse committed to the profession develops a nursing perspective on viewing and solving problems and "thinks like a nurse," having developed discipline-specific critical-thinking skills (Saarmann, Frietas, Rapps, & Riegel, 1992). How does one begin to understand if the socialization process is occurring? The measurement of such change can be accomplished in part by identifying the "students' conceptions of nursing activities at various critical periods during the role socialization process" (Coudret, Fuchs, Roberts, Suhrheinrich, & White, 1994, p. 342). Several academic institutions have sought to measure this in their own students. Two instruments frequently used by institutions in this work are the Corwin (1961) Role Conceptions Scale and Nursing Role Conceptions Questionnaire by Pieta (1976), which was adapted from Corwin's (1961) work. Both instruments examine a hypothetical statement/question and ask respondents to state the extent to which they believe the behavior **should** be practiced in nursing and then the extent to which they perceive the behavior is **actually** being practiced. The difference between ideal and real is termed role discrepancy, a source of personal and professional

Figure 52.1 – Kramer's Postgraduate Socialization Model

---

**Kramer's Postgraduate Resocialization Model**

Stage I Skill and Routine Mastery
The nurse focuses on developing technical expertise and mastering specific skills to overcome feelings of frustration and inadequacy. May not focus on other important aspects of nursing care.

Stage II Social Integration
The nurse's major concern is having peers recognize the nurse's competence and accept the nurse into the group.

Stage III Moral Outrage
The nurse recognizes incongruities between conceptions of the **bureaucratic** role, which is associated with the rules and regulations and loyalty to agency administration; the **professional** role, which is committed to continued learning and loyalty to the profession; and the **service** role, which is concerned with compassion and loyalty to the client as a person.

Stage IV Conflict Resolution
The nurse resolves conflicts of Stage III by surrendering behaviors and/or values or by learning to use both the values and behaviors of the professional and bureaucratic system in a politically astute manner.

---

Source: *Reality Shock: Why Nurses Leaving Nursing*, by M. Kramer, 1974. Reprinted with permission.

Figure 52.2 – Benner's Stages of Nursing Expertise

---

### Benner's Stages of Nursing Expertise

*Stage I: Novice*
No experience (e.g., nursing student). Performance is limited, inflexible, and governed by context-free rules and regulations rather than experience.

*Stage II: Advanced Beginner*
Demonstrates marginally accepted performance. Recognizes the meaningful **aspects** of a real situation. Has experienced enough real situations to make judgements about them.

*Stage III: Competent Practitioner*
Has two or three years of experience. Demonstrates organizational and planning abilities. Differentiates important factors from less important aspects of care. Coordinates multiple complex care demands.

*Stage IV: Proficient Practitioner*
Has three to five years of experience. Perceives situations as wholes rather than in terms of parts, as in Stage II. Uses maxims as guides for what to consider in a situation. Has holistic understanding of the client, which improves decision making. Focuses on long-term goals.

*Stage V: Expert Practitioner*
Performance is fluid, flexible, and highly proficient; no longer requires rules, guidelines, or maxims to connect an understanding of the situation to appropriate action. Demonstrates highly skilled intuitive and analytic ability in new situations. Is inclined to take a certain action because "it felt right."

---

*From Novice to Expert: Excellence and Power in Clinical Nursing Practice*, by P. Benner, 1984, Menlo Park, CA: Addison-Wesley Nursing, pp. 21-34. Reprinted with permission of the author.

conflict. It is the intent of the nursing programs using these measurements to have a low discrepancy rate. Both instruments have three areas that are measured: professional: loyalty to the profession of nursing, commitment to practice standards, and involvement in professional activities; service: welfare of the individual client, decisions made with the client as primary concern; and bureaucratic: hospital policies and procedures, loyalty to the employing institution. Additional measurement instruments include the Nursing Care Role Orientation Scale (NCROS), originally developed in 1978 by Stone and Knopke, and the Stone Health Care Professional Attitude (STONE) Inventory, modified by Lawler in 1978. The NCROS was designed to measure nurses' orientation to their role, and the STONE Inventory was designed to assess professionalism based on Dumont's (1970) paradigm (Nesler et al., 2001). Many programs modify the instruments as necessary to better address their own students. No matter which instrument is used, the research findings compel faculty to return to the drawing board and look at the ability of their curriculum to provide reality-based education and continue to stress the values and ideals of nursing.

## Educational Transition

The literature includes references to the first year of nursing school as the "ideal where you learn what should be, and the 2nd, 3rd, and 4th years as 'reality' when you learn what is" (Reutter, Field, Campbell, & Day, 1997, p. 151).The first year of nursing is one of discovery for most students. Finally in the field, they begin to determine for themselves what nursing is and how it is practiced. Influences such as those fostered by the media, family stories, and comments from upper-level students give way to seeing with their own eyes what nurses do and how they spend their time at work. Students place a high value on clinical knowledge almost from the beginning, wanting to "get in the real world" of clients. Tasks are incredibly seductive, and the desire to learn how to do it often supercedes any rationale for why the task is being done. Too often, classroom time is seen as "helpful but with little real application to the patient" (Reutter et al., 1997, p. 151). Time spent in comprehensive learning laboratory activities covering the basic principles of client care is seen as a rite of passage to get to the hospital. Nursing role conceptions are "changed and altered by learning along with work experiences and exposure to clinically experienced role models" (Coudret et al., 1994, p. 344).

Beginning with the second year, students begin to absorb not only the values they have been exposed to in the educational milieu but also those of others, including clients and caregivers (Tanner, 2000a). Opinions rather that values may carry more weight in the initial introduction to the practice area. The clinical nurses' perceptions, both spoken and observed of students, their faculty, and even their program, begin to color the novices views

(Thomka, 2001). The process of internalizing these observations and values formation begins as students continually reassess how and what others value in practice. In the second year of the nursing curriculum, there is a greater emphasis on applying theory to practice and on the performance aspect of socialization. Students are now required to cope with the **real** rather than the **ideal** situations (Reutter et al., 1997).

Throughout the literature, stories of real versus ideal and classroom versus clinical abound. Nursing continues to reinforce this dichotomy when students hear "but this isn't how we do it in the real world" (Davidson, 2001). In the clinical area, a student is suddenly faced with nurses who do not practice as the student was taught. Students observe carefully how the teacher explains this disconnect. For example, if students observe this disconnect discussed during a post-clinical conference instead of directly with the nurse, the seeds of nonconfrontative behavior are planted. Instead, the teacher, who encourages the students to communicate and question the clinical nurse when not comfortable with practice issues, teaches them from the very beginning that it is important to speak up. Often, a student may not be aware that there is more than one way to implement care. Having the clinical nurse explain what was done and why will add to the students' knowledge base. The students learn to dialogue, discern, and question, all important components of critical thinking. To students, the teacher is seen not just as the source of knowledge but also as a barometer for what is acceptable behavior on the clinical unit.

It is continually said that nurses eat their young; where did this idea begin? Unfortunately, socialization in nursing has for too many years been one of survivorship. A common method of initiation includes "jumping the hoop" as a way of acclimating one to the real world of nursing. For far too many nurses, this game was first played when they were students. Preparing students to care for clients included the students going to the hospital the afternoon/evening before clinical and acquiring their client assignments for the following morning. After reading the client's chart alone, each student then headed back to the dormitory/home armed with a pile of notes to begin to put the components of a care plan together. These were clients the students had never seen, spoken with, or auscultated. Yet they would be expected to have a care plan completed by the next morning (Tanner, 1986). This usually took students until 3:30 a.m., after which the students would fall across the bed in exhaustion only to have the alarm go off two hours later, signaling it was time to get ready for clinical practice. Lesson learned? That in practice, nurses need no sleep. This behavior is borne out again in practice as nurses on their way into a night shift are heard to say, "I hope it's not too busy tonight. I didn't sleep today." Where did nurses ever get the notion that they didn't need sleep? The roots of this behavior can be traced back to their days as a student.

Present-day nursing educators talk frankly with students about the need for adequate rest and point out frequently the importance of not following behaviors they see in the clinical setting that reinforce the idea of working when exhausted. Students are encouraged to sleep before their first day of clinical and prepare a care plan after they have cared for the client at least one day. This method also emphasizes the importance of listening to the client's story before planning nursing care (Wesorick, 1995).

Much emphasis has been placed on inculcating critical thinking into the curriculum. We also need educators who are able to think critically about their methods of clinical instruction and the rationale for assignments made.

Although changes in the healthcare environment require movement from traditional to more innovative ways of delivering nursing care, nurse educators are challenged to consider how they presently educate students. This includes determining what changes in the educational process are necessary to equip these students to function in this new environment (Elberson & Williams, 1996). Faculty "do not have the luxury of teaching their courses the way they always have" (Lindeman, 2000, p. 3).

Another example of jumping the hoop is seen immediately following a new nurse's orientation when assigned to care for the unit's most complicated client. Assignments made by giving the most difficult client to the nurse with the least amount of skill do nothing to enhance that neophyte's knowledge level and self-confidence. In fact, the effect it has on self-esteem is what leads many nurses to transfer from the area in which they started as soon as possible. Individuals do not forget how they were treated in the first weeks of practice, impacting professional behaviors throughout their entire career. Nursing should not be an exclusive club with rites of entry guaranteed only by shared misery. "Let's see if they can take it" is not an appropriate premise on which to build the socialization process. A novice given a client within the scope of beginning practice, supervised by colleagues and encouraged to share concerns and triumphs, is a nurse who will successfully socialize into the workplace (Haffner & Raingruber, 1998).

As this chapter is written, the latest statistics show that only two out of five new graduates will remain in nursing after the first year of practice (Aiken, Clarke, Sloane & Sochalski, 2001). Although this information is sobering in its implications to a profession in the midst of a shortage, it should also serve as a wake-up call to the current methods of socialization into the practice arena. Whether or not a neophyte is in the same position at the same institution a year after beginning employment is not an indicator of successful socialization into nursing. Socialization into the profession needs to include "the skills associated with working in a world of change and ambiguity" (Lindeman, 2000, p. 3).

For over a century, nursing practice was based on an apprenticeship model where beginners followed the experts learning skills, imitating behaviors (Lindeman, 2000). This was the height of institutional nursing, built on decades of the tradition of paternalism routinely thrusting the nurse into a subservient role to the physician (MacDonald, 2002). This handmaiden role was characterized by behaviors such as standing when a physician entered the nurses' station, offering one's chair to a physician, following a physician on rounds (a few steps behind), not speaking to the physician in front of the client, and serving coffee. As often happens with an oppressed group, unrealistic and unfounded fears based on folklore abounded (Roberts, 1997). Novices were often regaled with admonitions such as, "Don't ever call physicians during a night shift, despite the client's condition;" "Only a physician can attend a delivery so keep the laboring woman from giving birth at all costs;" "Never express your own thoughts; if you have an idea, present it to the doctor so the doctor will think he/she thought of it first."

With the average age of a nurse in middle to late 40s, socialization efforts must include an understanding that many practicing nurses were introduced to the profession with such an institutional mindset. They then have a tendency to pass this mindset on to each group of students on the clinical unit. It is critical that nursing educators make a concerted effort to help students identify these behaviors as negative influences on healthcare delivery.

The apprenticeship model in institutional nursing began with the admission interview for all predominantly female nursing applicants. These interviews not only helped clarify why an applicant chose nursing but also allowed for subjective inferences to be drawn regarding an applicant's ability to succeed in the program. Married students were not allowed because it was believed they were unable to devote the time to both their studies and being a "good wife." Once admitted, the female students were taken into the dormitory and nursing became their life. Clinicals, lectures, chapel, even social events were scheduled by the school (Lindeman, 2000).

Present-day programs do not have the luxury of asking personal and probing questions of its applicants. Public educational institutions cannot allow such criteria for admission without the threat of losing federal or state funding. Currently, colleges of nursing enroll nontraditional students who have multiple roles – family breadwinners, single parents, outside jobs, demanding personal lives, and program studies. The increasing diversity of nursing students has "forced a change in teaching styles and academic programs to adapt accordingly" (McBride, 1999, p. 115). Older students bring a wealth of life experiences to the classroom/clinical area that generic students frequently do not possess due to their youth. Often, nontraditional students bring values and behaviors from previous socialization in differing healthcare careers. These might include emergency medical technician, paramedic, respiratory therapist, or certified nursing assistant. Although socialization into these areas of health care have many commonalities, nursing does hold a set of values, beliefs, and knowledge germane to the profession. Faculty need to be cognizant of the strengths these students bring to the group and be aware that resocialization to nursing's specific values and beliefs needs to occur.

Students believe the two main factors that "facilitated their learning and professional socialization were the influence of clinical instructors and their peers" (Campbell, Larrivee, Field, Day, & Reutter, 1994, p. 1130). In present-day programs, often the only time a student spends with the teacher and peer group is in the classroom and at clinical experiences. This decrease in the amount of time together gives even less time for observing and assimilating values and attitudes formerly learned when together in the dormitory and the classroom (Nesler et al., 2001). It is essential that students spend time "working with faculty and others who can help them understand the professional role" (Tanner, 2000, p. 8). Study groups are an excellent method to use to increase time outside of the classroom for the group to be together. The important thing about belonging to such a group is that all members begin to realize that they share many of the same anxieties. "Collectively, they can identify their own feelings, verbalize frustrations, and share pride in accomplishments" (Brookfield, 1993, p. 205). Studies show that students gain insight into behavior, both their own and others', by coming to the realization that they "share similar fears and were at a comparable competence level" (Haffer & Raingruber, 1998, p. 65).

Figure 52.3 presents a comparison of the old paradigm based on a medical model to the new paradigm based on a healthcare model. When operating from the old paradigm, caregivers often fell into the trap of "find it, fix it," focusing on "just what ails you" – a specific body part or system. In the healthcare model, emphasis is placed on not just the ache or pain but on the individual's response to that ache/pain as a whole person. Institutional nursing does not lend itself well to a model based on health. In the newer model, practice has evolved into professional nursing. In the old paradigm, rules and regulations that were born out of hierarchal thinking were the hallmark of institutional nursing and were based on the unscientific belief that the healthcare provider knew what was best (Tanner, 2001). Two examples of institutional practice are restricted visiting hours for families; asking spouses, parents, or others to leave even though there was no reason; and feeding times for newborns every four hours with no feedings in-between.

As our culture changed, people were encouraged and often expected to take responsibility for their own health care. Institutional nursing met its demise. Although there are definite norms and parameters to follow, nursing care itself must be uniquely designed to meet the goals and needs of individual clients. Assumptions that doctors or nurses know best, making decisions on behalf of clients without involving them, and feeling threatened when clients have access to alternative sources of medical information are signs of paternalism that have no place in modern health care (Coulter, 1999).

Currently, our call as a profession is to continue to work at reversing this subservient role (Tanner, 2000) and assist new nurses to become practitioners who are able to clarify dependent, interdependent, and independent scopes of practice (see Figure 52.4). This suggests that the curriculum balance between time allocated to learning the dependent functions of the nurse and the independent functions "should mirror contemporary practice" (Lindeman, 2000, p. 3).

Diversity has played and will continue to play a part in the socialization of nurses. In the not-so-distant past, nurses were viewed as Caucasian females in uniform who spoke one language – English. Even presently, when looking at commercial language boards for aphasic clients, a nurse is often portrayed as a Caucasian female with a cap. Diversity

Figure 52.3 – Old Versus New Paradigms

| *Old Paradigm* | *New Paradigm* |
|:---:|:---:|
| Newtonian view | Quantum view |
| ↓ | ↓ |
| Medical care model | Healthcare model |
| ↓ | ↓ |
| "Absence of disease" | "Body, mind, and spirit in balance" |
| ↓ | ↓ |
| Physiological | Human response |
| (objective) | (subjective) |
| ↓ | ↓ |
| Mechanical view | Wholistic view |
| ↓ | ↓ |
| Life events: Medical | Live events: Balance |
| ↓ | ↓ |
| Fix: "Power over" | Ownership: "Power releasing" |
| ↓ | ↓ |
| Passive | Partnership |
| ↓ | ↓ |
| Episodic (short term) | Continuous (long term) |
| ↓ | ↓ |
| Limited strategies | Endless possibilities |
| ↓ | ↓ |
| Institutional service | Professional service |
| ↓ | ↓ |
| | Independent, process-dominated practice wherein the nursing service is based on the individual's human response to the present health status or situation. |
| Dependent, task-dominated practice wherein the nursing service is directed by physicians' orders and hospital policies and procedures. | |
| *"Doing things right"* | *"Being there at the right time, intervening in the right way with the right resources to support healing."* |

Note. From *The Closing And Opening Of A Millennium: A Journey From Old To New Thinking* (p. 41), by B. Wesorick, 1995, Grand Rapids, MI: Practice Field Publishing. Copyright 1995 by Bonnie Wesorick. Reprinted with permission of the author.

training in health care has been slow to capture the true diversity that is apparent in the present-day world. Generational differences, behaviors unique to one's culture, class distinctions, and religious beliefs are but a few of the areas that need to be addressed. Clients expect to have a caregiver who can speak their language. A two-hour *Spanish for the Healthcare Provider* class is not going to encourage a family to seek treatment at a facility where it is obvious no one can communicate with them. New nurses are acutely aware of this change in culture and expect a socialization process that honors diversity and does not seek homogeneity (Christman, 1998).

Figure 52.4 – Nursing's Unique Professional Services

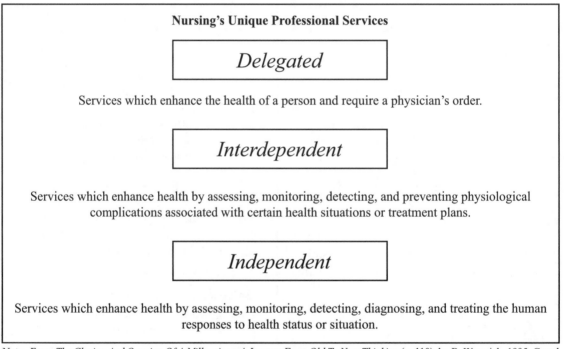

**Nursing's Unique Professional Services**

**Delegated**

Services which enhance the health of a person and require a physician's order.

**Interdependent**

Services which enhance health by assessing, monitoring, detecting, and preventing physiological complications associated with certain health situations or treatment plans.

**Independent**

Services which enhance health by assessing, monitoring, detecting, diagnosing, and treating the human responses to health status or situation.

# Values

In the past, values were often shared by society as a whole regarding health care and acute hospitalizations (Woodward, 1998). The explosion of healthcare technology, the opening of previously closed doors to information, and the sensational medical mishaps reported through the media have resulted in consumers creating a new set of values. These values may or may not correlate with those of a healthcare institution. Socialization of nursing students fosters students' awareness that people have different values and abilities to monitor and direct their own health care.

Insurance regulations and decreases in length of client stays have had an enormous impact on how nursing care is rendered. What is considered to be safe and adequate care in current curricula would not have been considered such at all in programs of the past (Tanner, 2000). That all-important race for the ever-shrinking capitated dollar means that nursing continues to view both acute and long-term settings as belonging to an ever-changing landscape.

Although students are able to delineate values of the profession, they are still limited in their abilities to elaborate their views in a way that indicates that these values have been fully internalized (Reutter et al., 1997). The values of the healthcare system can conflict with the traditional values of nursing (Lindeman, 2001). The profession of nursing has long espoused health, wellness, and wholeness as integral to its beliefs. Yet in practice, students see on a daily basis that the "majority of nurses are working in a disease state medical model system" (Wesorick, 1995, p. 40). From the beginning of their entry into the profession, they witness a disconnect between what is taught and what is actually practiced. In a world where high praise but few dollars are lent to prevention, a widening chasm evolves for the beginning practitioner to view.

# Errors

Mistakes by students and how they are handled are critical to their future practice. When treated poorly – yelled at, cussed at, charts bouncing around the desk – some students learn one thing and one thing only "making a mistake is so awful I do not want to let anyone know when I make another one." As individuals who respond to behavioral reinforcements, a negative experience can cause one to do anything not to repeat that experience. Opportunities to dialogue about an error must be available to students immediately after an error is made and later after they have had more time to process what happened. These conversations can also open up ways to deal with feelings and how to handle negative interactions with staff, faculty, or physicians (Haffner & Raingruber, 1998).

The nursing profession has an expectation that nurses be competent at all times. This is the ideal, something to strive toward. Although we must not lower our expectations of competency, "it would serve our nursing community better if we could turn our anger into understanding and supportive sharing" (Crisall, 1997, p. 4). Too often in the clinical area, "students go through a humiliating ordeal to communicate/correct their errors" (Miller & Malcolm, 1990, p. 71). By changing the way we view errors, we can respond with empathy and strategies for corrective action and constructive discipline. Such a message would be proactive and positive rather than destructive to the individual and ourselves and would maintain the integrity of the profession (Crisall, 1997). Although the need to minimize errors that have costly human consequences is recognized, faculty need to consider what this process does to students. Do students come out of these experiences with an enhanced ability to think critically or an overwhelming fear of making another mistake (Miller & Malcolm, 1990)? The ability of a neophyte to comprehend that even the simplest of tasks has a complex cognitive process beneath it, is an important component of successful socialization.

## Journaling

Reflective writing is a terrific way for an experienced nurse to see the day's activities through the eyes of a student. Often teachers are shocked to read that what was to their mind a successful morning of client care did, in fact, overwhelm students from the beginning. Many times, students view a clinical day on the unit as chaos unfolding before them. Encouraging the writing of lived experiences utilizes reflective learning and gives students the opportunity to clarify the knowledge underpinning their actions (Burton, 2000). Most importantly reflective writing encourages students to integrate theory with practice (Burton, 2000).

Journaling should be a part of each clinical day, and weekly summaries should be left with the clinical teacher for review. This process also promotes a sense of trust for nursing students and initiates a model for confidentiality. Students learn quickly that the thoughts and feelings they express on paper are safe with the teacher. Individual students' perception of a teacher's trustworthiness has been noted as an important factor in their ability to reflect (Burton, 2000). This is also an excellent way to allow neophytes to see the nurse as a secret sharer (Gordon, 1996).

The downside of journaling by students has been cited as postponed entries, thereby missing the moment; a decreased enthusiasm when it is seen as a chore; and a general unwillingness to reflect. Nursing teachers who are cognizant of these common pitfalls constantly strive to find alternative solutions to overcome them.

# Self-Confidence

Development of self-confidence and self-esteem are critical to the successful socialization of any new member to a profession. All too often, nursing students complete their program with less personal confidence than when they started the program (Lindeman, 2000). Lack of self-esteem and passive-aggressive behavior are characteristics noted in nurses (Roberts, 1997). For example, consider the student who is observing a practicing nurse working without eating or taking a break, in short, unable to delegate to peers and take some time for self. When questioned about this, the nurse may respond "If I don't do it, who will?" or "There is so much to do. I will have more time to get it done if I don't eat." Many students assume this behavior to be the norm and enter the profession thinking they, too, do not have time or are not worthy of taking time to eat, take a break, sit, or, most importantly, take time to think about their clients. Faculty members who point out the fallacy of this behavior and how it fosters poor self-esteem help novices begin to see which behaviors should not be imitated.

From the beginning of the clinical practice, faculty teach that the work is never done and that missing meals does not increase efficacy, stamina, or nurses' own well-being. By seeing that students take a break and learn to delegate their client care when off the unit, faculty members emphasize the importance of helping colleagues and also what delegation entails. Teachers need to constantly emphasize that when nurses are seated and discussing clients and their care, this is not time wasted but rather time well spent.

Students' awareness of their limited knowledge and experience may lead to a feeling of inadequacy, which is particularly stressful. Because they are still developing a sense of their own competence, students are very vulnerable to feedback. Negative comments from others about students' work decrease their professional self-esteem. Seeking validation just to **make sure** is an important aspect of their learning (Reutter et al., 1997). Problems can result when a novice's desire to learn how to **do it** is coupled with an experienced nurse's inability to emphasize the importance of reflection on work completed. This leads to a situation that leaves students awash in indecision and low self-esteem relative to their ability to render care correctly. Self-confidence and self-esteem can be developed through conscious attention to doing so. Nursing desperately needs faculty who are able "to reinforce students' strengths while also helping improve performance" (Lindeman, 2000, p. 4).

# Lifelong Learning

"The knowledge explosion has made outdated the notion that one can ever achieve mastery of a body of knowledge, so the focus has to be toward a preparation for lifelong learning" (McBride, 1999, p. 119). Too often, the novice looks at the end of college and the completion of the licensure examination as a chance to pack the books away. A foundation of socialization of the neophyte must include the premise of lifelong learning. Faculty need to introduce lifelong learning as a given to membership in the profession, not as a choice. This is demonstrated throughout the curriculum by witnessing practicing nurses returning for advanced degrees, journal/discussion groups at the clinical sites and at the academic institution, client care and grand rounds opportunities, etc. Actual ways that lifelong learning is demonstrated in a practice arena go beyond competency fairs and Joint Commission on Accreditation of Healthcare Organizations (JCAHO) drills. Students should listen for and be made aware of practicing nurses who:

- Subscribe to journals.
- Cite recent articles and research.
- Utilize the hospital website, internet access, and library options.
- Join professional organizations.
- Give presentations at staff meetings, continuing education programs, and regional and national conferences.

This is a golden opportunity for faculty to talk with students and point out that not only are these nurses sharing knowledge with others but that they are also expanding their own knowledge base. All nurses should share with novices how they update their own libraries, why they attend professional conferences and meetings, what resources they could not live without, and where good information is found. Students need to be constantly reminded that whether or not they learn rests solely on them.

Developing and teaching a curriculum that presents nursing coherently as both an art and a science and being a "guide at the side" (Tanner, 2000) are the responsibilities of faculty members. The ultimate goal for nurse educators is to educate nurses who, with experience and practice, will be clinical scholars capable of functioning in a multitude of settings (Elberson & Williams, 1996). Faculty who present the attitude that "every nurse needs to continually refresh, understand, and use their knowledge base assist students to see lifelong learning as a **life of learning**" (Davidson, 2001, p.2).

From the very beginning to the completion of the nursing students' clinical experiences, faculty need to continually point out when nurses take, and when they choose not to take, the opportunity to be a lifelong learner. The expert at the bedside is often the object of hero worship for novices. Teachers who are aware of this will encourage students to note if the nurse has earned certification in a nursing specialty. This is a wonderful example of lifelong learning as it presents the opportunity to discuss how certifications are obtained and **kept current** though additional education.

It is critical that neophytes see continuous learning as a component of professional socialization that is considered as important as the learning of clinical tasks. It is important that students are socialized by faculty to view nursing as a profession rather than a technical vocation, with its own body of knowledge, research, and theories (Tanner, 2000). It is imperative to the socialization process that faculty take into consideration the extent to which nursing is shaped by changes in healthcare delivery and academia – two major social systems in the process of reinventing themselves (McBride, 1999). Figure 52.5 looks at these changes in perception and shows the movement from traditional to a more expanded view of nursing and nursing education. Success in the current healthcare industry requires an intact sense of self-esteem and self-confidence. In the past, these qualities in nursing candidates were not sought after by hospital leadership. In fact, the behaviors rewarded were ones that relegated staff nurses to a subservient or victim role.

Figure 52.5 –  Shifting Paradigms

| Shifting Paradigms | |
| --- | --- |
| **Traditional View** | **Expanded View** |
| Healthcare delivery<br>  Nursing at bedside<br>  Process oriented (what professional is doing)<br>  Emphasis on meeting needs/<br>    oblivious to costs<br>  Emphasis largely on mortality<br>    and some on morbidity<br>  Nursing = direct care<br>  Nurse supports primary care provider<br>  Responsible for discharge planning<br><br>Academia<br>  Emphasis on teaching<br>  Place-bound<br>  Scholarship narrowly defined/congruent with<br>    personal interests<br>  Service perceived as quasi-charity<br>  Centralized administration | Healthcare delivery<br>  Nursing at patient's side<br>  Outcomes oriented (value of what professional is<br>    doing)<br>  Emphasis on triaging needs/mindful of costs<br>  Emphasis on mortality, limiting morbidity, and<br>    maximizing functioning/quality of life<br>  Nursing = direct care; promoting self-care; directing<br>    care given by others; designing population-based<br>    health programs; and managing patient services<br>  Nurse provides primary care<br>  Responsible for managing lifestyle change<br><br>Academia<br>  Emphasis on learning<br>  "Virtual University"<br>  Scholarship broadly defined/congruent with<br>    institutional mission<br>  Service valued for revenue generation<br>  Responsibility-centered management |

Note.  From "Breakthroughs in Nursing Education: Looking Back, Looking Forward," by A. B. McBride, 1999, *Nursing Outlook, 47* (3), 114-119. Copyright 1999 by Mosby, Inc.  Reprinted with permission of the author.

With the increasing popularity of obtaining magnet status as an indicator of how well an institution is doing, client care divisions are looking at and rewarding those individuals who demonstrate insight into their work behaviors and how attitudes affect others in the workplace. Students who have been socialized throughout their educational experiences to reflect on not just the work, but also on how the work affects them and others, will become the nurses who are successful and pursued for employment.

## Learning Activities

1. Write your own definition of Socialization and how you envision it happening in nursing.
2. Interview a nurse recruiter at a hospital. Where do they see their job ending...after the interview? hiring? orientation? internship? How do they see socialization occurring in their institution?
3. Interview a nursing faculty member and ask him or her to define socialization. How does it occur? How do they measure it? Where in the curriculum do opportunities for socialization occur?

## References

Aiken, L. H., Clarke, S. P., Sloane, D. M., & Sochalski, J., Center for Health Outcomes and Policy Research, School of Nursing, University of Pennsylvania (2001, May). Cause for Concern: Nurses' Reports of Hospital Care in Five Countries. *LDI Issue Brief,* pp. 1-4.

Benner, P. (1984). *From novice to expert*. Menlo Park, CA: Addison-Wesley.

Brookfield, S. (1993). On impostorship, Cultural suicide, and other dangers: How nurses learn critical thinking. *Journal of Continuing Education in Nursing, 24*, 197-205.

Burton, A. J. (2000). Reflection: Nursing's practice and education panacea? *Journal of Advanced Nursing, 31*, 1009-1017.

Campbell, I., Larrivee, L., Field, P. A., Day, R., & Reutter, L. (1994). Learning to nurse in the clinical setting. *Journal of Advanced Nursing, 20*, 1125-1131.

Christman, L. (1998). Who is a nurse? *Image: Journal of Nursing Scholarship, 30*, 211-214.

Clayton, G. M., Broome, M. E. & Ellis, L. A. (1989). Relationship between a preceptorship experience and roles socialization of graduate nurses. *Journal of Nursing Education, 28,* 72-75.

Corwin, R. G. (1961). Role conception and career aspiration: A study of identity in nursing. *Sociological Quarterly, 2*, pp.69-86.

Coudret, N. A., Fuchs, P. L., Roberts, C. S., Suhrheinrich, J.A., & White, A. H. (1994). Role socialization of graduating student nurses: Impact of a nursing practicum on professional role conception. *Journal of Professional Nursing, 10*, 342-349.

Coulter, A. (1999). Paternalism or partnership? *British Medical Journal, 319*, 719-720.

Crisall, S. J. (1997). AJNAGENDA. *American Journal of Nursing, 97*(3), 4.

Davidson, S. B. (2001). The secret of lifelong learning. *Oregon Nurse, 66*(2), 3.

Dumont, M. (1970). The changing face of professionalism. In L. Netzer (Ed.), *Education, administration, and change* (pp. 20-26). New York: Harper & Row.

Elberson, K. L., & Williams, S. A. (1996). Innovative strategies for promoting clinical scholarship: A holistic approach. *Holistic Nursing Practice, 10*(3), 33-40.

Haffer, A. G., & Raingruber, B. J. (1998). Discovering confidence in clinical reasoning and critical-thinking development in baccalaureate nursing students. *Journal of Nursing Education, 37*, 61-70.

Kramer, M. (1974). *Reality shock: Why nurses leave nursing.* St. Louis, MO: CV Mosby.

Lawler, T. G. (1988). Measuring socialization to the professional nursing role. In O. L. Strickland & C. F. Waltz (Eds.), *Measurement of nursing outcomes (Vol. 2): Measuring nursing performance: Practice, education, and research* (pp. 32-53). New York: Springer.

Lindeman, C. A. (2000). Nursing's socialization of nurses. *Creative Nursing, 6*(4), 3-4.

MacDonald, C. (2002). Nurse autonomy as relational. *Nursing Ethics, 9*(2), 194-201.

McBride, A. B. (1999). Breakthroughs in nursing education: Looking back, looking forward. *Nursing Outlook, 47*(3), 114-119.

Miller, M. A., & Malcolm, N. S. (1990). Critical thinking in the nursing curriculum. *Nursing and Health Care, 11*(2), 67-73.

Muff, J. (1982). *Socialization, sexism, and stereotyping: women's issues in nursing.* St. Louis, MO: The C.V. Mosby Company.

Nesler, M. S., Hanner, M. B., Melburg, V., & McGowan, S. (2001). Professional socialization of baccalaureate nursing students: Can students in distance nursing programs become socialized? *Journal of Nursing Education, 40*, 293-302.

Pieta, B. A. (1976). A comparison of role conceptions among nursing students and faculty from associate degree, baccalaureate degree, and diploma nursing programs and head nurses. *Dissertation Abstracts International, 37* (5604-B), 11B. (Publication No. 77-10,688).

Reutter, L., Field, P. A., Campbell, I. E., & Day, R. (1997). Socialization into nursing: Nursing students as learners. *Journal of Nursing Education, 36*, 149-155.

Roberts, S. J. (1997, Fall). Nurse executives in the 1990s: Empowered or oppressed? *Nursing Administration Quarterly*, 64-71.

Saarmann, L., Freitas, L., Rapps, J., & Riegel, B. (1992). The relationship of education to critical-thinking ability and values among nurses: Socialization into professional nursing. *Journal of Professional Nursing, 8*, 26-34.

Sheer, B. (1994). Reshaping the nurse practitioner image through socialization. *Nurse Practitioner Forum, 5*, 215-219.

Stone, H., & Knopke, H. (1978). *Data gathering instruments for evaluation educational programs in the health sciences.* Unpublished manuscript, University of Wisconsin, Madison.

Tanner, C.A. (1986). The Nursing Care Plan as a Teaching Method: Reason or Ritual. *Nurse Educator, 11*(4), 8-10.

Tanner, C. (2000a). Socializing students on the complexity of practice. *Creative Nursing, 6*(4), 8-11.

Tanner, C. A. (2000b). Editorial: Critical thinking: Beyond nursing process. *Journal of Nursing Education, 39*, 338-339.

Tanner, C.A. (2001). Competency-Based Education: The New Panacea. *Journal of Nursing Education, 40*(9), 387-388.

Thomka, L. A. (2001). Graduate nurses' experiences of interactions with professional nursing staff during transition to the professional role. *Journal of Continuing Education in Nursing, 32*, 15-19.

Wesorick, B. (1995). *The closing and opening of a millennium: A journey from old to new thinking.* Grand Rapids, MI: Practice Field Publishing.

Woodward, V. M. (1998). Caring, patient autonomy and the stigma of paternalism. *Journal of Advanced Nursing, 28* (5), 1046-1052.

# Chapter 53: BRIDGING THEORY TO PRACTICE

Carol "Candy" Gordon, BS, MS, RN, BC

*Transitioning roles from student nurse to practicing nurse is daunting, even for the most confident of graduates. Ms. Gordon walks us through the process of designing and implementing a program to effect successful transitioning for both employee and employer. Goals, benefits, and overall program satisfaction are explored as the gap is bridged between theory and practice. – Lynn Engelmann and Linda Caputi*

## Introduction

The bridge between education and clinical practice for newly graduated nurses is sometimes a long, steep upward climb, fraught with excitement and joy but also fear and frustration. The new nurse has left the safe shelter of the classroom and is taking the first, tentative steps toward the ultimate goal of becoming a confident, fully functioning professional.

## Educational Philosophy

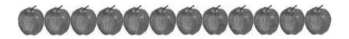

I believe that everyone is a teacher as well as a learner. The experience of learning should be centered around the students at whatever stage they are on the continuum of skills acquisition and educational level. Each student's unique educational needs must be addressed based on learning styles, experiences, and educational background. My goal as a teacher is to facilitate learning by assessing the students' learning styles and needs and providing a stimulating educational environment where those needs are met by varied instructional modes throughout the teaching-learning cycle. Learning is enhanced within an environment of mutual respect and trust that builds confidence, personal growth, and critical-thinking skills. My desire is to promote within each student a passion for continuous lifelong learning. – Carol Gordon

It is often apparent that the new graduates hired into nursing positions struggle with the transition into their new role. The challenge to make this transition a fulfilling and positive experience can be daunting, both for the new nurse and for the institution.

In May 1998, Central DuPage Hospital (CDH) decided to address this challenge and developed a 12-week New Graduate Program designed to meet the needs of new practitioners moving into their first professional experience. After only two years, the program was deemed so successful that it was enlarged to two sessions yearly to meet the needs of the winter graduates.

The program continues to be offered each winter and summer, with plans to add a third session to accommodate graduating nurses who choose to take a few months off before beginning their career. This chapter covers the process CDH used to study the need for a new graduate orientation program and its eventual design and implementation.

## Assessment of Need

As an outgrowth of the CDH Recruitment and Retention Committee, a group was formed to investigate the need for and feasibility of a program designed for nurses entering the profession. The impetus for studying the possibility of such a program was to provide a recruitment tool both for new graduates and experienced nurses, to promote retention among new nurses, and to provide a positive experience for nurses during the first months in their profession.

### *Questions and Analysis*

During the data-gathering process, resources were identified and contacted to assess the need and discuss the possibilities of a new graduate program. The following questions were asked.

#### *What Is the Current State?*

A great deal of discussion in the group related to how new graduates were welcomed and mentored into their new careers at CDH. Generally, the new graduates participated in the standard orientation program together with experienced nurses, with no additional support specific to the new graduate. During their clinical orientation, the newly employed nurses – experienced as well as inexperienced – were assigned preceptors and completed the competency validation tool with those preceptors. During the latter part of the orientation period, discussions were held with orientees, preceptors, and/or charge nurses or unit managers. At that time it was decided whether each orientee was capable of assuming the role without further orientation. The orientation period was extended by one to two weeks as necessary.

The entire orientation experience was no different for a new graduate than for an experienced nurse. Although the new graduates often required a slightly longer orientation period, there was no formal mechanism for any further support or additional learning opportunities.

## What Skills Are Needed for a Nurse to Do the Job?

Using the current competency lists as the starting point, skills specific to the new graduate were identified. Interpersonal skills as well as clinical skills were added to the list of skills to be considered. Additional attention was given to specialty unit skills in addition to general nursing skills.

## What Are the Gaps Seen Between Nursing Education and Practice?

Several people were consulted as resources to answer this question. These people identified a concern regarding the difficulty of moving from the school setting, with its emphasis on learning facts and tasks, to the reality of nursing, where the facts and tasks must be integrated into the actual care of the client. The transition from learning the specific nursing skills and facts to applying the entire body of knowledge to clients – and at the same time learning organizational and prioritizing skills – was frequently overwhelming. Although it is recognized that schools of nursing teach critical thinking at application and higher levels, the sheer number of occasions the graduate nurse must engage in this type of thinking on a daily basis is overwhelming.

Additional gaps identified included the difficulty in bringing together the clinical skills and knowledge gained in school and applying it in a comprehensive manner. A gap identified by most of the resources consulted was the difficulty in "looking at the big picture," which includes bringing together assessment skills; interpretation of data; and analysis of input from the client, other staff members, and physicians to plan and implement the care. The ability to prioritize, to anticipate and adjust to changes in clients' conditions, and to deal with rapidly changing responsibilities are all skills that are developed through experience and guidance/coaching by mentors.

## What Are the Biggest Challenges/Frustrations Seen in the First Months?

Evans (2001) described the expectations of new nurses as a process of separation, transition, and integration. Separation from student status, with its familiarity and security, to the uncertainty of autonomous, professional practice brings conflicting emotions. Transition to staff nurse status is described as the specific shock-like reactions to finding oneself in the situations for which one worked, studied, and prepared only to find one, in fact, does not feel prepared at all. Integration into the profession occurs through role models who provide recognition, positive feedback, and positive interactions.

## What Is Most Helpful to a New Graduate in the First Months?

The resource people who were consulted described the overall mentoring relationships with experienced nurses, even when not officially designated as such, as the one most helpful factor in the first months.

### Resources Consulted

Many various resources were consulted for their differing viewpoints and to determine their support for a new graduate program. These resources included the following.

### Managers/Administration

Input was solicited from managers and administrators for their opinions and suggestions and also to ensure administrative/managerial support for a new graduate program. The financial and staffing implications were significant. The support of managers and administrators was critical to the continuing exploration and ultimate implementation of a new graduate program.

### Staff Nurses

Staff nurses were identified as an excellent resource because they have experienced being new graduates and could provide valuable information on what was helpful and what was problematic as they transitioned into the role of a professional nurse. Additionally, staff nurses – particularly preceptors – were identified as critical to the success of both the program and the orientees themselves.

Staff nurses shared their perceptions of what would enhance the orientation process for new graduates and the types of additional classes they believed would add to the program. Generally, the nurses consulted were excited about the idea of a new graduate program and offered suggestions and input about what they believed would be helpful and/or not helpful to a new graduate participating in a formal program.

### Local Faculty Member

A faculty member from a local university – also a CDH employee – who taught students in their last semester provided additional input. This teacher offered insight into what could and could not be expected of new graduates relative to what they learned in their formal educational process. She also discussed the concerns and fears that graduating students had shared with her as they looked forward to their first nursing position.

## *Clinical Educators*

Clinical educators from within CDH, involved in the orientation of new nurses, brought their perspective and information about what was included in the orientation process currently offered. They assisted in identifying opportunities for further classes and experiences that could be tailored to meet the unique needs of the new graduates.

## *Literature*

The university faculty resource person provided textbooks and skills lists. These were used to identify skills and knowledge the students were required to master before graduation. Articles discussing the stresses on new nurses as they assumed their new roles were reviewed. Due to an extremely tight timeline, a complete literature search was not performed.

## Development of the Program

Once the decision was made to develop and implement the New Graduate Program for the summer of 1998, the process of developing and organizing was delegated to the Department of Clinical Education. What looked like an insurmountable task to complete in such a short amount of time became more manageable by breaking the larger task into smaller parts.

The first decision made before proceeding with development of the program was to determine how long the new-graduate orientation period would be. A 12-week, full-time program seemed to be a reasonable length of time that could be supported by all the client care units. Twelve weeks would offer enough time to include both classroom and clinical experiences. Three clinical educators were then designated to lead the development of the program. Following is a step-by-step description of how the program was developed, implemented, and evaluated.

### *Developing Overall Goals*

The overall goal of the program was to provide the newly graduated nurses with an orientation program that would include learning opportunities and support to become confident, competent, and caring professional nurses. Measurements of success would include:

- Length of time the new graduate remained employed.
- Ability of the new graduate to carry a full load on the assigned client care unit.
- Positive socialization, such as new-graduate interactions with other employees, communication with the entire team rather than just with the preceptor, assertive behaviors with other team members, ability to handle own disputes, other team members approaching the new graduate for input or advice, and participation in unit social functions.
- Feedback from preceptors, managers, charge nurses, physicians, other employees on the unit, and the new graduate.
- Competency list completed and filed in Human Resources.
- Decrease in open positions and in turnover/vacancy rates.

### *Consultants*

During the development of the program, many various resources were consulted for ideas, suggestions, encouragement, and expertise in all areas of planning.

### *Client Care Managers*

From the onset, client care managers were involved in providing suggestions related to what they had observed as gaps for new graduates transitioning to practice on their units. Ideas included:

- Classes that provide initial understanding of issues specifically related to this health system.
- Classes to refresh what had already been taught in the nursing school classroom.
- Other experiences that would include new information related to the specialty area.

Discussions occurred with managers on how they could best support the new graduates in the program. Check-ins were established. Check-ins are weekly meetings among the managers, preceptors, and orientees to provide a more formal type of feedback and to give orientees an opportunity to discuss progress toward goals. These check-ins were viewed as important not only for those involved but also to allow for correction or change in the program as needed, thereby serving a formative evaluation purpose as well.

Managers were enlisted to set the tone with their staff about how to support the new graduate and preceptor. Establishing expectations for the staff was key to promoting the enculturation of the new graduate into the unit.

## Staff Nurses

The staff nurses comprised a key group of employees for input and support. Mentoring and collegial relationships between staff nurses and the new graduates needed to be established. Staff nurses had a major influence on four areas identified as crucial to the success of the program and ultimately to the success of the new nurses. These four areas include:

- Input from the staff nurses about their experiences as new graduates entering the profession: what helped them, what caused problems for them, what they wish they had known, and what could have made things better for them. The nurses had a wide range of new graduate experiences, from those who had no orientation whatsoever (sink-or-swim mentality) to those who had a positive, nurturing orientation experience. Suggestions ranged from easily implemented ideas to impossibilities. These were evaluated and included as appropriate.

- Because the staff nurses would be functioning as preceptors and mentors to the new graduates, it was important to listen to their concerns and suggestions as well as to identify ways of supporting them in these roles. Although some staff had attended a full-day course about precepting, many of them had never oriented a new graduate. The needs of the preceptors were discussed and plans were made to meet those needs prior to implementing the program.

- In many cases, the staff nurses participated in teaching in the classroom. Many of them were excited about using their gifts in teaching and supporting the new graduates.

- The staff nurses who would not be precepting or teaching were considered to be a key component of the orientation program by their support – or lack of it – for the new graduates and the preceptors. Ideally, the preceptors were assigned a greatly reduced client care assignment, which meant the other staff nurses would need to pick up some extra client care responsibilities. The attitude of the non-precepting nurses toward the program would impact both the new graduates and the preceptors. A supportive, encouraging attitude was desirable from each member of the staff.

## Local Faculty

Ideas from faculty from colleges and universities affiliated with CDH were particularly helpful in designing the curriculum. They shared the concerns that had been voiced by their last-semester students surrounding their expectations and fears. The faculty also discussed some of the differences in curricula among the various colleges. For example, some of the schools' curricula included critical care classes with clinical experiences, but others did not. Most of the schools included classes on leadership and delegation, with opportunities to practice. However, at other schools those experiences were limited.

## Content Experts

Content experts were identified, including many of the institution's advanced practice nurses and experienced staff. These experts helped to determine the types and content of classes offered as part of the program.

## Human Resources

Hiring new graduates was delegated to the human resources department in cooperation with the client care managers. It was emphasized that the orientees would be expected to participate in the entire program on a full-time basis. If a new graduate was hired in a part-time position, that status would begin after completion of the 12-week program. Because the human resources recruiters would be the only ones interviewing potential members of the group and then making the hiring decisions, it was important that they understand the goals and components of the program.

## Clinical Educators

The clinical educators were responsible for the orientation of all nurses new to the health system. This orientation was general in nature and offered to all newly hired nurses. Prior to this program beginning, there was nothing offered specifically to the needs of new graduates. During the orientation period, the clinical educators frequently interacted with the new employees and were able to identify gaps and differences between new graduates and experienced nurses.

Once the decision was made to proceed with a new graduate program, the clinical educators, working as a team, led the development.

### Identifying Units that Can Accommodate New Graduates

Each client care manager was asked to consider the resources of the unit, the number of qualified preceptors, and any other factors that might impact the orientation of new nurses. Using this information, managers were asked to determine the number of new graduates the unit could effectively support. The decision was made by administration of the hospital that, even if a unit had no current budgeted openings, new graduates could be accepted as **overhires**, knowing that some turnover could occur before the end of the 12-week program.

During the first several weeks of the program, the new graduates would work only on the day shift. This required each unit accepting one or more new graduates to have enough preceptors on the day shift to meet the needs of the new graduates. Managers were faced with the challenge of scheduling enough preceptors to assist not only the new nurse graduates but also any other new employees joining the healthcare team. Discussions were held on the feasibility of having new graduates on specialty units. Some controversy accompanied these discussions because some staff members believed that new graduates should never be placed on a specialty unit without spending at least a year on a medical-surgical unit. Other staff members believed that given appropriate classes and support, new graduates could function well in a specialty area. Each manager of a specialty unit was asked to decide whether that unit would be able to accommodate a new graduate, considering the new graduates would receive additional support through classroom experiences.

### *Deciding on Hiring Prerequisites/Plan*

Due to the tight timeline, it was decided that the new graduates would be hired for a division – such as maternal/child or medical/surgical – rather than for a specific unit. The interview and hiring process was handled by the human resources department rather than by individual client care managers. At the end of the program, new graduates would be placed on a client care unit that might or might not be the unit where they would receive their orientation. At the end of the program, the managers would evaluate their openings and place the new graduates on the unit and shifts available, taking the requests of the new graduates into consideration.

Through a rigorous process, interviewers selected the most likely candidates from a pool of new graduate applicants, including some who were currently employed in other positions within the institution as they completed their studies.

### *Developing a List of General Knowledge*

### *Topics to be Addressed*

The clinical educator team developed a list of topics applicable to all units hiring new graduates. This list included topics such as delegation, administration of blood and blood products, IV administration, resuscitation procedures, computerized documentation, and wound/skin care. Many of the topics were included because the new graduates needed specific information about the implementation of these topics at this facility. For example, a class on care of the client with diabetes mellitus would include not only the latest on diabetes management but also the resources available at this facility and how the diabetes teaching occurs for the client at CDH.

The new graduates were expected to complete the same basic list of competencies as was expected for all nurses in each area. Educational opportunities were identified to meet the learning needs related to the competencies. Some of these opportunities included classroom instruction, self-learning modules, and other interactive sessions.

Clinical educators, in collaboration with content experts, defined measurable behavioral objectives for each class. Content outlines were developed, including time frames and teaching methodologies for each topic. Potential instructors were identified based on expertise, experience teaching, and interest in working with new graduates. Some of the topics included on this general top list for all new graduates included the following items.

### Interpersonal Skills and Professionalism

Topics to help the new graduates grow in their interpersonal skills and professionalism were included. Classes addressing listening skills, critical thinking, prioritizing, taking care of and honoring themselves and others, and dealing with difficult people were offered. A class dealing with interactions with the medical staff was facilitated by a physician. The presentation included ways to communicate with physicians and the kinds of information a physician is interested in knowing.

### Delegation

Classes on delegation were designed to present the principles of delegation, with examples to stimulate critical thinking. Discussions included the role of each member of the interdisciplinary team and information about the training period for each role. Guidelines for the types of tasks appropriate for unlicensed caregivers were given. Some of the new graduates had been working in an unlicensed role at CDH, so it was important to talk about the potential difficulties of transitioning from that role to the role of a licensed nurse.

A follow-up class was held several weeks after the initial delegation classes to provide an opportunity to discuss the successes and difficulties the new graduates encountered when delegating. Many of them were having difficulty delegating tasks because they thought they needed to do it all and viewed asking for help as a weakness. The session was led by a client care manager who was able to provide coaching and advice to help these new nurses delegate more effectively.

### Death and Dying

Typically, the new graduates had neither been present when a client died nor cared for a client in the dying process during their nursing school clinical experiences. A session was developed by the chaplain titled *Death, Dying, Grief, and Growth*. This session helped the new graduates process their feelings prior to caring for clients during this final stage of life. They explored their reactions to situations in their personal lives involving death and discussed what they had learned from those experiences.

## *Equipment*

An opportunity for hands-on practice with equipment and devices during the first week of orientation is a key component of the program. This practice ensures the preparedness of the new graduates to perform certain skills and to use certain pieces of equipment – IV pump, PCA pump, bladder scanner, automatic blood pressure machine, feeding pump – when needed. There were several reasons for this decision.

- New graduates voiced their lack of confidence when using these types of equipment. These skills laboratory sessions provided an opportunity to learn about and practice using these devices before doing so in a client care situation. The new graduates arrived on the unit feeling confident because they had demonstrated a level of competence with the equipment.
- The skills laboratory classes also gave new graduates an opportunity to practice specific nursing skills, such as nasogastric tube insertion and urinary catheter insertion. Because the opportunities to perform these skills varied among the different schools, some new graduates had not performed these skills. The skills laboratory provided the opportunity to practice in a nonthreatening situation with expert guidance immediately available.
- The time spent practicing skills in the laboratory saved time and effort by the preceptors on the unit. By the time the new graduates reached the unit, they had been able to demonstrate and practice the skills under the supervision of the staff nurses serving as instructors for the session. The preceptors were able to move directly to other topics knowing that the skills had already been introduced in the classroom/ simulated setting.

## *Developing a List of Specialty Subjects to Be Addressed*

After the list of general classes was developed, competency lists for the specialty areas open to receiving new graduates were studied. Classes in each specialty area were identified in the same manner as the general classes. Objectives, content outline, time frames, teaching methodologies, and potential instructors were identified. Classes scheduled for the critical care division included a basic EKG interpretation course of 7 classes, hemodynamic monitoring, titratable IV medications, care of the cardiac client, and neurologic assessment. Classes for the medical-surgical division included assessment of the older adult, emergency management of the medical-surgical client, and postoperative care. The maternal-child division classes included assessment of the pediatric client, preparing a child for procedures, assessment of the newborn including gestational age, labor support, and management of obstetrical complications.

### *Planning Schedule Based on Logical Flow of Material*

As the classes were being developed, the schedule for sequencing the classes was planned. The original schedule took on the following form:

- The first day of orientation for all employees covered the general, house-wide orientation program. This session covered the mission, vision, and values of the hospital; safety information; human resources information relative to benefits and personnel policies; and completion of individual tasks, such as assigning computer access codes, obtaining name badges, and distributing parking passes.
- Because most general classes apply to all the new graduates, working on any type of client care unit, those general classes were scheduled during the first four weeks. These classes focused on topics needed before the new graduates cared for clients in the clinical area. This also included sessions in the skills laboratory and learning computer documentation.
- The last day of the first week was assigned as a clinical day so the new graduates could care for clients on the clinical units and begin applying some of their knowledge.
- Over the following four weeks, classes were scheduled every Monday and Tuesday, with the rest of the week spent in the clinical area. The classes were maintained consistently on those days for ease in clinical scheduling. After the fifth week, classes were scheduled for every Monday. At this time, the classes focused on the specialty areas.

### *Preceptor Preparation*

One of the crucial pieces of the entire program is the quality and support of the preceptor/orientee relationship. Client care managers were given information and suggestions regarding how to select preceptors and were asked to be highly discriminating in their choices.

Managers were asked to follow the criteria developed by the education department for the selection of preceptors. It was requested that, before consideration, the potential preceptor attend the hospital preceptor workshop. Additionally, each preceptor should possess the following qualities:

- A willingness and interest in training new people.
- Competence in current position and employment in that position a minimum of six months.
- Good organizational skills.
- A demonstration of a team philosophy.
- A positive attitude.
- Good communication skills.
- Ability to be approachable.
- The position of full-time employee.

In addition, a preceptor selected to work with a new graduate should also:
- Verbalize a desire and commitment to the success of the new graduate.
- Believe in the value a new graduate can bring to the team.
- Be willing to precept on a full-time basis for up to six months.
- Be available to the new graduate for an indefinite period of time.
- Agree to attend the new graduate preceptor training to prepare for the additional responsibilities.
- Encourage team support of new graduates.
- Ensure that the new graduate attends all scheduled meetings and classes.

A special luncheon was given to honor the preceptors followed by a three-hour training session that focused on the unique needs of new graduates. The entire New Graduate Program was presented along with a description and listing of the classes offered.

The preceptors learned about the support they would be given. A presentation on the mentoring process followed by a discussion of Benner's (1984) model of skill acquisition. A local faculty member discussed the formal educational preparation the new graduate received during nursing school and suggested ideas for assignments and learning opportunities. Time was allowed for questions and an open forum to share thoughts and ideas on how best to work with a new graduate.

The preceptors were asked to talk through their thought processes as they cared for clients so the new graduates could learn about the preceptor's critical thinking and decision making. The preceptors were also instructed to encourage the new graduates to ask frequent questions whenever they were not sure how a decision had been made or an action had been chosen. Talking through the planning process and prioritization choices can greatly benefit the new graduates.

# Implementation of the Program

The first group of 18 new graduates launched their careers at CDH on June 25, 1998. Six were hired for the medical-surgical division, five for the maternal-child division, and seven for the critical care division, which includes step-down units. Each had been assigned a unit within their division. That unit would be responsible for orienting the new graduate for the first 12 weeks. After that time, the new graduate would receive a permanent assignment within the division, although not necessarily on that unit. Each new graduate would be assigned to a primary preceptor who would be assisted as needed by an alternate preceptor.

# Evaluation

A variety of evaluation methods were helpful in identifying successes as well as opportunities to improve the program.

## *Unit Meetings*

Meetings were scheduled regularly between the manager, preceptor, and new graduate to discuss the progress toward goals. These meetings provided a mechanism for discussions regarding:

- Opportunities for clinical experiences and questions and answers regarding any aspect of the experiences.
- Suggestions for ways to provide experiences.
- Feedback among all parties about any aspect of the clinical experience.

## *Classroom Evaluation*

Evaluations of the content, the presenter, and whether the participants were able to meet the objectives were completed at the end of each class by each participant. The presenter also evaluated the class relative to the time allowed to cover the subject matter, any changes that needed to be made to content, and any changes in handouts or other learning materials.

## *Check-In Sessions*

Every two to three weeks during the program, check-in sessions were held with the orientation group facilitated by a clinical educator. At that time, the group was asked to discuss the program, the clinical experiences, what additional learning experiences would meet their needs, and whether the classes were relevant to their practice. These sessions provided an opportunity for the facilitator to lead a discussion of strategies to address issues raised or to clarify information. Frequently a plus-delta approach was used (what was going well and what needed to change).

### Clinical Educator Meetings

As the orientation program progressed, the clinical educators met to discuss any changes that were needed related to needs or identified issues based on the discussions with the new graduates. Managers and staff educators were also consulted regarding general concerns as well as issues about individual orientees. Course corrections and supplemental learning opportunities were identified and implemented as appropriate.

### Final Evaluation

At the end of the program, overall evaluations were sent to new graduates, preceptors, and managers concerning both classroom and clinical experiences. The evaluations were overwhelmingly positive, with the new graduates relating that they felt "safer, more confident, and comfortable in clinical situations." Several of the new graduates stated they believed the program was "necessary for all new graduates – no new graduates should be without it."

A problem identified for the preceptors was the difficulty limiting their client care assignments during the first few weeks. The preceptors frequently felt rushed and stated they were not able to provide in-depth instruction to the orientees. The reality was that when a unit became busy, good intentions were not always the priority.

It was also difficult to maintain the one-preceptor guideline. The majority of staff nurses at CDH were employed part-time. Most orientees worked with a minimum of two preceptors. With several preceptors involved, communication became key. Communication skills among preceptors varied. It was important for preceptors to clearly communicate the orientee's progress toward goals with each other. However, a benefit of having more than one preceptor was the exposure to various approaches to organizing, prioritizing, and nursing care.

## Changes Based on Evaluations

### Hiring Patterns

Due to time constraints, the first group of new graduates was hired for a division rather than a specific unit. For some of them, the unit to which they were assigned was not the unit in which they received their orientation. The results of evaluating this type of hiring practice demonstrated dissatisfaction for the new graduates who found it difficult to build relationships on the unit, knowing they might be placed elsewhere. There was also dissatisfaction in not knowing what their final assignment would be and the fear of having to reorient after a short time. The staff on the units also were dissatisfied and reluctant to build relationships with the orientees, believing they were investing a lot of time and effort in someone who would be leaving to go to another unit. With the transfer to another unit, the new graduates had to be reoriented before their newly acquired skills and confidence were internalized.

Beginning with the second year of the program, the new graduates were interviewed by the client care managers and offered a specific position on a client care unit. The orientees were immediately recognized as permanent members of the staff, which resulted in much greater satisfaction for both the orientees and the staff on the unit. The staff were highly motivated to invest time and energy in someone who would become a peer.

Although new graduates continue to be hired to specialty units, the screening has become more stringent for those areas. In addition, most of the specialty units have extended the orientation period significantly beyond the 12-week new graduate orientation.

### *Additional Classes*

Several classes (both general and specialty) have been added, based on feedback from the program participants, instructors, preceptors, managers, and clinical educators. A few classes have been deleted, also based on feedback. The new graduates believed that some of the subjects had been covered in such depth in their nursing programs that the classes were redundant.

Other classes have been added based on changes implemented within the CDH system. For example, a pain management program has been added at the institution. A representative from the pain management program now addresses the new graduates and discusses the program and expectations regarding the assessment of and interventions for pain. To reinforce the information, each new graduate completes a web-based course about pain management.

A class outlining the various committees throughout the system was added. Included is a discussion of the benefits of involvement in committees and an opportunity to attend committee meetings of interest to the graduates. If they are interested in attending, they are introduced to a member of the committee and scheduled to attend with that person as their host.

## Tour of Affiliates

CDH is part of a healthcare system that includes convenient care sites, a rehabilitation/ extended care facility, an assisted living facility, a retirement home, a home care/hospice division, a physical therapy/cardiac rehabilitation facility affiliated with a health club, and multiple physician practices. Starting with the second group of new graduates, an entire classroom day is devoted to the continuum of care as practiced within the healthcare system. The day begins with a discharge planner discussing how decisions are made for the client's ongoing needs following discharge from the hospital. A home care/hospice nurse then discusses what is available through each affiliate. The rest of the day is spent touring and orienting to the various facilities, including information on what type of client care is delivered, how the interdisciplinary team works within each facility, and how each one interfaces with the rest of the healthcare system.

## Observational Experiences

Each new graduate is offered time in several different departments to gain insight into the client experience. The preoperative holding area and the post-anesthesia care units are visited by most of the participants. Additionally, nurses in cardiac units observe in the cardiac cathetherization laboratory, in surgery during an open-heart procedure, and in the cardiac rehabilitation program. Nurses on the orthopedic unit observe orthopedic surgery and physical therapy. Nurses in obstetrics spend a day with a lactation specialist, a day in the neonatal intensive care unit, and a day in the high-risk perinatal clinic. Mother/baby nurses spend a day in labor and delivery and vice versa. Additional experiences may include observing interventional radiology procedures, dialysis, or rehabilitation services.

New graduates are also given an opportunity to designate a department or person they would like to observe. This may include spending a day on a different unit to which they might like to cross-train in the future. Some new graduates requested spending a day with a chaplain, and others have requested a day with a respiratory therapist or time in the cardiology department, observing clients undergoing cardiac stress tests. Every effort is made to honor their requests.

## Benefits of Program

The new graduate program has proven beneficial for the graduates, the client care units, and the entire CDH healthcare system. Benefits specific to each are discussed below.

## *The Graduates*

Benefits to the new graduates include a strong support system as the transition is made from the student role to the professional role. New graduates are formally welcomed to the institution during an informal session with the vice president for Client Care Services/ chief nursing officer. This vice president spends a morning with the group interacting with them, asking and answering questions and reaffirming the commitment of the institution to their success. The new graduates are welcomed at a Meet-and-Greet Tea, which is held the afternoon before their first clinical day. Invited to the tea are managers, preceptors, staff educators, charge nurses, and previous new graduates. This is held with the specific purpose of providing a welcoming event along with exposure to the people on the unit with whom they will be working. They are able to meet and become familiar with people they will see on their first clinical day.

Another benefit is the development of a strong support group for each other. The group has served as a place to bring their experiences and receive feedback and encouragement from the rest of the new graduates. They become friends. Some of the groups have held reunions.

The new graduates benefit from the enhancement and practical application of the knowledge and skills they gained in school. Under the guidance of the preceptors and experienced staff nurses; they learn how to care for their clients; how to organize their responsibilities; what to expect as a practicing nurse; and how to interact with the clients, families, physicians, and other staff members.

During the orientation period, staff nurses and physicians include new graduates in interesting or unusual procedures. It is quite common for the staff and physicians to seek out the new graduates to observe when there is a new procedure or interesting case. This awareness of providing new experiences has lasted even beyond the official orientation period.

The orientation plan benefits the new graduates by allowing for individual differences in learning needs and level of confidence and competence. The opportunities for feedback, both in sessions with the managers and in the weekly check-in sessions, are helpful for identification of issues and needs, which are then addressed in a timely manner. The flexibility to extend the orientation period as necessary ensures that the new graduate is ready to assume the role and responsibilities before the orientation period is complete.

Staff nurses serving as instructors also provided the new graduates the opportunity to meet and get to know the nurses on all units. This facilitated a sense of belonging and identification with the hospital. It also provided another pool of coaches, resources, and mentors. An atmosphere of camaraderie and teamwork evolved from these interactions.

## The Client Care Unit

An immediate benefit to the client care units is the recruitment of new staff members. In times of a nursing shortage, the staff appreciates the influx of new nurses. Besides having the new graduates as colleagues, the fresh perspective and current knowledge base they bring benefits the entire unit. Many of the staff comment on how much fun it is to see the enthusiasm and excitement emanating from the new graduates. The new nurses frequently offer ideas and suggestions that they have seen work in other institutions they experienced during their school clinicals.

The new graduate program provides opportunities for professional growth for the nursing staff through precepting the new graduates, teaching classes, and becoming mentors. As the new nurses become fully functioning members of the team, many begin to move into leadership positions. Two of the earlier members of the new graduate programs are serving as charge nurses for their shift. Other previous new graduates have become preceptors so they can share the unique perspective of having successfully completed the program. Several previous new graduates are now active on unit-based nursing practice committees and other hospital committees.

As the new graduates assimilated into their profession, they demonstrated a loyalty to the unit and system that provided them the opportunities to succeed. The units have benefited from their enthusiasm. One interesting perspective is the idea of "get them young and train them right," which enables the new graduates to orient to the unit without having to unlearn bad habits or conflicting ways of providing care.

## The Health System

The New Graduate Program has become a major recruitment tool, with participants strongly recommending the program to friends. Many of the participants have stated that they applied to the program based on word-of-mouth information from a friend or previous classmate. Other new graduates learned about the program from other employees or through advertising.

Godinez, Schweiger, Gruver, and Ryan (1999) estimated that between 35% and 60% of new graduates change their places of employment within the first year. One of the measures of success designated during the development of the program was the length of time new graduates remained employed at CDH. The pool of 95 new nurses hired into the New Graduate Program since 1998 has been a great benefit to the health system, and retention of these nurses has been good. Retention rates at one year are all well above the 40%-65% rates cited above. Retention rates for the new graduate classes are:

| | |
|---|---|
| July 1998 | 72% retention at one year |
| June 1999 | 93% retention at one year |

| January 2000 | 75% retention at one year |
| June 2000 | 86% retention at one year |
| January 2001 | 66% retention at one year |
| June 2001 | 90% retention at one year |
| January 2002 | 86% retention at six months |

Of the 95 participants, 22 were employed as staff members in other positions at the time of their graduation from nursing school, representing upward mobility for most. Of those still employed at CDH, 89% continue to work on the same unit they were hired as a graduate. The other 11% have transitioned to another unit within CDH, representing nurses who stayed within the healthcare system.

Of those who left the healthcare system, 13 moved to other jobs, seven left due to dissatisfaction, four moved out of the area, three were discharged, three left for personal reasons (staying home with children, etc.), and one left to enter medical school.

## Conclusion

The New Graduate Program at CDH has been a success. Seven groups of exceptional, motivated, and eager new graduates have enrolled in the program. The majority of these graduates have become outstanding members of the healthcare team at CDH. By all measures established at the beginning, its goals have been met, and there have been many opportunities to improve the program to better meet the needs of the new graduates. The combination of classroom and clinical has created a foundation that enables the transition to the role of professional nurse. With recruitment and retention always a challenge, this approach is helping CDH fill staffing needs with competent, capable, and caring nurses.

## Learning Activities

1. Discuss the four most helpful things to you in your first weeks as a new graduate.
2. Discuss the four least helpful things to you in your first weeks as a new graduate.
3. Develop a list of classes that would support a new graduate during the initial weeks of orientation for general nursing skills (medical/surgical), or specialty skills.

# References

Benner, P. (1984). *From novice to expert: Excellence and power in clinical nursing practice.* Menlo Park, CA: Addison-Wesley.

Evans, K. (2001). Expectations of newly qualified nurses, *Nursing Standard, 15*(41), 33-38.

Godinez, G., Schweiger, J., Gruver, J., & Ryan, P. (1999). Role transition from graduate to staff nurse: A qualitative analysis. *Journal for Nurses in Staff Development, 15*(3), 97-110.

# Index

# Tables

# Figures

# Appendices